DATE DUE

Neurobiology of Stereotyped Behaviour

Neurobiology of Stereotyped Behaviour

Edited by

Steven J. Cooper

School of Psychology, University of Birmingham, UK

and

Colin T. Dourish

Merck Sharp & Dohme Research Laboratories,
Neuroscience Research Centre, Harlow, UK

CLARENDON PRESS · OXFORD
1990

Oxford University Press, Walton Street, Oxford OX2 6DP

Oxford New York Toronto
Delhi Bombay Calcutta Madras Karachi
Petaling Jaya Singapore Hong Kong Tokyo
Nairobi Dar es Salaam Cape Town
Melbourne Auckland
and associated companies in
Berlin Ibadan

Oxford is a trade mark of Oxford University Press

Published in the United States
by Oxford University Press, New York

British Library Cataloguing in Publication Data
Neurobiology of stereotyped behaviour.
1. Man. Behaviour. Neurobiological aspects
I. Cooper, S. J. (Steven J.) II. Dourish, Colin T.
612.8
ISBN 0–19–852160–X

Library of Congress Cataloging in Publication Data
Neurobiology of stereotyped behaviour / edited by Steven J. Cooper and Colin T. Dourish.
Includes index.
1. Stereotyped behavior (Psychiatry) 2. Stimulants—Physiological effect.
3. Dopamine—Receptors. 4. Brain chemistry. I. Cooper, S. J.
II. Dourish, Colin T.
[DNLM: 1. Stereotyped Behavior—drug effects. 2. Stereotyped
Behavior—physiology. QV 77 N4945]
RC569.5.S74N48 1989 616.85'227—dc20 89–16391
ISBN 0–19–852160–X

Set by Colset Private Limited, Singapore
Printed in Great Britain by
Courier International Ltd
Tiptree, Essex

Preface

We are all used to treating the hallmarks of rational behaviour as normal: of laying particular value upon the organized, the planned, the goal-directed, and the intelligible. Rational behaviour is functional, complex, and open to change as a consequence of experience. From this point of view, stereotyped behaviour is seen as an aberration: apparently purposeless, repetitive and invariant, and not under self-control. Stereotyped behaviour is familiar in psychiatry and neurology, where it may be treated as an indication of abnormality. Not only do simple and more complex motor responses exhibit stereotyped features, but also thoughts, utterances and courses of action can show a repetitive, apparently inexplicable, character. Institutionalized individuals, as well as farm and zoo animals, maintained in restricted and impoverished physical and social environments, can succumb to an inescapable loop of repeated acts.

The present volume is the first to consider the question of stereotyped behaviour from a broad biological and clinical perspective. As psychopharmacologists, we became familiar with the induction of often intense stereotyped behaviour through our work with drugs, especially those which affect the dopaminergic and 5-hydroxytryptaminergic systems of the brain. Why do these drugs, and many others, have these effects? Are the stereotyped forms of behaviour, which some drugs induce, signs of abnormality that lack any relevance to normal function? Are they merely a convenience for describing and categorizing the effectiveness of centrally active drugs? Or, will closer study of stereotyped behaviour, in all its guises, tell us something of importance with regard to the functions and attributes of brain systems, and of the organization and manifestation of behaviour? We feel that the last possibility, optimistic as it might seem, provides the real justification for the present volume.

We have been joined, as authors of the following chapters, by a group of eminent neuro- and psychopharmacologists, physiological and experimental psychologists, neurologists and psychiatrists. After some deliberation, we, as editors, decided not to seek a highly integrated, comprehensive account of all aspects of stereotyped behaviour: instead, authors were encouraged to be individualistic in their approach and to treat chosen aspects of stereotyped behaviour from their own points of view, reflective of their own specialist interests. In this way, several, sometimes contrasting, approaches to the question of stereotyped behaviour have emerged. We hope that this patchwork creates interest for the reader, but also that it will encourage fresh thought and investigation into an intriguing, and still poorly understood, field of biological and clinical enquiry

The first chapter, by ourselves, is an historical introduction to the neuro-pharmacological experiments that forged the links between the brain dopamine system and certain forms of drug-induced stereotyped behaviour. The second is a chapter by Trevor Robbins and his colleagues, who deal in depth with the theoretical issues raised by the effects of stimulant drugs, and which also considers the neuropsychological significance of these studies. John Waddington and his colleagues then address the question of the roles of the D-1 and D-2 receptor subtypes in relation to stereotyped and non-stereotyped forms of behaviour. This is followed by a second chapter of ours which deals with yawning and associated responses that are elicited by numerous drugs. Robert Isaacson and Willem Gispen then describe studies on grooming responses that are elicited by a number of neuropeptides, and they argue that, in fact, the grooming responses represent an adaptive response to the experience of stress. Gerald Curzon's chapter reviews experimental work on stereotyped responses mediated by the brain's 5-hydroxy-tryptaminergic system. Philip Teitelbaum and his colleagues offer first of all a sophisticated approach to the description and analysis of stereotyped behaviour, but also argue that often what are observed as stereotyped responses are isolated and fragmented components of behaviour that are normally meshed together in an integrated way. Reid and Staddon offer a more formal and mathematical approach to the analysis of behavioural responses induced by some schedules of reinforcement in operant tasks. In the concluding two chapters, Chris Frith and D. J. Done consider forms of stereotyped behaviour in human individuals, and their place in psychiatry, while Jon Stoessl provides details of stereotyped acts and gestures as studied by the neurologist. This volume, then, is a compendium of several different kinds of approach to the study of stereotyped behaviour. Read together, the chapters should remove any impression that stereotyped forms of behaviour reflect simple underlying mechanisms, which have little relevance to a better appreciation of other states and modes of behaviour.

This volume should appeal to a wide audience, but perhaps most especially to pharmacologists, psychiatrists, psychologists, neurologists, and all students of behaviour who have acquired an interest in stereotyped behaviour, in all its manifestations.

The gestation period of this volume has been gargantuan. We express our sincere thanks to the contributors for their authoritative and interesting chapters, and for their patience. Their reward, and ours, will be the appreciation of all those who would learn more about stereotyped behaviour.

Birmingham, UK   S. J. C.
Harlow, UK   C. T. D.
September 1989

Contents

Contributors   ix

1 An introduction to the concept of stereotypy and a historical perspective on the role of brain dopamine   1
Steven J. Cooper and Colin T. Dourish

2 The neuropsychological significance of stereotypy induced by stimulant drugs   25
T. W. Robbins, G. Mittleman, J. O'Brien, and P. Winn

3 Aspects of stereotyped and non-stereotyped behaviour in relation to dopamine receptor subtypes   64
John L. Waddington, Anthony G. Molloy, Kathy M. O'Boyle, and Mark T. Pugh

4 Neural basis of drug-induced yawning   91
Colin T. Dourish and Steven J. Cooper

5 Neuropeptides and the issue of stereotypy in behaviour   117
Robert L. Isaacson and Willem H. Gispen

6 Stereotyped and other motor responses to 5-hydroxytryptamine receptor activation   142
Gerald Curzon

7 Disintegration into stereotypy induced by drugs or brain damage: a microdescriptive behavioural analysis   169
Philip Teitelbaum, Sergio M. Pellis, and Terry L. DeVietti

8 Mechanisms of schedule entrainment   200
Alliston K. Reid and J. E. R. Staddon

9 Stereotyped behaviour in madness and in health   232
C. D. Frith and D. J. Done

10 Stereotyped motor phenomena in neurological disease   260
A. J. Stoessl

Index   293

Contributors

COOPER, S.J.
School of Psychology, University of Birmingham, Birmingham B15 2TT, UK.

CURZON, G.
Department of Neurochemistry, Institute of Neurology, University of London, Queen Square, London WC1N 3BG, UK.

DeVIETTI, T.L.
Department of Psychology, Central Washington University, Ellensburg, Washington 98926, USA.

DONE, D.J.
Clinical Research Centre, Division of Psychiatry, Harrow, Middlesex HA1 3UJ, UK.

DOURISH, C.T.
Merck Sharp & Dohme Research Laboratories, Neuroscience Research Centre, Terlings Park, Harlow, Essex CM20 2QR, UK.

FRITH, C.D.
Clinical Research Centre, Division of Psychiatry, Harrow, Middlesex, HA1 3UJ, UK.

GISPEN, W.H.
Rudolf Magnus Institute and Institute of Molecular Biology, State University of Utrecht, 3521 GD Utrecht, The Netherlands.

ISAACSON, R.L.
Department of Psychology, University Center at Binghamton, State University of New York, Binghamton, New York 13901, USA.

MITTLEMAN, G.
Department of Experimental Psychology, University of Cambridge, Downing St., Cambridge CB2 3EB, UK.

MOLLOY, A.G.
Department of Clinical Pharmacology, Royal College of Surgeons in Ireland, St Stephen's Green, Dublin 2, Ireland.

O'BOYLE, K.M.
Department of Clinical Pharmacology, Royal College of Surgeons in Ireland, St Stephen's Green, Dublin 2, Ireland.

O'BRIEN, J.
Department of Experimental Psychology, University of Cambridge, Downing St., Cambridge CB2 3EB, UK.

PELLIS, S.M

Department of Psychology, University of Florida, Gainesville, Florida 32611, USA.

PUGH, M.T.

Department of Clinical Pharmacology, Royal College of Surgeons in Ireland, St Stephen's Green, Dublin 2, Ireland.

REID, A.K.

Department of Mathematics and Computer Science, Eastern Oregon State College, La Grande, Oregon 97850, USA.

ROBBINS, T.W.

Department of Experimental Psychology, University of Cambridge, Downing St., Cambridge CB2 3EB, UK.

STADDON, J.E.R.

Departments of Psychology and Zoology, Duke University, Durham, North Carolina 27706, USA.

STOESSL, A.J.

Department of Clinical Neurological Sciences, St Josephs Hospital, 268 Grosvenor Street, London, Ontario N6A 4V2, Canada.

TEITELBAUM, P.

Department of Psychology, University of Florida, Gainesville, Florida 32611, USA.

WADDINGTON, J.L.

Department of Clinical Pharmacology, Royal College of Surgeons in Ireland, St Stephen's Green, Dublin 2, Ireland.

WINN, P.

Department of Experimental Psychology, University of Cambridge, Downing St., Cambridge CB2 3EB, UK.

An introduction to the concept of stereotypy and a historical perspective on the role of brain dopamine

STEVEN J. COOPER and COLIN T. DOURISH

Early studies on psychomotor stimulants and behavioural stereotypy

Psychosis associated with the use of amphetamine (benzedrine) was first described by Young and Scoville (1938). Following the Second World War, amphetamine abuse became prevalent, and it was not uncommon for individuals to take large doses of the drug. Cases of amphetamine-induced psychosis ceased to be rarities, and Connell highlighted the problem with the publication of his now classic monograph (Connell 1958). Connell put forward the important proposal that the clinical features of amphetamine psychosis were difficult to distinguish from acute or chronic paranoid schizophrenia. Subsequently, Ellinwood (1967) provided a detailed behavioural description of amphetamine psychosis in individuals who had been taking large daily doses of the drug, and identified the presence of paranoid psychosis, with hallucinations and thought disorder.

Attempts were made to discover if amphetamine abuse exacerbated symptoms in predisposed individuals, or could provoke psychotic reactions in non-schizophrenic individuals. Griffith and his colleagues made the first attempt to induce amphetamine psychosis in non-schizophrenic volunteer subjects in a controlled hospital setting (Griffith *et al*. 1968). 10 mg of D-amphetamine was administered hourly, and an abrupt onset of paranoid delusions occurred, but in the absence of thought disorder or hallucinations. Recognizing that amphetamine abusers often took very large doses, Angrist and his colleagues increased the dosage schedule to 50 mg/hour and were able to document hallucinatory phenomena and some forms of thought disorder, in addition to paranoia (Angrist *et al*. 1974). They concluded that amphetamine psychosis can replicate symptoms of schizophrenia in nearly every respect.

In patients experiencing a schizophrenic episode, and in patients with partial remission of schizophrenia, small doses of the psychostimulants, methylphenidate, D- or L-amphetamine dramatically intensified pre existing psychotic symptoms (Davis 1974; Segal and Janowsky 1978). In contrast, normal volunteers showed no significant psychotic symptoms when challenged with small doses of stimulants.

These observations and experimental results provided one of the major foundations for the dopamine theory of schizophrenia (Snyder *et al.* 1974). The report by Connell (1958), amongst other evidence, inspired the study of effects of larger doses of amphetamine in laboratory animals in order to determine their behavioural consequences. The stimulant effect of amphetamine in animals (e.g. increased locomotor activity) was already well known, but Randrup *et al.* (1963) also observed, in rats, activity 'of a grossly abnormal stereotyped character'. Since this paper helped to initiate a considerable research effort devoted to amphetamine-induced stereotyped behaviour, its findings will be described in some detail.

D-amphetamine (in doses of 1.5 and 3 mg/kg) was injected into rats housed individually in cages made from wire netting. After the larger dose, rats sniffed constantly but only covered a small part of the cage floor or lower part of the walls. Mouth movements, and licking or biting the wire netting also occurred. Locomotor activity was absent, and so too were grooming, eating and drinking. This form of stereotyped behaviour developed after 30 min and lasted for 2–3 hours. After injection of the smaller dose, rats sniffed constantly, and showed a tendency to remain at one point in the cage. In the same article, the authors described a preliminary pharmacological analysis of the behavioural effect produced by D-amphetamine. Neither α- nor β-adrenergic antagonists had any effect on the response but three 'tranquillizers' proved to be effective antagonists: chlorpromazine, haloperidol, and ethoxybutamoxone (Randrup *et al.* 1963). A second report followed, in which Randrup and Munkvad (1965) showed that perphenazine antagonized amphetamine-induced stereotypy. Most importantly, they recognized the possible relationship between drugs which were effective in treating symptoms of schizophrenia, and those which antagonized amphetamine-induced stereotyped behaviour in rats.

The utility of simple animal behavioural tests to screen for drugs which might be effective clinically in the treatment of schizophrenia had already engaged the attention of Janssen and his colleagues. They used antagonism of apomorphine-induced gnawing as a screening test, and also antagonism of the behavioural effects of 10 mg/kg of amphetamine (Janssen *et al.* 1960, 1965, 1967). The behavioural effects of the amphetamine treatment which they observed—stereotyped mouth and tongue movements (chewing, gnawing, licking)—were consistent with Randrup and Munkvad's observations.

'Compulsive' gnawing induced in rodents by apomorphine had, in fact, been reported much earlier (Amsler 1923; Harnack 1874). Ernst (1967) also compared apomorphine and D-amphetamine in rats that had been pretreated with the monoamine oxidase (MAO)-inhibitor, iproniazid. He reported that both apomorphine and D-amphetamine produced similar effects to those described by Randrup *et al.* (1963): at its most intense, the compulsive gnawing syndrome involved animals remaining in the same location for 5–10 minutes or longer, while gnawing the wire caging and clinging to the wires with their teeth. Ernst (1967) introduced a rating scale to provide a means of ranking the intensity of the behavioural response produced by the drug treatments (see also Janssen *et al.* 1967). In his paper, Ernst (1967) also drew a distinction between the mechanisms of action of apomorphine and D-amphetamine, and suggested that D-amphetamine induced gnawing compulsion by causing release of endogenous dopamine, while apomorphine may mimic the effect of dopamine at its receptors. Interestingly, Ernst's investigations had been inspired by the discovery that much of the dopamine in the brain is found in the extrapyramidal system (Bertler and Rosengren 1959; Sano *et al.* 1959), and by observations that reserpine decreased the level of dopamine in the brain, produced catatonia in rats, and a parkinsonian syndrome in man (Carlsson 1959). He proposed that apomorphine was able to mimic dopamine's effects and might prove therapeutically useful in treating patients with Parkinson's disease (Ernst 1969). In effect, he was advocating that the induction of stereotyped behaviour could be used as a means to detect dopamine agonist activity, in the development of drugs for use in treating parkinsonian patients.

Many, though not all, psychostimulant drugs, given in large enough doses, will induce behavioural stereotypy in rats. Fog (1969) reported that, in addition to D-amphetamine and apomorphine, methamphetamine, pipradol, methylphenidate, pemoline, and cocaine could induce the effect, although caffeine and nikethamide did not.

Dopamine neuroanatomy and stereotyped behaviour

Discovery and description of dopamine-containing pathways

Research into the distribution of dopamine in the brain, and the function of dopamine as a neurotransmitter began with reports that dopamine is a normal constituent of mammalian brain (Carlsson *et al.* 1958; Montagu 1957; Weil-Malherbe and Bone 1957). Although the concentration of dopamine in the brain was about the same as that of noradrenalin, its distribution was quite different, suggesting that dopamine might have a neurotransmitter action of its own. Bertler and Rosengren (1959), in a report from Carlsson's laboratory, showed that most of the brain's dopamine was found in the corpus striatum. A similar result was published by Sano and colleagues (1959) using post-mortem human brain tissue. Significant amounts of dopamine were later detected in the substantia nigra (Bertler 1961). Carlsson (1959) proposed that dopamine was involved in extrapyramidal motor functions, and could also be implicated in such disorders as Parkinson's disease and Huntington's chorea.

In Vienna, Hornykiewicz responded to these reports, and began post-mortem studies of dopamine concentrations in the brains of parkinsonian patients. Ehringer and Hornykiewicz (1960) found that there was an almost complete absence of dopamine in the caudate and putamen of parkinsonian patients. This result led immediately to a clinical trial with L-dopa, which was known from animal studies to increase brain dopamine levels after depletion by reserpine (Carlsson 1959). Birkmayer and Hornykiewicz (1961) identified L-dopa as an effective antiparkinsonism drug, while analogous results were obtained by Barbeau and his colleagues (1962) in Canada. Later, Cotzias et al. (1967, 1969) introduced the clinically useful treatment of Parkinson's disease using large oral doses of L-dopa. The rapid and undoubted success of this treatment greatly stimulated research into the function of dopamine in the brain, with particular emphasis on its role in the extrapyramidal system.

Further advances occurred during this early period of dopamine research, which resulted in revelations concerning the distribution of dopamine-containing neurones in the brain. Falck et al. (1962) developed a method to visualize monoamines, including dopamine, in tissue sections under a fluorescence microscope. Using this method, the occurrence of dopamine in nerve cell bodies and terminals was demonstrated (Carlsson et al. 1962; Dahlstrom and Fuxe 1964; Fuxe 1965). The largest dopamine-containing neuronal pathway identified originated from cell bodies located in the pars compacta of the substantia nigra, and terminated in the caudate and putamen (the neostriatum), accounting for the high concentrations of dopamine in these regions (Andén et al. 1964). Degeneration of this nigrostriatal pathway is the major cause of morphological and biochemical lesions in Parkinson's disease. Another major dopamine pathway originates in the ventral tegmental area and projects to the nucleus accumbens, olfactory tubercle, and regions of the limbic cortex (mesolimbic pathway) (Andén et al. 1966). It would be inappropriate to carry this discussion into any further neuroanatomical detail, since the behavioural experiments which will now be reviewed were carried out at a time when a relatively simple distinction was drawn between nigrostriatal and mesolimbic dopamine systems.

Neural substrates of psychomotor stimulant-induced stereotyped behaviour

Following the descriptions of stereotyped behaviour induced by amphetamine (Randrup and Munkvad 1965; Randrup et al. 1963), Fog et al. (1967) undertook an experiment to determine the possible role of the corpus striatum in producing this response. They found that dopamine and methylscopolamine injected into the corpus striatum restored amphetamine-induced stereotyped behaviour in α-methyl-paratyrosine treated rats. Fog et al. (1967) concluded that brain amine metabolism in the corpus striatum was crucial for amphetamine stereotypy. This was consistent with the findings of Ernst and Smelik (1966) that crystalline L-dopa or apomorphine placed in the caudate nucleus or globus pallidus of rats evoked compulsive gnawing behaviour, which, as we have already noted, is similar to the stereotyped behaviour described by Randrup et al. (1963).

These seminal studies were followed by many others in which central injection of drugs was used to identify sites of action within dopamine-rich terminal areas involved in producing stereotypy. Cools and van Rossum (1970) injected D O P A, dopamine, and D-amphetamine unilaterally into the caudate nucleus in cats, and observed stereotyped head movements which were blocked by haloperidol. Fog and Pakkenberg (1971) injected either para-hydroxyamphetamine or dopamine bilaterally into the caudate nucleus of rats and observed stereotyped behaviour. Since injections of noradrenalin had no effect, they concluded that stereotyped behaviour depends on dopaminergic mechanisms in the corpus striatum.

Costall et al. (1972) noted a 'mild form' of stereotyped behaviour, characterized by sniffing but not gnawing or biting, in response to bilateral injections of D-amphetamine into either the caudate–putamen or the globus pallidus. In the same study, they demonstrated that intrastriatal or intrapallidal injection of haloperidol markedly inhibited the stereotyped behaviour produced by systemically administered amphetamine. Pijnenburg et al. (1975b) conducted a similar experiment, and attenuated the effect of systemically administered apomorphine or D-amphetamine by injecting haloperidol bilaterally into the caudate nucleus or nucleus accumbens.

Jackson et al. (1975) reported that rats, pre-treated with reserpine and the MAO-inhibitor nialamide, exhibited stereotyped head movements, gnawing, and chewing when dopamine was injected bilaterally into the neostriatum. Similarly, stereotyped head-dipping was observed by Makanjuola et al. (1980) when dopamine was injected bilaterally into the caudate–putamen of nialamide pre-treated rats, and the animals were exposed to a hole-board apparatus.

Such results implicate dopaminergic neurones in the corpus striatum and globus pallidus in mediating stereotyped behaviour produced by stimulants. A major reason for investigating the role of the corpus striatum is that it contains most of the brain's dopamine and was judged to be the site of action of amphetamine and apomorphine in producing stereotyped behaviour. Nevertheless, a further series of studies focused attention on mesolimbic dopamine neurones and discovered that these too may mediate some of the behavioural effects of psychomotor stimulants. An interest arose in mesolimbic meurones, in part because it was proposed that symptoms of schizophrenia may be associated with their dysfunction. Hence the antipsychotic effect of neuroleptics was attributed to an action on mesolimbic dopamine pathways (Andén 1972; Matthysse 1973).

When small doses of D-amphetamine are administered systemically, an increase in locomotor activity occurs, in the absence of intense gnawing or licking. Pijnenburg and van Rossum (1973) injected dopamine bilaterally into the nucleus accumbens and observed a strong stimulation of activity. The effect of dopamine could be antagonized by haloperidol (Pijnenburg *et al*. 1975*c*), fluphenazine, pimozide, and by the atypical neuroleptics, clozapine, thioridazine, and sulpiride (Costall and Naylor 1976*a,b*). These results suggested that dopamine in the nucleus accumbens may be associated with amphetamine-induced locomotor stimulation.

Support for this hypothesis came from Pijnenburg *et al*. (1975*a*) who reported that bilateral injection of haloperidol into the nucleus accumbens blocked amphetamine-induced hyperactivity. Furthermore, bilateral injections of D-amphetamine , apomorphine, or dopamine into the nucleus accumbens increased locomotor activity, but did not elicit head movements, gnawing, or chewing (Jackson *et al*. 1975). Similarly, Pijnenburg *et al*. (1976) reported that bilateral intra-accumbens injections of dopamine or D-amphetamine produced a strong stimulation of locomotor activity. Interestingly, in this study, Pijnenburg *et al*. (1976) also reported that dopamine, D-amphetamine, or apomorphine injected into the olfactory tubercle (another mesolimbic terminal site) stimulated locomotor activity.

In parallel with attempts to localize the effects of drugs using central injection techniques, brain-lesioning techniques were also employed. In the first instance, suction or electrolytic lesions were used to remove or damage, respectively, parts of the brain (e.g. Costall and Naylor 1973, 1974; Fog *et al*. 1970; Naylor and Olley 1972; Simpson and Iversen 1971). However, such lesions are non-selective, and more specific central lesions are obtained using the chemical neurotoxin, 6-hydroxydopamine (6-OHDA), which causes long-lasting depletion of brain catecholamines (Evetts *et al*. 1970). Direct injection of 6-OHDA into specific brain sites could be used, therefore, to identify dopamine pathways which may be critical in mediating stereotypy induced by psychomotor stimulants.

Thus, Creese and Iversen (1974) achieved severe dopamine depletion in either the caudate nucleus or the olfactory tubercle following bilateral injections of 6-OHDA. Hyperactivity produced by a small dose of D-amphetamine was not affected by either lesion, but stereotyped behaviour induced by a large dose of the drug was abolished by the caudate lesion. Neither lesion reduced the stereotyped behaviour elicited by apomorphine. Creese and Iversen (1974) concluded that dopamine in the striatum is critical for amphetamine-induced stereotypy. Similar findings were reported by Asher and Aghajanian (1974). Since 6-OHDA damages presynaptic catecholamine terminals, leaving postsynaptic receptors intact, the response to apomorphine (a direct dopamine agonist) should not have been diminished.

Kelly *et al.* (1975) examined the hypothesis that stereotyped behaviour induced by high doses of amphetamine depends on dopamine innervation of the striatum, whereas locomotor stimulation associated with a small dose of amphetamine requires the integrity of the nucleus accumbens. Bilateral injections of 6-OHDA were therefore made into the nucleus accumbens or the caudate nucleus, causing substantial depletion of dopamine. The results were consistent with the hypothesis: D-amphetamine (1.5 mg/kg) induced the locomotor response in the caudate-lesioned animals but did not do so in nucleus accumbens-lesioned rats. Conversely, D-amphetamine (5 mg/kg) elicited stereotyped behaviour in the latter group, but not in the former. Neither lesion abolished the behavioural effects of apomorphine, and, in fact, postsynaptic supersensitivity was observed in both groups, as had previously been described by Ungerstedt (1971). Subsequently, rats with selective lesions of dopamine terminals in the nucleus accumbens produced by 6-OHDA proved valuable in the study of directly-acting dopamine receptor agonists (e.g. Kelly *et al.* 1976; Woodruff *et al.* 1976).

The report of Kelly *et al.* (1975) therefore provided support for a neuroanatomical dissociation between dopamine pathways mediating hyperactivity and stereotyped behaviour induced by amphetamine (see review by Kelly 1977). Further experiments defined more specifically the role of the caudate nucleus (Iversen and Koob 1977). Lesions of the ventral caudate nucleus, but not of the dorsal region, markedly attenuated stereotyped behaviour induced by D-amphetamine.

As far as mesolimbic dopamine and stereotypy are concerned, most attention has focused on the nucleus accumbens. Nevertheless, there is evidence which indicates that dopamine innervation of the olfactory tubercles is also of importance. Costall and Naylor (1974) found that electrolytic lesions of the olfactory tubercles abolished sniffing, while injection of dopamine into the olfactory tubercles induced sniffing and locomotion (Costall and Naylor 1975a). Using a method described by Ljungberg and Ungerstedt (1977a) to quantify locomotion and stereotyped behaviour, Ungerstedt (1979) reported that local injection of dopamine into the nucleus accumbens of nialamide pre-treated rats elicited a strong locomotor effect. In contrast, local injection of dopamine into the olfactory tubercles produced intense sniffing and repetitive head and limb movement.

The question of the respective functions of the nucleus accumbens and olfactory tubercles in dopamine-mediated behavioural responses has been examined extensively by Cools (1986). Cools showed that bilateral injections of dopamine or apomorphine into the olfactory tubercles increased locomotor activity: this effect could be antagonzied by haloperidol. In contrast, injections into the nucleus accumbens produced only inconsistent effects. Cools concluded that dopamine within the lateral olfactory tubercle has an excitatory function with regard to locomotion, and, on the basis of other pharmacological data, suggested that dopamine in the nucleus accumbens may be inhibitory.

The question of neuroanatomical mediation of locomotion in normal rats and of the hyperactivity produced by stimulant drugs remains open, therefore. Despite the efforts which have been invested, it is clear that selective manipulations of the many dopamine projections within the mesolimbic/mesocortical system have not been attempted. Most attention has focused on the nucleus accumbens, although there are serious methodological problems surrounding attempts to study its functions and those of other dopamine projection areas. For example, it is difficult to control the extent of lesions or the spread of injected chemicals in solution. Refinement of methods to achieve greater precision and a more extended survey of dopamine terminal fields should provide valuable information about the roles that dopamine plays in relation to locomotor activity and stereotyped behaviour.

We shall conclude this section with a brief reference to a recently introduced technique which has been used to study dopaminergic mechanisms. Intracerebral dialysis allows the investigation of regional dopamine release in awake animals (Ungerstedt 1984). Using this approach, it has been possible to correlate the behavioural effects produced by drugs with dopamine release in the corpus striatum or nucleus accumbens (e.g. Sharp *et al.* 1986). These authors reported that 2-mg/kg D-amphetamine caused a marked increase in striatal dopamine release, which correlated positively with stereotyped behaviour but not locomotor activity. Dopamine release in the nucleus accumbens tended to be associated with locomotor activity (although the correlation was not statistically significant). Further studies with smaller doses of D-amphetamine may clarify relationships between increased locomotor response and regional dopamine release.

Pharmacological analysis of stereotyped behaviour

Antagonism of apomorphine- or amphetamine-induced stereotypy was quickly recognized as a property of neuroleptic drugs (e.g. chlorpromazine, haloperidol, pimozide), which are clinically effective antipsychotics (Janssen *et al.* 1960, 1965, 1967; Niemegeers and Janssen 1979). Hence, antagonism of drug-induced stereotyped behaviour was introduced as a simple *in vivo* method to screen for neuroleptic drugs. Ernst (1967, 1969) proposed that apomorphine caused stereotyped gnawing by acting directly at dopamine receptors, whereas amphetamine acted indirectly by increasing dopamine release. It followed that an important part of the action of neuroleptic drugs might be to block dopamine receptors.

Biochemical studies on the dopamine-blocking actions of neuroleptics date back to Carlsson and Lindqvist (1963), who observed that low doses of chlorpromazine and haloperidol stimulated the accumulation of the O-methylated metabolites of dopamine and noradrenalin following inhibiton of MAO. They suggested that neuroleptics blocked catecholamine receptors and, through a feedback mechanism, produced a compensatory activation of catecholamine neurones. Extensive work by Andén and co-workers (1970) on 15 neuroleptics, drawn from phenothiazine, thioxanthene, dibenzazepine, butyrophenone, and diphenylbutylamine classes, established blockade of dopamine receptors as a common mechanism of action of neuroleptic drugs. All the drugs tested increased the rate of dopamine turnover, although their effects on noradrenalin turnover were less consistent. Further evidence indicated that apomorphine prevented most of the increased dopamine turnover produced by neuroleptics (Di Chiara *et al.* 1976; Lahti *et al.* 1972). Wilk and Stanley proposed that antipsychotic efficacy could be predicted on the basis of a drug's ability to elevate the levels of dopamine metabolites (Stanley and Wilk 1977; Wilk and Stanley 1977). Contemporary work, in which dopamine release and metabolism has been studied using *in vivo* dialysis, confirms that neuroleptics increase brain dopamine metabolism (Zetterstrom *et al.* 1984; Imperato and Di Chiara 1985).

Our understanding of drug action at dopamine receptors has been considerably improved as a result of the development of new assay procedures. An important step forward came with the discovery that the effects of agonists acting at dopamine receptors may involve cyclic AMP (Kebabian and Greengard 1971; Kebabian *et al.* 1972). The dopamine receptor appeared to regulate the activity of an enzyme, adenylate cyclase, stimulation of which leads to the formation of cyclic AMP. Using this assay, it has been possible to show that neuroleptics act as antagonists at the dopamine receptor which regulates adenylate cyclase activity, and it has been suggested that antagonism at this receptor may contribute to the antipsychotic effects of neuroleptics (Kebabian 1978).

However, it soon became clear that there were drugs which produced apparently anomalous results in this biochemical test of dopamine-receptor antagonism. Most interestingly, a group of drugs, described as substituted benzamides (sulpiride, sultopride, tiapride, clebopride, and metoclopramide), proved to be inactive in the dopamine-sensitive adenylate cyclase assay (Elliott *et al.* 1977; Jenner *et al.* 1978). Yet they acted as dopamine antagonists (Worms 1982), and antagonized apomorphine-induced effects on behaviour.

The resolution of this apparent paradox came when a distinction was drawn between the dopamine D-1 receptor subtype (agonist activity at which enhances adenylate cyclase stimulation of cyclic AMP) and the dopamine D-2 receptor subtype (Kebabian and Calne 1979). Substituted benzamides, like sulpiride, were recognized as being highly selective dopamine D-2 receptor antagonists (Stoof and Kebabian 1984). Since sulpiride proved to be effective in clinical trials as an antipsychotic drug (Peselow and Stanley 1982), it appears possible that antagonism at the D-2 receptor may be necessary for antipsychotic effects of neuroleptic drugs.

This brings us to the question of the effects of substituted benzamides on drug-induced stereotyped behaviour. Initial studies indicated that apomorphine or amphetamine stereotyped behaviour could be antagonized by sulpiride and other substituted benzamides (Costall and Naylor 1975*b*; Jenner *et al.* 1978; Niemegeers and Janssen 1979; Worms 1982). Nevertheless, additional data qualified these observations and suggested that sulpiride and some other antipsychotic drugs selectively antagonize hyperlocomotion induced by psychomotor stimulants.

Thus, Ljungberg and Ungerstedt (1978) reported that haloperidol antagonized the compulsive gnawing induced by a large dose of apomorphine in rats, whilst sulpiride and two 'atypical' neuroleptics, clozapine and thioridazine, predominantly antagonized apomorphine-induced locomotor hyperactivity. Similarly, Ljungberg and Ungerstedt (1985) reported that clozapine and sulpiride antagonized only the locomotion induced by amphetamine, while Robertson and MacDonald (1984, 1985) have shown that these two compounds actually *enhanced* amphetamine-induced stereotyped behaviours (repetitive head movements, sniffing, and gnawing). In experiments with mice, the two substituted benzamides, sulpiride and amisulpiride, have been shown to potentiate apomorphine-induced stereotyped licking and sniffing (Vasse *et al.* 1985). These data, obtained using substituted benzamides, which act selectively as dopamine D-2 receptor antagonists, indicate that there is a complex relationship between drug action at dopamine receptors and the occurrence of stereotyped behaviour. (For further discussion of dopamine receptors and stereotypy see Waddington *et al.*, Chapter 3, this volume.)

Behavioural processes involved in stereotyped behaviour

In experimental work, the term 'stereotypy' has very frequently been taken to mean a *response* which is elicited by drug treatments, in the same sense that 'gnawing', 'licking', or 'sniffing' are terms used to describe observable behavioural responses. This misuse of the term 'stereotypy' has been particularly prevalent in pharmacological studies in which mimicking or antagonism of drug-induced 'stereotypy' has been used to screen for novel drugs. The misinterpretation of 'stereotypy' as a response has been reinforced through the use of stereotypy rating scales (e.g. Creese and Iversen 1973; Ellinwood and Balster 1974; Ernst 1967; Janssen *et al.* 1967; Naylor and Costall 1971).

As Randrup and Munkvad (1967) made clear, 'stereotyped' is descriptive and can be applied to any type of behavioural response. A response is stereotyped in character if it is performed repetitively, with little variation, and without apparent purpose. 'Stereotypy' is therefore not the name of a response, but can be invoked as a description of the recurrence and temporal distribution of behavioural responses which are of interest. The behaviour in question can range from simple motor patterns to complex patterns and sequences of behaviour, and include cognitive tasks as well as directly observable motor responses. Problems which arise with the use of stereotypy rating scales are:

1. Measurement of behavioural responses themselves (e.g. gnawing, rearing, sniffing) is confused with an assessment of the *stereotyped nature* of the behaviour.

2. The intensity of the stereotypy is assumed to be on a continuum which is directly related to the dose of the drug administered (i.e. a monotonic dose–response relationship) (Fray *et al.* 1980; Rebec and Bashore 1984; Dourish 1987; Robbins *et al.*, Chapter 2, this volume; Teitelbaum *et al.*, Chapter 7, this volume).

Stereotyped behaviour which is induced by amphetamine, apomorphine, and other psychostimulants became a focus for intensive study, in part because it can appear to be strikingly dissimilar from the normal activity of laboratory animals, and is therefore easily observed and recognized. The apparent simplicity of the responses induced by larger doses of these drugs recommended 'stereotyped behaviour' as a useful and economical index of the effects of drugs on particular neurotransmitter systems. The discovery of amphetamine- and apomorphine-induced stereotyped behaviour occurred at a time when interest in pharmacological treatments of schizophrenia and parkinsonism was gathering momentum, and when it was perceived that central dopamine neurotransmission might be particularly important with regard to the pathologies and treatments of both disorders.

Nevertheless, from a behavioural perspective, the apparent 'simplicity' of the performance of laboratory animals, following injections of large doses of psychostimulants, is only superficial. Investigations which have concentrated upon environmental and behavioural factors, as distinct from studies with a primary interest in pharmacological or neuroanatomical analysis, have revealed considerable complexity in phenomena of stereotyped behaviour. It has required a good deal of imaginative theorizing and experimentation to analyse the processes which may help to mediate the expression of repetitive forms of behaviour. In this section we shall consider briefly some of the relevant studies on behavioural processes at work in stereotyped behaviour.

We shall refer again to the early studies on amphetamine- and apomorphine-induced stereotyped behaviour, and consider descriptions of changes which take place in animals' behaviour following the drug treatments. The report of Randrup et al. (1963) illustrates some important points about drug dosage and the time course of drug effects. When a smaller dose of D-amphetamine (1.5 mg/kg) was injected into rats, the pattern of behaviour consisted of constant sniffing at the wire netting of the enclosure. The area covered in the course of locomotion about the cage became progressively more restricted. At a higher dose (3.0 mg/kg), abnormal behaviour became evident about 30 min after drug injection, and consisted of constant sniffing, mouth movements, and progressively more restricted locomotion until locomotor activity became absent altogether. This pattern of behaviour lasted for 2–3 hours.

Very detailed observations were made by Schiørring (1971, 1979) of rats' behaviour in an open-field apparatus. During the 'stereotypy-phase', which followed injection of 5 mg/kg of D-amphetamine, the behaviour of animals became limited to persistent sniffing, licking, and biting, together with side-to-side, or up-and-down, head movements. Prior to the development of that phase, forward locomotion and rearing upwards against the enclosure wall were increased, while grooming activity was decreased. As animals moved about the enclosure in this phase of locomotor hyperactivity, the paths traced by the animals became more restricted, and instead of moving extensively and irregularly about the enclosure as normal animals do, the rats followed a circular route close to the perimeter of the enclosure. Such studies emphasized that the induction of stereotyped behaviour by drugs involves increases in frequency or duration within restricted categories of behaviour, at the expense of responses in other categories. Furthermore, the behaviour which is observed depends, in part, upon the dose of the drug which is given, and the time after administration.

A number of other factors are known to affect the occurrence of stereotyped behaviour, and, indeed, its characteristics. For example, Ljungberg and Ungerstedt (1977*b*) reported that different effects could be induced by apomorphine, depending upon how the drug was administered. Subcutaneous injection of the drug in the flank produced compulsive gnawing, whereas subcutaneous injection in the scruff of the neck elicited increased locomotion sniffing and repetitive head movements. In another study, male Wistar rats responded to apomorphine with stereotyped gnawing, while animals of the same strain, but from a different supplier, responded predominantly with stereotyped climbing (Szechtman *et al.* 1982). In a comparison between rats reared in social conditions with an enriched environment and rats reared individually in an impoverished environment, amphetamine was found to induce more intense stereotypy (as measured by a rating scale) in the socially-deprived rats (Sahakian *et al.* 1975).

Familiarity with the test environment can also be an important determinant of the nature of stereotyped responses elicited by psychostimulant drugs. Thus, rats and guinea-pigs show reduced levels of stereotyped behaviour in response to amphetamine when tested in a novel cage, compared to testing in a familiar one (Einon and Sahakian 1979; Sahakian and Robbins 1975). Amphetamine-treated rats make more exploratory responses in a novel apparatus, but exhibit more intense stereotyped behaviour when they have been habituated to the apparatus (Mumford *et al.* 1979). The short-acting stimulant, β-phenylethylamine, elicited stereotyped rearing in rats tested in a novel environment but not in rats tested in a familiar environment (Dourish and Cooper 1984).

The type of apparatus used can help to determine the pattern of response which is exhibited in response to drug treatments. While stereotyped locomotor activity can be elicited in an empty open field (e.g. Schiørring 1971), stereotyped climbing and rearing can be elicited in rats and mice by stimulant drugs when subjects are tested in apparatus with a reduced floor area but which provides an opportunity to climb (Costall *et al.* 1978, 1981; Protais *et al.* 1976, 1984; Szechtman *et al.* 1982). Apomorphine-induced gnawing in rats has also been found to be influenced by the design of the test box (Ljungberg and Ungerstedt 1977*c*).

Such examples convey the strong impression that stereotyped behaviour is not immutable, but that its expression will be influenced, not only by the species of animal used or the drug injected, but also by behavioural and environmental factors present in the experimental situation. Properly understood, therefore, 'stereotyped behaviour' as a phenomenon becomes much more than a behavioural assay for testing centrally-active drugs; it may also contribute to our understanding of relationships between behaviour, neurochemistry, and responses to brain injury or brain dysfunction. The following sections highlight some recent work, that will be dealt with in greater detail in other chapters of this volume, which contributes to a better comprehension of the behavioural significance of stereotypy.

Analysis of changes in movement components

The variety of stereotyped responses exhibited by rodents following the administration of amphetamine or apomorphine is bewildering, and observations, however detailed, seem to offer no explanation of why gnawing predominates in one situation, locomotor activity in a second, and rearing in a third. However, considerable insight into the patterns of stereo-typed behaviour which develop in drug-treated animals has come from the application of the Eshkol–Wachman Movement Notation (Eshkol and Wachman 1958) to the analysis of movement components in rodents. Using this approach Teitelbaum and his colleagues have recently shown that apparently unrelated stereotyped acts produced by apomorphine in rats consist of composite behaviours which depend on particular values of three component variables (Szechtman et al. 1982, 1985; Teitelbaum et al., Chapter 7, this volume).

These three variables are continuous snout contact, forward progression, and turning. A sequence of events which follow administration of the drug can be established, and described in terms of changing values of the three variables. At the start of the drug's effects, rearing in the air is abolished, and forward progression begins, as the animal establishes snout contact with the ground. Then turning begins, growing in amplitude as forward progression diminishes. Forward walking changes into circling, then into revolving, and finally into pivoting. When the hindlimbs become immobile, side-to-side movements of the head are observed.

Continuous snout contact appears to be a fundamental component of apomorphine's behavioural effects (Szechtman et al. 1982). Combined with forward progression, it accounts for locomotion without rearing in the open field apparatus, climbing in an enclosed space, and 'cliff-jumping' (Weismann 1971).

A particularly important insight which derives from this type of approach to the study of drug-induced changes in movement is the relationship between pharmacological effects, on the one hand, and the ontogeny of movement in developing animals, as well as the recovery of function in brain-damaged animals, on the other. Apomorphine appears to produce a regression in behavioural competence and a progressive 'shut-down' in locomotion (Szechtman et al. 1985). This sequence is opposite to the increase in control of movement seen during ontogeny and recovery from bilateral lateral hypothalamic lesions which produce akinesia (Golani et al. 1979, 1981).

Szechtman *et al.* (1985) likened the shrinkage in environmental space which is explored by apomorphine-treated animals to the reduction in attention to external stimuli seen in human psychosis induced by amphetamine (Ellinwood 1967) (see Teitelbaum *et al.*, Chapter 7, this volume for further discussion of movement notation analysis of stereotypy).

Behaviour at the onset of stereotypy

One hypothesis which has been advanced to account for the variability observed in stereotyped behaviour is that stimulant drugs strengthen the behaviour which is being displayed at the onset of the drug action (Cools *et al.* 1977; Ellinwood and Kilbey 1975). Since the animal's behaviour will vary as a function of previous experience, including its degree of familiarity with the test environment, the design of the apparatus, and whether it is alone or with other animals, considerable variation may, in principle, occur.

Lyon and Randrup (1972) reported an operant conditioning study, the results of which have a bearing on this issue. Two groups of rats were tested under two schedules of reinforcement, in which termination of electric shock provided reinforcement in both cases. However, in one group, each lever-press delayed the onset of shock, whereas, in the second group, release of the lever was followed immediately by shock. Their results indicated an inter-action between performance under the reinforcement schedules, and behavioural stereotypy produced by increasing doses of D-amphetamine. At 1 mg/kg of D-amphetamine, lever pressing to delay shock was enhanced; in contrast, performance deteriorated in the group of animals which were trained to keep the lever depressed continuously to avoid shock. At higher doses, however, intermittent responding (shock delay) disappeared in some animals, while continuous responding in the second group remained largely unaffected.

Lyon and Randrup (1972) interpreted their results in terms of the development of behavioural stereotypy produced by amphetamine, and postulated that 'the increasing stereotypy yields increasingly higher rates of activity, but in a decreasing number of response categories' (p. 344). These results illustrate that large doses of a stimulant which induce stereotypy may actually improve performance on a task that involves perseverative responding. Experiments reported by Teitelbaum and Derks (1958), and by Collins *et al.* (1979) yield results which are consistent with this viewpoint. (For a full theoretical development of this position, see Lyon and Robbins 1975, and Robbins *et al.*, Chapter 2, this volume.)

Under other circumstances, however, drug effects may block ongoing behaviour. Szechtman (1986) reported that apomorphine did not strengthen ongoing copulation by male rats but, within a short time of injection, animals ceased to mate and began to exhibit the stereotyped behaviour which is typical for apomorphine-treated rats. Szechtman (1986) interpreted his results in terms of 'a shift of attention', i.e. response to selected categories of sensory input, but a neglect of others.

A report by Beck et al. (1986) emphasized a temporal gradient of decreasing responsivity to environmental change following drug administration. At first, amphetamine-treated rats incorporated body postures and movements which were environmentally dependent into their forms of stereotyped behaviour. However, at 30 min postinjection, amphetamine-treated animals were quite unresponsive to alterations in the environment, in contrast to control animals.

Taken together, the results of the studies surveyed here indicate that:

1. Ongoing behaviour has to be sufficiently compatible with drug-induced stereotyped responses for it to be maintained, albeit in a stereotyped form.

2. As the action of the drug develops (as a function of dose and time since injection), stereotyped behaviour becomes increasingly inflexible and unresponsive to environmental change.

Summary

The purpose of this first chapter is to provide a brief, historical introduction to stereotyped behaviour, placing particular emphasis on drug treatments that affect central dopamine activity. In addition to the descriptions of early pharmacological and neuroanatomical studies, we also refer to some of the important psychological variables which are involved in the expression of stereotyped behaviour. The point is made that the term 'stereotyped' is a descriptive one, and can be used to describe any form of behaviour that is repetitive, invariant, and non-adaptive. It does not indicate a type of response itself, but the form in which the response is manifested. Following our historical overview, the theme of dopamine and stereotyped behaviour is continued in greater depth in the succeeding three chapters.

References

Amsler, C. (1923). Beiträge zur Pharmakologie des Gehirns. *Naunyn-Schmiedebergs Arch. exp. Path. Pharmak*. **97**, 1–14.

Andén, N.E. (1972). Dopamine turnover in the corpus striatum and the limbic system after treatment with neuroleptic and anti-acetylcholine drugs. *J. Pharm. Pharmacol*. **24**, 905–6.

Andén, N.E., Carlsson, A., Dahlström, A., Fuxe, K., Hillarp, N.A., and Larsson, K. (1964). Demonstration and mapping out of nigro-striatal dopamine neurons. *Life Sci*. **3**, 523–30

Andén, N.E., Dahlström, A., Fuxe, K., Larsson, K., Olson, L., and Ungerstedt, U. (1966). Ascending monoamine neurones to the telencephalon and diencephalon. *Acta physiol. scand.* **67**, 313–26.

Andén, N.E., Butcher, S.G., Corrodi, H., Fuxe, K., and Ungerstedt, U. (1970). Receptor activity and turnover of dopamine and noradrenaline after neuroleptics. *Eur. J. Pharmacol.* **11**, 303–14

Angrist, B., Sathananthan, G., Wilk, S., and Gershon, S. (1974). Amphetamine psychosis: behavioural and biochemical aspects. *J. psychiat. Res.* **11**, 13–23.

Asher, I.M. and Aghajanian, G.K. (1974). 6-hydroxydopamine lesions of olfactory tubercles and caudate nuclei: effect on amphetamine-induced stereotyped behaviour in rats. *Brain Res.* **82**, 1–12.

Barbeau, A., Sourkes, T.L., and Murphy, G.F. (1962). Les catecholamines dans la maladie de Parkinson. In *Monoamines et systeme nerveux centrale* (ed. J. de Ajuriaguerra), pp. 247–62. Georg, Geneve and Masson, Paris.

Beck, C.H.M., Chow, H.L., and Cooper, S.J. (1986). Initial environment influences amphetamine-induced stereotypy: subsequently environment change has little effect. *Behav. neural Biol.* **46**, 383–97.

Bertler, A. (1961). Occurrence and localization of catecholamines in the human brain. *Acta physiol. scand.* **51**, 97–107.

Bertler, A. and Rosengren, E. (1959). Occurrence and distribution of dopamine in brain and other tissues. *Experientia* **15**, 10–11.

Birkmayer, W. and Hornykiewicz, O. (1961). Der L-Dioxyphenylalanin (L-DOPA)-Effekt bei der Parkinson-Akinese. *Wien. Klin. Wschr.* **73**, 787–8.

Carlsson, A. (1959). The occurrence, distribution and physiological role of catecholamines in the nervous system. *Pharmacol. Rev.* **11**, 490–3.

Carlsson, A. and Lindqvist, M. (1963). Effect of chlorpromazine and haloperidol on formation of 3-methoxytyramine and normetanepherine in mouse brain. *Acta pharmacol. toxicol.* **20**, 140–4.

Carlsson, A., Lindqvist, M., Magnusson, T., and Waldeck, B. (1958). On the presence of 3-hydroxytyramine in brain. *Science* **127**, 471.

Carlsson, A., Falck, B., and Hillarp, N.-A. (1962). Cellular localization of brain monoamines. *Acta physiol, scand.* **56** (Suppl. 196), 1–27.

Collins, J.P., Lesse, H., and Dagon, L.A. (1979). Behavioural antecedents of cocaine-induced stereotypy. *Pharmacol. Biochem. Behav.* **11**, 683–7.

Connell, P.H. (1958). *Amphetamine psychosis*. Maudsley Monographs, No. 5, Oxford University Press, London.

Cools, A.R. (1986). Mesolimbic dopamine and its control of locomotor activity in rats: differences in pharmacology and light/dark periodicity between the olfactory tubercle and nucleus accumbens. *Psychopharmacology* **88**, 451–9.

Cools, A.R. and van Rossum, J.M. (1970). Caudal dopamine and stereotype behaviour of cats. *Arch. int. Pharmacodyn.* **187**, 163–73.

Cools, A.R., Broekkamp, C.L.E., and van Rossum, J.M. (1977). Subcutaneous injection of apomorphine, stimulus generalization and conditioning: serious pitfalls for the examiner using apomorphine as a tool. *Pharmacol. Biochem. Behav.* **6**, 705–8.

Costall, B. and Naylor, R.J. (1973). The role of telencephalic dopaminergic systems in the mediation of apomorphine-stereotyped behaviour. *Eur. J. Pharmacol.* **24**, 8–24.

Costall, B. and Naylor, R. J. (1974). Extrapyramidal and mesolimbic involvement with the stereotypic activity of D- and L-amphetamine. *Eur. J. Pharmacol.* **25**, 121–9.

Costall, B. and Naylor, R. J. (1975*a*). The behavioural effects of dopamine applied intracerebrally to areas of the mesolimbic system. *Eur. J. Pharmacol.* **32**, 87–92.

Costall, B. and Naylor, R. J. (1975*b*). Detection of the neuroleptic properties of clozapine, sulpiride and thioridazine. *Psychopharmacologia* **43**, 69–74.

Costall, B. and Naylor, R. J. (1976*a*). Antagonism of the hyperactivity induced by dopamine applied intracerebrally to the nucleus accumbens septi by typical neuroleptics and by clozapine, sulpiride and thioridazine. *Eur. J. Pharmacol.* **35**, 161–8

Costall, B. and Naylor, R. J. (1976*b*). A comparison of the abilities of typical neuroleptic agents and of thioridazine, clozapine, sulpiride and metoclopramide to antagonize the hyperactivity induced by dopamine applied intracerebrally to areas of the extrapyramidal and mesolimbic systems. *Eur. J. Pharmacol.* **40**, 9–19.

Costall, B., Naylor, R. J. and Nohria, V. (1978). Climbing behaviour induced by apomorphine in mice: a potential model for the detection of neuroleptic activity. *Eur. J. Pharmacol.* **50**, 39–50.

Costall, B., Naylor, R. J. and Nohria, V. (1981). Use of the intracerebral injection technique to elucidate mechanisms of apomorphine climbing and its antagonism in the mouse. *Psychopharmacology*, **73**, 91–94

Costall B., Naylor, R. J., and Olley, J. E. (1972). Stereotypic and anticataleptic activities of amphetamine after intracerebral injections. *Eur. J. Pharmacol.* **18**, 83–94.

Cotzias, G. C., Van Woert, M. H., and Schiffer, I. M. (1967). Aromatic amino acids and modification of Parkinsonism. *New Engl. J. Med.* **276**, 374–9

Cotzias, G. C., Papavasiliou, P. S., and Gellene, R. (1969). Modification of parkinsonism—chronic treatment with L-DOPA. *New Engl. J. Med.* **280**, 337–45.

Creese, I. and Iversen, S. D. (1973). Blockage of amphetamine induced motor stimulation and stereotypy in the adult rat following neonatal treatment with 6-hydroxydopamine. *Brain Res.* **55**, 369–82.

Creese, I. and Iversen, S. D. (1974). The role of forebrain dopamine systems in amphetamine induced stereotyped behaviour in the rat. *Psychopharmacologia* **39**, 345–57.

Dahlström, A. and Fuxe, K. (1964). Evidence for the existence of monoamine-containing neurons in the central nervous system. I. Demonstration of monoamines in the cell bodies of brain stem neurones. *Acta physiol. scand.* **62** (Suppl. 232), 1–55.

Davis, J. M. (1974). A two factor theory of schizophrenia. *J. psychiat. Res.* **11**, 25–9.

Di Chiara, G., Porceddu, M. L., Vargiu, L., Argiolas, A., and Gessa, G. L. (1976). Evidence for dopamine receptors mediating sedation in the mouse brain. *Nature* **264**, 564–7.

Dourish, C. T. (1987). Effects of drugs on spontaneous motor activity. In

Experimental psychopharmacology (ed. A. J. Greenshaw and C. T. Dourish), pp. 153–211. Humana Press, Clifton, New Jersey.

Dourish, C. T. and Cooper, S. J. (1984). Environmental experience produces qualitative changes in the stimulant effects of β-phenylethylamine in rats. *Psychopharmacology* **84**, 132–5.

Ehringer, H. and Hornykiewicz, O. (1960). Verteilung von Noradrenalin und Dopamin (3-hydroxytyramin) im Gehirn des Menschen und ihr Verhalten bei Erkrankungen des extrapyramidalen Systems. *Klin. Wschr.* **38**, 1236–9.

Einon, D. F. and Sahakian, B. J. (1979). Environmentally induced differences in susceptibility of rats to CNS stimulants and CNS depressants: evidence against a unitary explanation. *Psychopharmacology* **61**, 299–307.

Ellinwood, E. H. (1967). Amphetamine psychosis: I. Description of the individuals and process. *J. nerv. ment. Dis.* **144**, 273–83.

Ellinwood, E. H. and Balster, R. L. (1974). Rating the behavioural effects of amphetamine. *Eur. J. Pharmacol.* **28**, 35–41.

Ellinwood, E. H. and Kilbey, M. (1975). Amphetamine stereotypy: the influence of environmental factors and prepotent behavioural patterns on its topography and development. *Biol. Psychiat.* **10**, 3–16.

Elliott, P. N. C., Jenner, P., Huizing, G., Marsden, C. D., and Miller, R. (1977). Substituted benzamides as cerebral dopamine antagonists in rodents. *Neuropharmacology* **16**, 33–342.

Ernst, A. M. (1967). Mode of action of apomorphine and dexamphetamine on gnawing compulsion in rats. *Psychopharmacologia* **10**, 316–23.

Ernst, A. M. (1969). The role of biogenic amines in the extra-pyramidal system. *Acta physiol. pharmacol. Neerl.* **15**, 141–54.

Ernst, A. M. and Smelik, P. G. (1966). Site of action of dopamine and apomorphine on compulsive gnawing behaviour in rats. *Experientia* **22**, 837–8.

Eshkol, N. and Wachmann, A. (1958). *Movement notation*. Weidenfeld and Nicolson, London.

Evetts, K. D., Uretsky, N. J., Iversen, L. L., and Iversen, S. D. (1970). Effect of 6-hydroxydopamine on CNS catecholamines, spontaneous motor activity and amphetamine induced hyperactivity in rats. *Nature* **225**, 961–2.

Falck B., Hillarp, N.-A., Thieme, G., and Torp, A. (1962). Fluorescence of catecholamines and related compounds condensed with formaldehyde. *J. Histochem, Cytochem.* **10**, 348–54.

Fog, R. (1969). Stereotyped and non-stereotyped behaviour in rats induced by various stimulant drugs. *Psychopharmacologia* **14**, 299–304.

Fog, R. and Pakkenberg, H. (1971). Behavioural effects of dopamine and p-hydroxyamphetamine injected into corpus striatum of rats. *Exp. Neurol.* **31**, 75–86.

Fog., R. L., Randrup, A., and Pakkenberg, H. (1967). Aminergic mechanisms in corpus striatum and amphetamine-induced stereotyped behaviour. *Psychopharmacologia* **1**, 179–83.

Fog, R. L., Randrup, A., and Pakkenberg, H. (1970). Lesions in corpus striatum and cortex in rat brains and the effect of pharmacologically induced stereotyped, aggressive and cataleptic behaviour. *Psychopharmacologia* **18**, 346–56.

Fray, P. J., Sahakian, B. J., Robbins, T. W., Koob, G. F., and Iversen, S. D. (1980). An observational method for quantifying the behavioural effects of dopa mine agonists: contrasting effects of D-amphetamine and apomorphine. *Psychopharmacology* **69**, 253–9.

Fuxe, K. (1965). Evidence for the existence of monoamine neurons in the central nervous system. IV. Distribution of monoamine nerve terminals in the central nervous system. *Acta physiol. scand.* **64**, (Suppl. 247), 39–85.

Golani, I., Wolgin, D. L., and Teitelbaum, P. (1979). A proposed natural geometry of recovery from akinesia in the lateral hypothalamic rat. *Brain Res.* **164**, 237–67.

Golani, I., Bronchti, G., Moualem, D., and Teitelbaum, P. (1981). "Warm-up" along dimensions of movement in the hypothalamic rat. *Brain Res.* **164**, 237–67.

Griffith, J. J., Oates, J., and Cavanaugh, J. (1968). Paranoid episodes induced by drugs. *J. Am. med. Ass.* **205**, 39–46.

Harnack, E. (1874). Über die Wirkungen des Apomorphines am Saugethier und am Frosch. *Naunyn-Schmiedeberg's Arch. exp. Path. Pharmak.* **2**, 255–306.

Imperato, A. and Di Chiara, G (1985). Dopamine release and metabolism in awake rats after systemic neuroleptics as studied by trans-striatal dialysis. *J. Neurosci.* **5**, 297–306.

Iversen, S. D. and Koob, G. F. (1977). Behavioural implications of dopaminergic neurons in the mesolimbic system. In *Advances in biochemical psychopharmacology, Vol. 16* (ed. E. Costa and G. L. Gessa), pp. 209–14. Raven Press, New York.

Jackson, D. M., Andén, N.-E., and Dahlström, A. (1975). A functional effect of dopamine in the nucleus accumbens and in some other dopamine-rich parts of the rat brain. *Psychopharmacologia* **45**, 139–49.

Janssen, P. A. J., Niemegeers, C, and Jagenau, A. (1960). Apomorphine-antagonism in rats. *Arzneimittel-Forschung* **10**, 1003–5.

Janssen, P. A. J., Niemegeers, C. J. E., and Schellekens, K. H. L. (1965). Is it possible to predict the clinical effects of neuroleptic drugs (major tranquillizers) from animal date? (Part I). *Arzneimittel-Forschung* **15**, 104–17.

Janssen, P. A. J., Niemegeers, C. J. E., Schellekens, K. H. L., and Leanerts, F. M. (1967). It is possible to predict the clinical effects of neuroleptic drugs (major tranquillizers) from animal data? (Part IV). *Arzneimittel-Forschung* **17**, 841–54.

Jenner, P., Clow, A., Reavill, C., Theodorou, A., and Marsden, C. D. (1978). A behavioural and biochemical comparison of dopamine receptor blockade produced by haloperidol with that produced by substituted benzamide drugs. *Life Sci.* **23**, 545–50.

Kebabian, J. W. (1978). Dopamine-sensitive adenylyl cyclase: a receptor mechanism for dopamine. In *Advances in biochemical psychopharmacology*, vol. 19 (ed. P. J. Roberts, G. N. Woodruff, and L. L. Iversen), pp. 131–54. Raven Press, New York.

Kebabian, J. W. and Calne, D. B. (1979). Multiple receptors for dopamine. *Nature* **277**, 93–6.

Kebabian, J. W. and Greengard, P. (1971). Dopamine-sensitive adenyl cyclase: possible role in synaptic transmission. *Science* **174**, 1346–9.

Kebabian, J.W., Petzold, G.L., and Greengard, P. (1972). Dopamine-sensitive adenylate cyclase in caudate nucleus of rat brain, and its similarity to the "dopamine receptor". *Proc. nat. Acad. Sci., USA* **69**, 2145-9.

Kelly, P.H. (1977). Drug-induced motor behaviour. In *Handbook of psychopharmacology*, Vol. 8 (ed. L.L. Iversen, S.D. Iversen, and S.H. Snyder), pp. 295-331. Plenum Press, New York.

Kelly, P.H., Seviour, P.W., and Iversen, S.D., (1975). Amphetamine and apomorphine responses in the rat following 6-OHDA lesions of the nucleus accumbens septi and corpus striatum. *Brain Res.* **94**, 507-22.

Kelly, P.H., Miller, R.J., and Neumeyer, J.L. (1976). Aporphines 16. Action of aporphine alkaloids on locomotor activity in rats with 6-hydroxydopamine lesions of nucleus accumbens. *Eur. J. Pharmacol.* **35**, 85-92.

Lahti, R.A., McAllister, B., and Wozniak, J. (1972). Apomorphine antagonism of the elevation of homovanillic acid induced by antipsychotic drugs. *Life Sci.* **11**, 605-13.

Ljungberg, T. and Ungerstedt, U. (1977a). A new method for simultaneous registration of 8 behavioural parameters related to monoamine neurotransmission. *Pharmacol. Biochem. Behav.* **8**, 483-9.

Ljungberg, T. and Ungerstedt, U. (1977b). Different behavioural patterns induced by apomorphine: evidence that the method of administration determines the behavioural response to the drug. *Eur. J. Pharmacol.* **46**, 41-50.

Ljungberg, T. and Ungerstedt, U. (1977c). Apomorphine-induced locomotion and gnawing: evidence that the experimental design greatly influences gnawing while locomotion remains unchanged. *Eur. J. Pharmacol.* **46**, 147-51.

Ljungberg, T. and Ungerstedt, U. (1978). Classification of neuroleptic drugs according to their ability to inhibit apomorphine-induced locomotion and gnawing: evidence for two different mechanisms of action. *Psychopharmacology* **56**, 239-47.

Ljungberg, T. and Ungerstedt, U. (1985). A rapid and simple behavioural screening method for simultaneous assessment of limbic and striatal blocking effects of neuroleptic drugs. *Pharmacol. Biochem. Behav.* **23**, 479-85.

Lyon, M. and Randrup, A. (1972). The dose–response effect of amphetamine upon avoidance behaviour in the rat seen as a function of increasing stereotypy. *Psychopharmacologia* **23**, 334-47.

Lyon, M. and Robbins, T.W. (1975). The action of central nervous stimulant drugs: a general theory concerning amphetamine effects. In *Current developments in psychopharmacology*, Vol. 2 (ed. W.B. Essman and L. Valzelli), pp. 79-163. Spectrum Publications, New York.

Makanjuola, R.O.A., Dow, R.C., and Ashcroft, G.W. (1980). Behavioural responses to stereotaxically controlled injections of monoamine neurotransmitters into the accumbens and caudate–putamen nuclei. *Psychopharmacology* **71**, 227-35.

Matthysse, S. (1973). Antipsychotic drug action: a clue to the neuropathology of schizophrenia. *Fed. Proc.* **32**, 200-5.

Montagu, K.A. (1957). Catechol compounds in rat tissues and in brains of different animals. *Nature* **180**, 244-5.

Mumford, L., Teixeira, A.R., and Kumar, R. (1979). Sources of variation in locomotor activity and stereotypy in rats treated with D-amphetamine. *Psychopharmacology* **62**, 241-5.

Naylor, R. J. and Costall, B. (1971). The relationship between the inhibition of dopamine uptake and the enhancement of amphetamine stereotypy. *Life Sci.* **10**, 909-15.

Naylor, R. J. and Olley, J. E. (1972). Modification of the behavioural changes produced by amphetamine in the rats by lesions in the caudate–putamen and globus pallidus. *Neuropharmacology* **11**, 91-9.

Niemegeers, C. J. E. and Janssen, P. A. J. (1979). A systematic study of the pharmacological properties of dopamine antagonists. *Life Sci.* **24**, 2201-16.

Peselow, E. D. and Stanley, M, (1982). Clinical trials of benzamides in psychiatry. In *the benzamides: pharmacology, neurobiology, and clinical aspects* (ed. J. Rotrosen and M. Stanley). pp. 163-94. Raven Press, New York.

Pijnenburg, A. J. J. and van Rossum, J. M. (1973). Stimulation of locomotor activity following injection of dopamine into the nucleus accumbens. *J. Pharm. Pharmacol.* **25**, 1003-5.

Pijnenburg, A. J. J., Honig, W. M. M., and van Rossum, J. M. (1975a). Inhibition of D-amphetamine-induced locomotor activity by injection of haloperidol into the nucleus accumbens of the rat. *Psychopharmacologia* **41**, 87-95.

Pijnenburg, A. J. J., Honig, W. M. M., and van Rossum, J. M. (1975b). Effects of antagonists upon locomotor stimulation induced by injection of dopamine and noradrenaline into the nucleus accumbens of nialamide-pretreated rats. *Psychopharmacologia* **41**, 175-80.

Pijnenburg, A. J. J., Honig, W. M. M., and van Rossum, J. M. (1975c). Antagonism of apomorphine- and D-amphetamine-induced stereotyped behaviour by injection of low doses of haloperidol into the caudate nucleus and the nucleus accumbens. *Psychopharmacologia* **45**, 65-71.

Pijnenburg, A. J. J., Honig, W. M. M., van der Heyden, J. A. M., and van Rossum J. M. (1976). Effects of chemical stimulation of the mesolimbic dopamine system upon locomotor activity. *Eur. J. Pharmacol.* **35**, 45-58.

Protais, P., Costentin, J., and Schwartz, J. D. (1976). Climbing behaviour induced by apomorphine in mice—a simple test for the study of dopamine receptors in striatum. *Psychopharmacology* **50**, 1-6.

Protais, P., Bonnett, J.-J., Costentin, J., and Schwartz, J.-C. (1984). Rat climbing behaviour elicited by stimulation of cerebral dopamine receptors. *Naunyn-Schmiedeberg's Arch. Pharmacol.* **325**, 93-101

Randrup, A and Munkvad, I. (1965). Special antagonism of amphetamine-induced abnormal behaviour. *Psychopharmacologia* **7**, 416-22.

Randrup, A. and Munkvad, I (1967). Stereotyped activities produced by amphetamine in several animal species and man. *Psychopharmacologia* **11**, 300-10.

Randrup, A., Munkvad, I., and Udsen, P. (1963). Adrenergic mechanisms and amphetamine induced abnormal behaviour. *Acta pharmacol. toxicol.* **20**, 145-57.

Rebec, G. V. and Bashore, T. R. (1984). Critical issues in assessing the behavioural effects of amphetamine. *Neurosci. Biobehav. Rev.* **8**, 153-9.

Robertson, A. and MacDonald, C. (1984). Atypical neuroleptics clozapine and thioridazine enhance amphetamine-induced stereotypy. *Pharmacol. Biochem. Behav.* **21**, 97–101.

Robertson, A. and MacDonald, C. (1985). Opposite effects of sulpiride and metoclopramide on amphetamine-induced stereotypy. *Eur. J. Pharmacol.* **109**, 81–9.

Sahakian, B. J. and Robbins, T. W. (1975). The effects of test environment and rearing condition on amphetamine-induced stereotypy in the guinea pig. *Psychopharmacologia* **45**, 115–17.

Sahakian, B. J., Robbins, T. W., Morgan, J. J., and Iversen, S. D. (1975). The effects of psychomotor stimulants on stereotypy and locomotor activity in socially deprived and control rats. *Brain Res.* **84**, 195–205.

Sano, I., Gamo, T., Kakimoto, Y., Taniguchi, K., Takesade, M., and Nishinuma, K. (1959). Distribution of catechol compounds in human brain. *Biochim. Biophys. Acta* **32**, 586–7.

Schiørring, E. (1971). Amphetamine-induced selective stimulation of certain behaviour items with concurrent inhibition of others in an open-field test with rats. *Behaviour* **39**, 1–17.

Schiørring, E. (1979). An open field study of stereotyped locomotor activity in amphetamine-treated rats. *Psychopharmacology* **66**, 281–7.

Segal, D. S. and Janowsky, D. S. (1978). Psychostimulant-induced behavioural effects: possible models of schizophrenia. In *Psychopharmacology: a generation of progress* (ed. M. A. Lipton, A. DiMascio, and K. F. Killam), pp. 1113–23. Raven Press, New York.

Sharp, T., Zetterström, T., Herrera-Marschitz, M., Ljungberg, T., and Ungerstedt, U. (1986). Intracerebral dialysis—a technique for studying dopamine release in the rat brain in relation to behaviour. In *Monitoring neurotransmitter release during behaviour* (ed. M. H. Joseph, M. Fillenz, I. A. MacDonald, and C. A. Marsden), pp. 94–104. Ellis Horwood, Chichester.

Simpson, B. A. and Iversen, S. D. (1971). Effects of substantia nigra lesions on the locomotor and stereotypy responses to amphetamine. *Nature New Biology* **230**, 30–2.

Snyder, S. H., Banerjee, S. P., Yamamura, H. I., and Greenberg, D. (1974). Drugs neurotransmitters, and schizophrenia. *Science* **184**, 1243–53.

Stanley, M. and Wilk, S. (1977). The effects of antipsychotic drugs and their clinically inactive analogs on dopamine metabolism. *Eur. J. Pharmacol.* **44**, 293–302.

Stoof, J. C. and Kebabian, J. W. (1984). Two dopamine receptors: biochemistry, physiology and pharmacology. *Life Sci.* **35**, 2281–96.

Szechtman, H. (1986). Behaviour performed at onset of drug action and apomorphine stereotypy. *Eur. J. Pharmacol.* **121**, 49–56.

Szechtman, H., Ornstein, K., Teitelbaum, P., and Golani, I. (1982). Snout contact fixation, climbing and gnawing during apomorphine stereotypy in rats from two substrains. *Eur. J. Pharmacol.* **80**, 385–92.

Szechtman, H., Ornstein, K., Teitelbaum, P., and Golani, I. (1985). The morphogenesis of stereotyped behaviour induced by the dopamine receptor agonist apomorphine in the laboratory rat. *Neuroscience* **14**, 783–98.

Teitelhaum, P. and Derks, P. (1958). The effect of amphetamine on forced drinking in the rat. *J. comp. physiol. Psychol.* **51**, 801–10.

Ungerstedt, U. (1971). Postsynaptic supersensitivity after 6-hydroxydopamine induced degeneration of the nigro-striatal dopamine system. *Acta physiol. scand.* **83**, (Suppl. 367), 69–93.

Ungerstedt, U. (1979). Central dopamine mechanisms and unconditioned behaviour. In *The neurobiology of dopamine* (ed. A.S. Horn, J. Korf, and B.H.C. Westerink), pp. 577–96. Academic Press, London.

Ungerstedt, U. (1984). Measurement of neurotransmitter release by intracranial dialysis. In *Measurement of neurotransmitter release in vivo* (ed. C.A. Marsden), pp. 81–105. John Wiley, Chichester.

Vasse, M., Protais, P., Costentin, J., and Schwartz, J.-C. (1985). Unexpected potentiation by discriminant benzamide derivatives of stereotyped behaviours elicited by dopamine agonists in mice. *Naunyn-Schmiedeberg's Arch. Pharmacol.* **329**, 108–16.

Weil-Malherbe, H. and Bone, A.D. (1957). Intracellular distribution of catecholamines in the brain. *Nature* **180**, 1050–1.

Weismann, A. (1971). Cliff jumping in rats after intravenous treatment with apomorphine. *Psychopharmacology* **21**, 60–5.

Wilk, S. and Stanley, M. (1977). Perlapine and dopamine metabolism: prediction of antipsychotic efficacy. *Eur. J. Pharmacol.* **41**, 65–72.

Woodruff, G.N., Kelly, P.H., and Elkhawad, A.O. (1976). Effects of dopamine receptor stimulants on locomotor activity of rats with electrolytic or 6-hydroxydopamine-induced lesions of the nucleus accumbens. *Psychopharmacology* **47**, 195–8.

Worms, P. (1982). Behavioural pharmacology of the benzamides as compared to standard neuroleptics. In *The benzamides: pharmacology, neurobiology and clinical aspects* (ed. J. Rotrosen and M. Stanley), pp. 7–16. Raven Press, New York.

Young, D. and Scoville, W.B. (1938). Paranoid psychosis in narcolepsy and the possible dangers of benzedrine treatment. *Med. Clin. N. Am.* **22**, 637–43.

Zetterström, T., Sharp T., and Ungerstedt, U. (1984). Effect of neuroleptic drugs on striatal dopamine release and metabolism in the awake rat studied by intracerebral dialysis. *Eur. J. Pharmacol.* **106**, 27–37.

2

The neuropsychological significance of stereotypy induced by stimulant drugs

T. W. ROBBINS, G. MITTLEMAN, J. O'BRIEN, and P. WINN

Introduction

The purpose of this chapter is to discuss the neuropsychological significance of stereotyped behaviour, in particular that induced by psychomotor stimulant drugs such as amphetamine. Behavioural stereotypy is a phenomenon with connotations in wide aspects of psychology, including animal learning theory, ethology, human experimental psychology, particularly in analyses of skilled or automatic performance, and in neuropsychological studies of brain-damaged patients. Stereotypy is also frequently observed in the psychopathology of man and other animals. There is, of course, no guarantee that all of these forms of stereotypy are related by common psychological processes and this will be one of the questions to be addressed below. We will be concentrating on the behavioural and neural mechanisms underlying stereotypy, because these aspects have previously been somewhat neglected in favour of a more neuropharmacological approach.

The basic pharmacology of stereotyped behaviour has been the subject of many reviews (e.g. Moore 1978; Groves and Rebec 1976; Robbins and Sahakian 1981) and will not be considered here in any great detail. (See Curzon, Chapter 6, this volume and Waddington et al., Chapter 3, this volume for further discussion.) The prime phenomena of interest for behavioural pharmacologists have been the repetitive orofacial responses and head movements induced by high doses of the phenylethylamine class of drugs, including amphetamine, methylphenidate, and β-phenylethylamine, and by dopamine receptor agonists such as apomorphine. Stereotypy of various forms can be induced by drugs outside this class, including the anticholinergic atropine, the hallucinogens LSD and phenylcyclidine, and the narcotic opiate morphine, but it is likely that these effects are all eventually mediated by interactions of other neurotransmitter systems with the dopaminergic projections or with associated basal ganglia structures. The great advantage of the pharmacological approach, as we shall see, has been the ease of constructing dose-effect curves, which enable the development of stereotypy to be monitored quite closely. Focusing upon the pharmacology of such a limited set of behavioural responses, however, has occasionally obscured the possible neuropsychological significance of drug-induced stereotyped behaviour.

There are several approaches one can adopt in studying the behavioural nature of stereotypy, including its detailed behavioural description and its environmental determinants. We shall deal with both of these and also attempt to relate stimulant-induced stereotypy to other forms of behaviour that have been suggested to arise in part from processes akin to psychomotor stimulation, including the stimulus-bound behaviour elicited by electrical stimulation of the hypothalamus in rats and other animals and the 'adjunctive' behaviour, including polydipsia, induced by the intermittent scheduling of small aliquots of food.

We also intend to examine whether the types of behavioural processes to be discussed can map adequately on to what is known of the neural basis of stereotyped behaviour and whether its mediation can provide some clues about the interaction of certain neural systems, including the basal ganglia, limbic system, and prefrontal cortex.

Function or purpose in stereotyped behaviour?

Stereotypy is a description of the nature of behaviour, rather than a specific response. (See Robbins and Sahakian 1981 and Cooper and Dourish, Chapter 1, this volume, for a discussion of conceptual problems of definition and related ones of measurement.) Although a definition, such as repetition in an invariant sequence of movements captures the topographical features of stereotypy, it fails to address those additional properties of behavioural autonomy which make the behaviour apparently inappropriate with respect to its environmental context.

The problem of inappropriateness is indeed central to the concept of stereotypy. Is this behaviour truly without purpose, or at least, without adaptive function? Hutt and Hutt (1965) in their definition neatly avoided the issue by stating that there was 'no observable goal' of stereotypy. Lyon and Robbins (1975) also regarded stereotypy as an inevitable concomitant of extreme psychomotor stimulation, and did not consider that it had any particular function. Others have speculated that it is rewarding, or that it serves to regulate arousal, or that it is a coping strategy to alleviate stress. These possibilities will now be considered.

Lyon–Robbins hypothesis

This states that amphetamine with increasing dose produces an increasing response rate within a progressively narrowing response repertoire. This could be seen as a description of what actually occurs, but it is also postulated that the observed behavioural effect results from the drug increasing the rate of all responses having a minimal tendency. This stimulation leads initially to reductions in pausing, and then at higher doses to enhanced behavioural competition among different response sequences. Eventually, the performance, especially the completion, of surviving response sequences is hindered by competition even among the response elements constituting the sequence. At this point overt behaviour is dominated by the repetitive performance of out-of-context motor elements, when the animal is essentially immobilized due to over-excitation. Behavioural stereotypy, as commonly defined, is then seen as the culmination of a process of heightened activation, mediated primarily by dopamine release in the basal ganglia, in which responses are initiated at increasingly rapid rates. Evidence for this position, schematically shown in Fig. 2.1, is reviewed by Lyon and Robbins (1975) and Robbins and Sahakian (1983). We will now briefly review here the main points of the theory which relate particularly to stereotyped behaviour.

Narrowing of the response repertoire   This is of course very obvious at high doses of amphetamine (i.e. 5–15 mg/kg). However, it is important to realize that the tendency is already present at lower doses. For example, Nieto *et al.* (1979) observed how behaviour generated by a fixed-time, 60-s schedule of food presentation in hungry rats was affected by increasing doses of D-amphetamine. They showed that the typical polydipsia and 'exploratory' behaviour normally occurring in the middle of the 60-s periods were replaced by premature and well-nigh exclusive orientation to the food magazine, in doses as low as 3.6 mg/kg. The tendency towards narrowing continues even after the behaviour has become quite severely stereotyped, as shown in elegant observational studies of the progressive effects of apomorphine (1.25 mg/kg subcutaneously) by Szechtman *et al.* (1985). Thus, in an unstructured environment, the normal pattern of pivoting (or turning) around its hindquarters, walking, rearing, and head-rising is replaced progressively in the rat by sliding snout contact with the ground coupled first with forwards progression and then with turning in the absence of progression until the rat pivots around only one hindlimb. Eventually even the lateral body movements disappear and the rat is essentially immobile. (See Teitelbaum *et al.*, Chapter 7, this volume, for further details.)

Behavioural competition Although behavioural competition could be inferred from the narrowing of the response repertoire, firmer evidence of it is derived from three criteria: (1) shortening in time of particular responses and the occurrence of abortive response sequences; (2) enhanced switching between response sequence; and (3) enhanced rate of performance of certain responses when competing responses are blocked. The effects of amphetamine satisfy each of these criteria (see Robbins and Sahakian 1983). The most obvious evidence of competition is between the locomotor effects of the drug and the intense head movements and sniffing stereotypy (e.g. Segal 1975).

Baseline-dependent effects From Fig. 2.1 it can be observed that the Lyon–Robbins hypothesis postulates that amphetamine will fail to stimulate any form of behaviour not already prepotent in the animal's repertoire. Further, it suggests that, although all responses have the same bell-shaped dose–effect curve, the maxima for these curves occur at different doses of the drug. Moreover, those responses occurring at initially high rates (e.g. under fixed ratio schedules or eating in deprived animals) have peak effects at much lower doses than those responses occurring at low rates (e.g. under DRL schedules, or sniffing in a familiar environment). There is some evidence to support these premises (Robbins and Sahakian 1983); their relevance to stereotyped behaviour can be seen by reference to Fig. 2.1. This is essentially a representation of the Yerkes–Dodson (1908) principle relating the optimal performance of tasks varying in difficulty to different hypothetical levels of arousal. The 'difficult' tasks are typically performed optimally at lower levels of arousal than the 'easy' ones. Stereotypy is seen as the maximal performance of responses (such as sniffing) which are relatively automatic or easy to execute, requiring for example little sensory feedback or planning. It is, of course, recognized that the organization of even relatively 'simple' responses such as sniffing and grooming can, in fact, be quite complex, involving the precise sequencing of several elements and hierarchical levels of control (cf. Szechtman *et al.* 1985; Fentress 1983).

Environmental control A corollary statement of the Lyon–Robbins hypothesis is that animals under amphetamine or other stimulants do not primarily suffer from deficits in sensory input. Indeed, it is maintained that stimulus control, including contingencies of reinforcement, will continue to influence behaviour until the drugged animal is prevented from responding appropriately by its increasingly stereotyped mode of behaviour. This

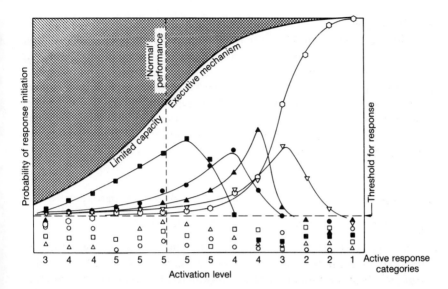

Fig. 2.1. A schematic diagram to illustrate the Lyon–Robbins hypothesis. Ordinate probability of response initiation; abscissa, activation level. This hypothetical process increases in strength from left to right and is equivalent to increasing dose of amphetamine or increasing dopaminergic activity. The numbers on the abscissa refer to the number of active (or behaviourally expressed) response categories at each activation level. Depicted are 'dose–response curves' for several responses in the rat, such as operant lever-pressing, locomotion, and sniffing as a function of activation level (or dose of amphetamine, or dopaminergic activity). The diagram shows how: (1) each response has its own characteristic inverted-U-shaped function and the family of curves is directly analogous to the Yerkes–Dodson principle; (2) some response categories, in the absence of any altered contingencies which would result in them becoming supra-threshold, are below the threshold for activation and hence not susceptible to stimulating effects; (3) there is a 'limited capacity' for the behavioural expression of the stimulated categories; (4) at normal levels of activation the responses occur at different baseline rates which help to determine the drug effect; (5) with increasing activation, there is an increasing probability of initiation within a reduced number of response categories; and (6) this results in a particular disruption of sequences of behaviour involving more than one response category.

implies that stereotyped behaviour can be under a degree of environmental control, including the previous learning and experience of the organism. The implication is of psychopathological significance because it shows, at least over a limited range of doses, how a considerable degree of individual variation in stereotypy, as well of complexity of response output, can potentially occur, even in the rat.

Examples of environmental modification of amphetamine stereotypy have been elegantly described by Ellinwood and Kilbey (1975) in the cat and monkey, and Sahakian and Robbins (1975a) reported an example of stereotyped social behaviour in a guinea-pig treated with 5 mg/kg D-amphetamine which continuously pursued a particular cage-mate, gnawing at a particular location on its fur. To understand the significance of these phenomena, in terms of both their behavioural and neural processes of organization, it is useful to consider the three main ways in which environmental factors interact with the frank stereotypy of simple movements produced by amphetamine:

(1) interruption or disruption;

(2) competition, resulting in a 'blending' of behavioural patterns;

(3) stereotypy of conditioned behaviour or learned habits.

Types (1) and (2) can be illustrated by the effects of high doses of amphetamine on performance in spatial tasks such as the 'Morris water-maze', in which the animal is trained to swim to the location of a submerged platform in opaque water. This procedure obliterates local cues and makes the animal dependent upon extra-maze ones instead. As Mittleman (unpublished results) has recently found, some rats treated with 5 mg/kg of amphetamine, remarkably, are still able to swim directly to the location of the platform, even though the dose produces a strong stereotypy in the home cage which occludes other forms of behaviour. The goal of escaping from the water-maze is apparently sufficiently compelling to enable the animal to interrupt its stereotypy, at least temporarily. In contrast, other animals exhibiting similarly strong stereotypy in the home cage, are unable to escape from the water-maze within the allowed time, and swim repetitively around the perimeter of the circular maze instead. This stereotyped swimming is often accompanied by repetitive forelimb movements and sniffing which would be normally shown in the home cage. This example illustrates how environmental demands can modify the form of stereotyped behaviour rather than interrupt it. Both types of environmental influence have been observed in other situations. Thus, novel stimuli can disrupt amphetamine stereotypy (Sahakian and Robbins 1975a) in a way analogous to the interruption exhibited by some rats in the water-maze. Lyon and Randrup (1972) were among the first to show how stereotyped forms of behaviour become blended, often quite effectively, with instrumental behaviour in a shock escape–avoidance situation. The overall, wide variability in response to the drug has also been seen by Ranje and Ungerstedt (1974) in a water Y-maze escape task.

The third type of interaction of environmental factors with stereotypy occurs when operant behaviour itself appears to become stereotyped in nature in response to the drug. The often-reported dissociation of instrumental and consummatory behaviour, in which the former is performed in a perseverative fashion, may be an example of this. Evenden and Robbins (1983a,b) have observed how behaviour under a two-lever random ratio schedule of reinforcement may have perseverative properties, in which the rat may continue to switch between two levers without pausing to collect food reinforcement following treatment with D-amphetamine. Occasionally, such behaviour occurs after the end of the session when, of course, no further reinforcement is programmed (see the cumulative record depicted as fig. 6 in Robbins and Sahakian 1983). Barrett and Stanley (1982) have reported similar perseveration of a lever-lifting operant in rabbits. Further evidence that the operant behaviour under this schedule becomes autonomous of its control by food reinforcement following amphetamine can be seen from the fact that the lever-pressing operant behaviour is maintained even though the presentation of food or its omission lose their capacity to produce respectively 'win–stay' and 'lose–shift' behaviour (Evenden and Robbins 1983a).

The 'perseverative switching' observed by Evenden and Robbins (1983b) again emphasizes how quite long sequences of behaviour can become stereotyped after amphetamine in rats, but evidence of further breakdown into long perseverative runs of response on a single lever was not easy to find. This makes the effects of apomorphine on this operant schedule of even greater interest. In fact, following systemic apomorphine over a range of doses, behaviour became restricted almost entirely to one of the two levers (Robbins 1980). The enhancement of switching seen with amphetamine was absent following apomorphine; this drug appeared to induce a much more intense form of stereotypy, perhaps under less environmental or experiential control than that of amphetamine. Stereotyped operant behaviour has also been observed following apomorphine with brain stimulation reward as the primary reinforcer in rats (Broekkamp et al. 1973) and in monkeys working for food (Dooley and Bowden 1983). Analogous results have been reported by Abelson and Woods (1980) for the effects of apomorphine in pigeons. It is possible that the apomorphine-induced lever-pressing (or key-pecking) represents some interaction between the unconditioned effects of the drug (e.g. to elicit rearing and approach to a protruding object in the rat, or pecking in the pigeon) and the operant requirement. Untrained rats may also show increases in 'stereotyped' lever-pressing following apomorphine, although the effect is much smaller than when the rats have received training under the two-lever schedule (T. W. Robbins, unpublished results).

Such phenomena in animals are of course predicted by the often complex forms of stereotypy shown by human amphetamine abusers. Many of these stereotypies involve complex routines such as motor-care maintenance, TV repair, or even artistic design, speech, and thought (Rylander 1971; Kramer et al. 1967). Bleuler's (1950) emphasis upon the occurrence of stereotypy at several levels of organization in schizophrenics thus also appears to hold for animal and human subjects treated with amphetamine.

Repeated treatment and amphetamine   Chronic or sub-chronic treatment with amphetamine can enhance certain aspects of response to the drug (sensitization), while producing apparent tolerance to others (see Eichler *et al.* 1980; Segal and Schuckit 1983; Mittleman *et al.* 1985). Thus, whereas sniffing, head, and limb movements tend progressively to increase following repeated treatment, licking and gnawing decline in frequency. The mechanisms underlying these changes are still unclear. On the one hand, neuropharmacological factors probably contribute to sensitization, but the possible additional influence of conditioning should not be ruled out. However, the basic description used by Lyon and Robbins to describe the acute effects of increasing doses of stimulants also appears broadly to hold for the cumulative effects of repeated treatment.

Stereotypy as a reward

Amphetamine and related stimulants are abused agents and are self-administered by animals. Hence they can, by definition, act as reinforcers. To what extent are the stereotyped effects related to the reinforcing action? Hill (1970) speculated that amphetamines enhanced the effects of conditioned reinforcement and, furthermore, that stereotyped behaviour was the ultimate expression of such an action: stereotyped sniffing in the rat, for instance, represents enhanced approach to olfactory incentives. There are certainly some circumstantial indications that this hypothesis should be taken seriously. First, there are anecdotal reports that stereotyped behaviour in amphetamine abusers can have pleasurable (though hardly euphoric) subjective effects (Rylander 1971). Second, if one equates time spent in particular activities as a reflection of their reinforcing efficacy (cf. the Matching Law of Herrnstein; see Heyman 1983), then it is obvious (though somewhat circular) to say that stereotyped behaviour represents the action of a powerful reinforcer. It is also obvious that one of the effects of reinforcers is selectively to increase the repetition of contingent behaviour (Schwartz 1980), which would lead to increased rate of performance of a reducing number of response categories, as mooted by Lyon and Robbins in describing the effects of amphetamine. Several authors have pointed out that, if for example, dopamine release is the basic mechanism of the reinforcing effect of amphetamine, then whatever responses are occurring at the time of onset of amphetamine's effects will be automatically reinforced, and hence repeated (e.g. Ellinwood and Kilbey 1975). Some of the perseverative effects of the drug on operant behaviour, whether maintained normally by unconditioned (Teitelbaum and Derks 1958) or merely by conditioned reinforcer (Robbins 1976), could conceivably arise from just such an action. The suggestion would be that even the kinaesthetic feedback of operant behaviour can become a conditioned reinforcer enhanced by the drug, hence making the behaviour self-sustaining (see Robbins and Sahakian 1983 for a fuller discussion).

Although the reinforcement hypothesis would account for important idiosyncratic aspects of stereotypy at relatively low doses of stimulants, it fails to adequately explain why stereotypy ultimately takes a similar form for different individuals within a species, whether rat, monkey, or man. Even human amphetamine addicts tend to show a preference towards manipulative forms of stereotypy (Rylander 1971). Hence, rather than postulating the nature of the response as the ultimate determinant of the form of stereotyped behaviour (as do Lyon and Robbins 1975), one has to postulate an absolute hierarchy of putative reinforcers, with olfactory and oral stimulation or proprioceptive and kinaesthetic feedback in the rat being in some way more basic sources of reinforcement than, say, gustatory, somaesthetic, auditory, or visual aspects of unconditioned or conditioned reinforcers. While it has been shown that such comparably simple behaviour as stimulus-bound gnawing elicited by electrical stimulation of the motor root of the trigeminal nerve has reinforcing properties (Van der Kooy and Phillips 1979), the problems of testing the relative rewarding properties of different stereotyped activities remain formidable.

There are two other major difficulties for a monolithic account of the effects of amphetamines in terms of reinforcement. First, even when the drug is self-administered by animals it appears that there is at least some crude regulation of plasma concentration of the drug (Wise 1981) so that the high levels which induce stereotyped behaviour are presumably less reinforcing than intermediate ones. Lethal overdosing by cats self-administering amphetamine (Ellinwood and Kilbey 1975) would seem more likely to arise from stereotyped operant behaviour overriding interoceptive signals of toxic effects rather than from the drug's rewarding action *per se*. Second, amphetamines often have aversive effects in animals and can lead to subjective paranoia in human subjects (Connell 1958). Thus, these drugs can hardly be said globally to enhance the positively reinforcing effects of environmental stimulation. For these reasons, it may be more correct, though less parsimonious, to say that reinforcement contingencies play some role in determining the form of amphetamine-induced stereotyped behaviour, but that stereotypies do not arise solely from an exaggeration of central reinforcement mechanisms.

Stereotypy as a coping response to stress

Another possible instrumental contingency is that stereotypy serves to reduce the aversive effects of stimulants. Related to this notion is the possibility that these drugs are stressors and that stereotypy represents a coping response to their stressful effects (Antelman and Chiodo 1983). In examining this hypothesis, it is important to bear in mind three distinct, though related, questions:

1. Is stereotypy a response to stress?

2. Are stimulants stressors?

3. Does stimulant-induced stereotypy reduce stress?

There is a good deal of evidence that certain stressful environmental conditions, such as housing singly or rearing in isolation, produce stereotypy in captive or laboratory animals (Meyer-Holzapel 1968; Ridley and Baker 1982; Fentress 1983). The adaptive significance of this behaviour is far from clear. Fitzgerald (1967) raised the possibility that stereotypies increase sensory input in times of sensory deprivation—a hypothesis, with its emphasis on 'self-stimulation', clearly related to the concept of stereotypy as a reinforcer, but almost diametrically opposed to the idea that stereotypy is a coping response which reduces stimulus input during stress. Ridley and Baker (1982) consider that, although cage stereotypy could conceivably act to increase stimulus input, it is most unlikely that the abnormal and lasting effects of early social isolation (either for monkeys or man, in the case of autism) have any discernible function, resulting instead from pathological changes in the central nervous system. These authors also showed that the stereotypies shown by vervet monkeys, when treated with amphetamine, resembled to a greater degree those induced by early social isolation than by separate caging. Thus it is clear that stereotypies produced by different conditions in the same animal can be morphologically distinct. This questions to some extent the notion that the different conditions can be simply subsumed by the term stress, although it is possible that the different forms of the stereotyped behaviour could arise from different degrees of stress acting like different doses of amphetamine.

The rigidity of behaviour in response to stimuli as diverse as electrical stimulation of the hypothalamus, mild pinching of the tail, social isolation, and intermittent schedules of reinforcement has suggested to many investigators that the stimulation is stressful and that the behaviour is stereotyped in nature. These conditions in the rat can all lead to repetitive oral or locomotor activities which resemble, but which are not identical to, behaviour induced by amphetamine. Several links, however, have been shown to exist between amphetamine-induced stereotypy and these other responses. For example, rats reared in isolation exhibit both enhanced stereotyped sniffing in response to amphetamine- and enhanced tail-pinch-induced oral behaviour (Sahakian *et al.* 1975; Sahakian and Robbins 1977). Moreover, rats positive for stimulus-bound eating or drinking following electrical stimulation of the hypothalamus exhibit more sensitization to amphetamine-induced stereotyped head and limb movements than rats screened as negative (Mittleman *et al*. 1986). The tendency towards schedule-induced polydipsia and electrically-elicited, non-regulatory ingestive behaviour is quite highly correlated (Mittleman and Valenstein 1984), as is the relationship between schedule-induced drinking and amphetamine stereotypy (Mittleman and Valenstein 1985). Furthermore, the individual differences in 'stereotypy' can be related to properties of the dopamine system and its response to stress. Thus, those rats exhibiting the strongest non-regulatory ingestive responses are those also showing the largest response in their dopamine systems to repeated footshock (Mittleman *et al*. 1986).

Many stressors, including severe food deprivation, cold, immobilization, and exposure to inescapable electric shocks, do not seem to lead to stereotyped behaviour and so the generality of the proposition that stress increases stereotypy is somewhat in doubt. It remains possible that certain forms of stress produce stereotypy because of their special characteristics. One striking common feature of the different stressors that do elicit stereotypy is that they often lack clear-cut environmental cues. Whereas exposure to electric shock or changes in temperature involve quite specific stimulation in addition to the stressful state, treatments such as isolation rearing or housing, electrical stimulation of the hypothalamus, mild tail-pinching, and indeed, amphetamine, all lack strong exteroceptive properties. Hebb's distinction between 'cue' properties of stimuli (such as their spatio-temporal aspects) and their intensive or 'arousal' properties is germane. Stereotypy appears most likely to be elicited in conditions involving high levels of arousal having no obvious external focus or cause.

The specific proposition that amphetamine is a stressor has been well argued by Antelman and Chiodo (1983) from a comparative review of the physiological, neuroendocrine, and neuropharmacological effects of stimulants and more conventionally accepted stressors. One of their main assumptions is that stressors should act in an additive and substitutable way in combination with amphetamine so that: (1) the presence of stress should move the dose–response curve for stereotypy to the left, and (2) sensitization to its effects by previous experience of the drug could be replaced by previous experience of other stressors. They cite as supporting evidence that previous experience of either tail-pinch stimulation, foot-shock, or food deprivation enhances amphetamine stereotypy. Possible problems of interpretation for these findings are that, in general, stereotypy rating scales only were used to measure the effects and full dose–response curves were not determined. In comparing the conclusions of Antelman and Chiodo (1983) with both previous and more recent literature, there is certainly evidence that the stressors they describe alter the behavioural response to amphetamine and related drugs, although the picture may be more complex than they indicate. For example, MacLennan and Maier (1983) have shown that exposing rats to a prior regimen of severe electric shocks does appear to enhance the response to amphetamine (4 mg/kg), but only if the shocks are uncontrollable, thus precluding 'coping responses'. Rats receiving the same amount of shock as controls, but allowed to escape from it, showed no greater stereotypy than unshocked controls. The enhanced response in the uncontrollable group in fact consisted of a transition from 'intermittent' stereotyped sniffing to head movements and continuous stereotypy over a wide area, an effect also consistent with elevated locomotor activity.

Previous evidence has certainly indicated that food deprivation enhances the locomotor effect of amphetamine (Campbell and Fibiger 1971) and apomorphine (Sahakian and Robbins 1975*b*) and, from the rating scale measures alone, it is difficult to ascertain if this was the same type of response seen in the studies reviewed by Antelman and Chiodo (1983). This is a salient concern because it is apparent that the response of rats to both amphetamine and apomorphine is somewhat differently affected by the 'stressors' of isolation rearing and food deprivation (Campbell and Fibiger 1971; Sahakian *et al.* 1975; Sahakian and Robbins 1975*b*). Considerations such as these are not necessarily antithetical to the Antelman and Chiodo position but they do show that there is much more to explain about the relationship of specific aspects of the amphetamine response and stress, especially since it is evident that different aspects of the amphetamine response may depend on different neuroanatomical substrates (Kelly *et al.* 1975).

A study by Einon and Sahakian (1979) has further exposed the difficulties of asserting that different environmental conditions merely act upon a single hypothetical construct such as 'stress' (although their investigation was directed at 'arousal'). They examined the separate and combined effects of several variables upon the amphetamine response in both male and female rats, including day–night cycle, isolation-rearing experience, and novelty of the test cage. The effects could not be readily explained in terms of a single intervening variable such as 'arousal' (or, by extension, 'stress'). Of particular importance was the confirmation of an earlier finding (by Sahakian and Robbins 1975*a*, using guinea-pigs) that amphetamine stereotypy was disrupted by environmental novelty. Thus, the focused sniffing in a restricted location was not made any more intense, but rather was replaced by sniffing over a wider area of the cage and locomotor activity typical of lower doses of the drug. Given that novelty is a major determinant of arousal (Berlyne 1960) and a stressor (Friedman and Ader 1967), it is apparent that increments in 'arousal' and 'stress' do not always act in the same direction as increasing doses of amphetamine. Faced with a similar problem, of explaining the different effects of combined stressors upon human performance, Broadbent (1971) was moved to postulate instead two 'arousal mechanisms'. This is somewhat beyond our present scope, but it is possible that the animal evidence may warrant a similar division (see Robbins 1984). Another factor of probable importance is the cue versus arousal distinction referred to above. Novel environmental stimulation clearly depends for its arousing effects upon analysis of its cueing properties. The effects of novelty upon amphetamine stereotypy may then not be inconsistent with the suggestion that stereotypy is promoted in conditions involving high arousal by interoceptive rather than exteroceptive cues.

The final question to be considered—whether stereotypy acts as a coping response—is the most difficult and one about which there is relatively little information. The most direct evidence would involve demonstrating that the induction of stereotyped behaviour by amphetamine reduces the neuroendocrine concomitants of the 'stressful' effects of the drug, such as elevated corticosterone and β-endorphin output. It is immediately apparent that this is a very difficult task. If the stereotyped behaviour were blocked, for example, by novel test conditions or by pharmacological means, then presumably this hypothesis would predict that plasma corticosterone levels would be elevated above normal for that dose of amphetamine. A recent experiment has confirmed this prediction by demonstrating attenuation of amphetamine-induced stereotypy following DA depletion from the caudate-putamen (Jones et al. 1989). This effect was manifested as a prolongation of the plasma corticosteroid response to the drug, which strikingly resembled a similar enhanced endocrine response to uncontrollable footshock (Swenson and Vogel 1983). By contrast, DA depletion from the ventral striatum antagonized the locomotor response to the drug, but merely retarded the plasma corticosterone response. Further analysis is required of the neuro-endocrine sequelae of these effects.

Given that some of the other forms of behaviour induced by 'non-specific' means may be related to stimulant-induced stereotypy, it could well prove easier to use these to test the hypothesis that such behaviour is stress-reducing. The evidence is not compelling, to date, although several authors support the idea, for example, Fentress (1983) in discussing displacement behaviour, Valenstein (1976) for behaviour induced by electrical stimulation of the brain, Rowland and Marques (1980) and Antelman and Chiodo (1984) for tail-pinch-induced eating, and Brett and Levine (1979) for schedule-induced polydipsia. Only the latter study employed endocrine measures and was indeed successful in showing that schedule-induced drinking was correlated with a suppression in the activity of the pituitary–adrenal system. Even this result, however, may be open to alternative interpretations. A related hypothesis concerning the effects of tail-pinch-induced stimulation is that the elicited behaviour reduces pain produced by the pinch (Morley and Levine 1980). But all the available evidence seems to indicate is that the tail-pinch stimulation may release opioids such as β-endorphin, which secondarily promote oral behaviour (e.g. Morley and Levine 1980). Again, no one seems to have shown conclusively that such oral behaviour reduces the neuroendocrine response to stress.

The studies reviewed in this section suggest that there is a common state or intervening variable underlying the effects of different stressors. Whether this is called 'stress' or 'arousal' or (as we prefer) 'activation' seems not to be particularly important. However, it is crucial to note that accepting the idea that non-specific states such as stress or activation can produce stereotyped behaviour does not necessarily entail support for the notion that the stereotypy regulates that state.

Stereotypy as a loss of volition

Kraepelin (1919) in attempting to explain the stereotypies of psychiatric patients felt that they might arise from the removal of a volitional influence that normally held primitive automatisms in check. This hypothesis has a neural analogue from the writings of Hughlings Jackson which would assert that stereotypies result from loss of inhibition of higher brain centres over lower ones. Modern research has identified the neural systems involved in stimulant-induced stereotypies, as well as related syndromes, but has not provided a model of how the systems interact to generate the behavioural phenomena we have described.

Neural basis of stimulant-induced stereotypy

The early work of Randrup and his collaborators strongly suggested that amphetamine-induced stereotypy was mediated by the central dopamine systems (Randrup and Munkvad 1970), but the crucial evidence came from studies in which the catecholamine neurotoxin 6-hydroxydopamine was infused locally into dopamine-containing brain regions to identify the critical neural substrates. Thus Creese and Iversen (e.g. 1975), in a succession of papers, were able to show that selective depletion of dopamine (DA) from the caudate–putamen in the rat reduced the stereotyped head-movements produced by amphetamine but enhanced the gnawing and licking responses to the DA receptor agonist apomorphine (because of the development of 'supersensitive' receptors in response to the presynaptic denervation). This important result was followed by the discovery that amphetamine-induced locomotion depended, not upon the nigrostriatal DA pathway, but upon the related mesencephalic DA projection from the ventral tegmental DA pathway to the nucleus accumbens (Kelly *et al.* 1975). The latter result was substantiated by the findings of Pijnenburg and colleagues (1976) that infusions of amphetamine into the nucleus accumbens, and also into the olfactory tubercle, elicited hyperactivity in the rat.

Many of the other effects of activating circumstances mentioned above have similarly been shown to depend upon the central DA systems, including the behaviour evoked by electrical stimulation of the hypothalamus and tail-pinch stimulation (Phillips and Fibiger 1976; Antelman and Szechtman 1975; Rowland *et al.* 1980) as well as schedule-induced drinking (Robbins and Koob 1980; Wallace *et al.* 1983). The effects of stressors such as electric shock and isolation have similarly been linked to changes in the central DA projections (see Bannon and Roth 1983). One problem for the hypothesis that all of these effects, including stereotypy, result from 'stress' is that different aspects of the central DA systems seem to be implicated in the various effects. Thus, according to Bannon and Roth, the effects of stressors are seen mainly in the mesolimbicocortical DA system rather than in the nigrostriatal DA projection. And tail-pinch-induced eating is unaffected by DA depletion from the nucleus accumbens (G.F. Koob and L. Stinus, personal communication) whereas schedule-induced drinking is attenuated by such treatment.

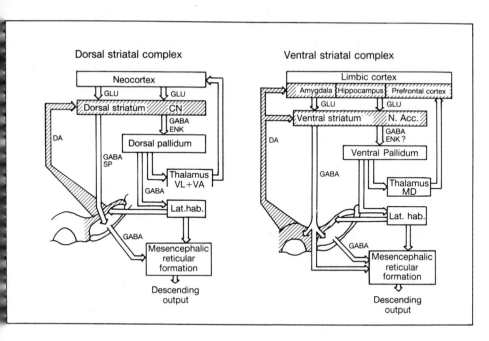

Fig. 2.2. Schematic diagram showing the neural connections of the dorsal and ventral striatum. Not shown are the details of the projections of substantia nigra, pars reticulata. GLU = glutamate. ENK = enkephalin. (For a review, see Nauta and Domesick 1984).

There have been great strides made in elucidating the neuroanatomical connections of the nucleus accumbens and caudate–putamen (see Fig. 2.2 and Nauta and Domesick 1984), although the significance of these for the mediation of the amphetamine response and, indeed, for any functional response is far from clear. Further advances made in elucidating the mechanisms underlying stereotypy have been largely neuropharmacological in nature, for example in specifying modulatory influences of other transmitters such as 5-HT, GABA, acetylcholine, noradrenalin (NA), and opioid neuropeptides (e.g. Robbins and Sahakian 1981) and will not be considered further. We raise instead some unsolved puzzles, first in terms of the precise way in which the DA systems mediate stereotypy and then in terms of the interactions of these systems with other forebrain influences, including the limbic system and neocortex, and also with the neural mechanisms efferent to the striatum. We will not be proposing definite answers to any of the problems posed, but raise them to stimulate further interest and research.

Outstanding problems for the dopamine hypothesis

Mediation of stereotypy at the neuronal level   Kuczenski (1983) and Groves and Tepper (1983) have recently provided important theoretical reviews on how the striatum mediates amphetamine stereotypy at the neuronal level. Kuczenski questions the hypothesis that the transition from locomotor activity in the rat to stereotypy reflects simply progressively increasing dopaminergic activity in the striatum on the basis of biochemical and electrophysiological date. In biochemical terms there is a lack of precise correlation between the occurrence of stereotypy and degree of striatal DA release or amphetamine concentration. Electrophysiological studies of single cells in the substantia nigra and striatum in anaesthetized animals show that doses of amphetamine below about 2.5 mg/kg reduce, whereas higher doses in contrast elevate, striatal firing rate (Rebec and Segal 1978). They suggest that there is a qualitative shift in the way in which the nigrostriatal projection regulates impulse-dependent DA release at terminals in the striatum. Specifically, the inhibitory influence of the pre-synaptic DA autoreceptors in the substantia nigra is suggested to be overridden at higher doses of amphetamine, leading to random DA bombardment of the post-synaptic cell and hence to diminished information transfer. Perhaps then, amphetamine stereotypy can be seen as resulting from a combination of DA activation and impaired information transfer. This model would explain why the form of amphetamine stereotypy can evidently be affected by environmental and experiential factors at lower doses, but becomes increasingly autonomous and independent of the environment at higher ones.

Behavioural differences between amphetamine and apomorphine   There are several major differences in the behavioural effects of apomorphine and amphetamine, although the implication of the early work was that these, respectively, direct and indirect agonists exerted their effects at the same DA receptors. Thus, in operant situations apomorphine increases response repetition, whereas amphetamine also enhances response switching (Evenden and Robbins 1983b; Robbins 1980). Amphetamine increases responding maintained specifically by conditioned reinforcement, whereas the rate-increasing effects of apomorphine are evidently independent of it (Robbins *et al.* 1983). Finally, the effects of these drugs on unconditioned behaviour in both the rat and pigeon are quite different (Fray *et al.* 1980: see Robbins and Sahakian 1981 for a review). A recent demonstration of this difference in the rat is shown in Fig. 2.3. The behavioural effects of various doses of systemically administered amphetamine or apomorphine were quantified for 1 hour in a simple observation chamber with a wire grid floor. The response categorization technique of Fray *et al.* (1980) was employed as well as a standard stereotypy rating scale (Creese and Iversen 1975), with time-sampling of behaviour at 5-min intervals. At 8 mg/kg (intraperitoneal) of D-amphetamine, the predominant responses are sniffing in restricted locations, combined with lateral head-movements, with the head oriented

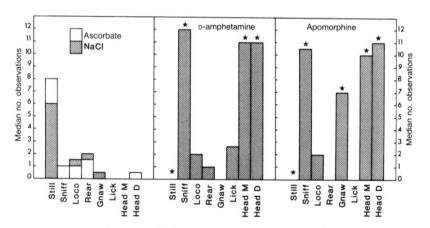

Fig. 2.3. Comparative effects of intraperitoneal D-amphetamine (8 mg/kg) and subcutaneous apomorphine 5 mg/kg) upon various components of unconditioned behaviour measured according to the method of Fray *et al.* (1980). Head M = lateral head movements. Head D = Head oriented down towards the floor of the cage. Loco = locomotor acitivity or movement of all four limbs. The rats (*n* = 8) were observed in wire cages (approx. 30 × 30 cm) for 60 min, about 5 min after injection. The measures are the scores of the median of 12 time-sampled periods of observation made at 5-min intervals. The rats received saline and ascorbate vehicle injections on control days. The asterisks show significant differences from control values, using non-parametric tests. (J. O'Brien, P. Winn, and T.W. Robbins, unpublished results.)

downwards at the floor. In contrast, 5 mg/kg of apomorphine also induces a strong gnawing response (which was not seen at any dose of amphetamine tested, even at doses of 15 mg/kg). The other major difference is that apomorphine produces much less locomotor activation than amphetamine at lower doses (Fray *et al.* 1980).

The behavioural differences between amphetamine and apomorphine might arise from a number of factors, acting either alone or in combination.

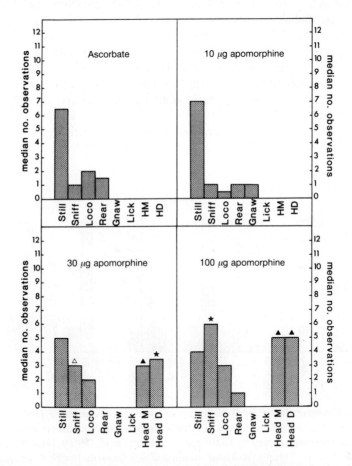

Fig. 2.4. Dose-dependent effects of apomorphine following bilateral microinjection into the head of the caudate–putamen in the rat. Infusions were made in a volume of 2 μl. The co-ordinates for the injection were + 2.0 from bregma, ± 3.0 from the midline, and − 5.5 mm from the dura (Pellegrino and Cushman 1967). See legend to Fig. 2.3 for further details. (J. O'Brien, P. Winn, and T. W. Robbins, unpublished results.)

For example, amphetamine affects other neurotransmitter systems (e.g. noradrenalin and 5-HT) which could well modulate its primarily DA action. It is conceivable that the different effects of the two drugs arise from actions at different receptors or at different neural sites. Alternatively, they could arise from their presynaptic versus postsynaptic modes of action: because of this, the behavioural effects of amphetamine might well be more susceptible to influences of the environment or previous conditioning. To attempt to answer some of these questions, we followed these simple experiments by injecting doses of the two drugs directly into their proposed central sites of action, in the caudate–putamen and nucleus accumbens, via bilateral stainless-steel cannulae, using standard procedures (see Taylor and Robbins 1984). Some of our results have surprised us because they have not readily fitted into the simple scheme that the caudate–putamen mediates amphetamine and apomorphine stereotypy.

In Fig. 2.4, it is immediately apparent that apomorphine failed to elicit gnawing when administered over a wide range of doses bilaterally into the posterior head of the caudate nucleus, although some repetitive head movements and the 'head-down' posture were observed. The volume injected was high ($2\mu l$) and should have ensured access to the bulk of the striatum. Our experiences with D-amphetamine were even more disappointing. We were unable to replicate the stereotypy typical of a peripheral dose of about 8 mg/kg with low doses (3–30 μg) in the same volume. Driven to using even higher, possibly neurotoxic doses, we did begin to find evidence of a very weak form of stereotypy, consisting of sniffing, with locomotion and head movements (Fig. 2.5). On the Creese–Iversen scale this corresponded to a median score of only 2 (discontinuous stereotypy), whereas the peripheral dose of 8 mg/kg produced ratings with a median of 4.0 (continuous stereotypy in a restricted location).

Failure to find significant effects with central injections of drugs such as amphetamine and apomorphine should of course always be regarded with suspicion. The drugs are lipophilic and will diffuse rapidly from their site of action; there is further the problem of reflux along the shaft of the cannula. Thus, attaining the concentration of a drug in a central site appropriate to that reached following systemic injection may be difficult to achieve. But there are considerations which reduce the impact of such objections. First, it is possible to produce significant biasing effects of amphetamine upon a head-movement operant following unilateral striatal infusions of doses as low as 10 μg (M. Carli and T.W. Robbins, unpublished results). Second, we have found it particularly easy to elicit locomotor activity from the nucleus accumbens in doses as low as 3 and 10 μg/2 μl, confirming the results of Pijnenberg et al. (1976). Indeed, the locomotor response was greater by far than any we have seen to occur following peripherally administered doses of the drug (J. Taylor, J. O'Brien, P. Winn, and T.W. Robbins, unpublished

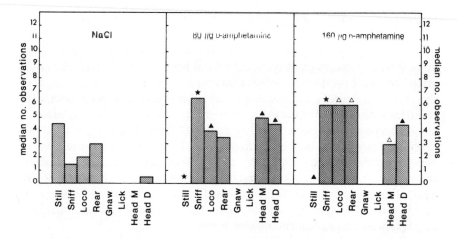

Fig. 2.5. Dose-dependent effects of bilateral microinjections of D-amphetamine into the caudate–putamen in the rat. For further details, see legend to Figs. 2.3 and 2.4. (J. O'Brien, P. Winn, and T. W. Robbins, unpublished results.)

results). Thus, it is difficult to argue that the central effect of the drug will be dissipated by diffusion or spread; the effects of the same centrally administered doses of amphetamine are greater at one site, but weaker at the other, than the effects of the peripherally administered drug. For these reasons, we believe that is may be profitable to at least consider an alternative hypothesis, that DA activation of the caudate–putamen may be a necessary, but not sufficient condition for amphetamine stereotypy.

A critical comparison of our results with others in the literature shows that our results do not disagree to any great extent. Five studies claim to have shown amphetamine or apomorphine stereotypy following intrastriatal infusions (Ernst and Smelik 1966; Fuxe and Ungerstedt 1970; Fog and Pakkenberg 1971; Costall *et al.* 1972; Staton and Solomon 1984). However, the evidence is far from convincing, either because of technical drawbacks in the microinjection procedures used or because of problems of behavioural measurement. For example, some of the studies have used very large volumes (5 μl) or crystalline implants which may have led to substantial diffusion of the drug or non-specific damage, respectively. The measurement of stereotypy was all-or-none in the earlier studies, but the use of stereotypy rating scales in the later ones revealed surprisingly weak effects. For example, Costall *et al.* (1972) observed a maximum average rating of about 1.9 on their scale on which 2.0 only reflected 'continuous sniffing and small head movements with periodic exploratory activity'. The experiment of Staton and Solomon (1984) reported quantitatively similar results. In looking for some signs of stereotypy, each of these studies seems to have ignored the remarkably weak nature of the effects actually observed and hence their significance. A recent study on the effects of intracerebral amphetamine in the marmoset (Annett *et al.* 1983) has provided further evidence to support our case. These authors carefully administered a series of doses of amphetamine into either the nucleus accumbens or more dorsally, into the caudate. They found that intra-accumbens injections dose-dependently increased not only locomotion, but also the incidence of small stereotyped head movements (or 'checking') that were only seen at the highest intracaudate doses. Thus, in this species, the nucleus accumbens, rather than the caudate, appeared to be the main site of action for the locomotor and also the more stereotyped effects of the drug.

In resolving the apparent discrepancy between the effects of caudate DA depletion upon amphetamine stereotypy and the relative lack of effect of intracaudate amphetamine, the most obvious possibility is that the stereotypy elicited by systemic amphetamine depends upon other actions of the drug in addition to its effect on caudate DA. The most prominent of these other actions would appear to be DA release into other telencephalic regions, including the amgydala, prefrontal cortex, and the nucleus accumbens.

Co-ordinated functioning of the caudate–putamen and nucleus accumbens Crucial to our understanding of the neural substrates of the amphetamine response is the relative contribution of these two structures. They can be considered as parts of the dorsal and ventral striatum, respectively, with largely independent outputs through the dorsal and ventral pallidum (see Fig. 2.2). However, because of the neuroanatomical relationships between the two structures (see Fig. 2.2), the nucleus accumbens is in a position to alter functioning in the nigrostriatal projection, whereas the reciprocal possibility is absent (Nauta and Domesick 1984). As previously mooted (Robbins and Everitt 1982), this provides possibilities of competition between parallel, independent output pathways on the one hand as well as direct interactions on the other, either of interrupting nigrostriatal activity or in some way boosting or amplifying it. The available evidence does not allow one to mediate easily among these alternatives.

The Lyon–Robbins hypothesis clearly predicts competition between the two systems and we have already considered some evidence that the locomotor and overtly stereotyped effects of the drug do appear to compete at the behavioural level. There is further, even stronger evidence of competition from the experiments of Joyce and Iversen (1984) on the effects of DA-depletion from the posterior head of the caudate nucleus on various aspects of the amphetamine response. They showed that the anorectic effects of amphetamine were reduced at high doses, when stereotyped behaviour was reduced. However, an even more relevant finding was the very high levels of locomotor activity shown in response to 5 mg/kg of amphetamine, far greater than seen at any dose of the drug in intact animals. The clear implication of this result is that the stereotypy produced by the drug in some way competes with the locomotor effects, masking further, dose-dependent increases. If one assumes that the locomotor effect is largely mediated by the ventral striatum, in particular, by the nucleus accumbens, then this is clear evidence of a competitive relationship between the two responses and neural systems.

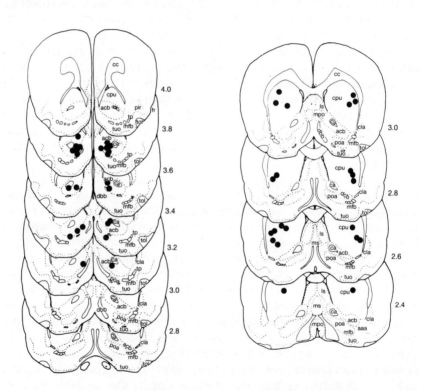

Fig. 2.6. Sites of microinjections in rats receiving bilateral, simultaneous microinjections into nucleus accumbens and head of the caudate–putamen in the rat. acb = nucleus accumbens. cpu = caudate–putamen. Other abbreviations are defined in Pellegrino and Cushman (1967) from which these sections are taken. The numbers refer to AP (anterior–posterior) co-ordinates rostral to bregma, in mm. The tips of the cannulae were confirmed following analysis of cresyl violet stained sections and are marked with a filled circle. Co-ordinates for the intended sites were: caudate–putamen—AP from bregma + 2.0, L ± 3.5, V − 5.5 from dura; nucleus accumbens—AP from bregma 3.4, L ± 1.5, V − 7.2 from dura. (J. O'Brien, P. Winn, and T.W. Robbins, unpublished results.)

The question of competition between the nucleus accumbens and caudate seems somewhat less clear-cut when considering some of the more elaborate forms of stereotypy we have discussed, including the stereotyped locomotor patterns and the complex perseverative behaviour. Indeed, there is some evidence that DA in both the caudate and nucleus accumbens contributes to the perseverative responding with conditioned reinforcement produced by the stimulant pipradrol (see Robbins and Everitt 1982). Furthermore, if the rotation produced by amphetamine in rats with unilateral depletion of DA in the caudate can be taken as a form of stereotyped locomotion, there is clear evidence that both structures again participate. For example, Kelly and Moore (1976) showed that, whereas the unilateral depletion of DA from the head of the caudate determined the direction of rotation, additional depletion from the nucleus accumbens determined its rate. This led to the proposal that the accumbens DA projection somehow 'gain-amplified' the bias produced by the caudate imbalance, although it is also possible to interpret the results simply as the co-ordination of head turning and whole body locomotion.

The 'gain-amplification' hypothesis is compatible with the possibility that the intensity of stereotyped behaviour is determined by DA projections throughout the striatum, including the nucleus accumbens itself. A test of the hypothesis would be simultaneously to infuse amphetamine bilaterally into both structures and this we have attempted in a number of recent studies modelled along the lines of the central infusion work described above. Rats were equipped with two sets of bilateral cannulae into the sites depicted in Fig. 2.6. The design of the experiment requires rather complex controls and we adopted a set of comparisons of a single, high dose of amphetamine into either the accumbens or the caudate versus the effect of half that dose into both structures. The prediction is that the latter condition would exhibit the strongest signs of stereotypy.

The main results of the experiment are shown in Fig. 2.7. The strongest effects were certainly found in the 'divided dose' condition, in particular for head movements and the head-down posture. However, even at these massive doses the level of stereotypy observed was still not great by comparison with that seen following 8 mg/kg of systemic amphetamine, the median Creese–Iversen rating being 3.0 rather than 4.0.

There are other reasons for being cautious in interpreting these data. As can be readily seen from Fig. 2.7, the caudate sites are actually somewhat anterior and it is possible that stronger effects would be seen at more posterior sites (i.e. $< +2.0$ from bregma). Pilot experiments in our laboratory (C. Ksir and J. Taylor, unpublished results) have indicated that it is possible to elicit stereotyped movements from such regions, although again the effects are not particularly strong, and include a form of grooming not seen with systemic treatment. The present results are also consistent with

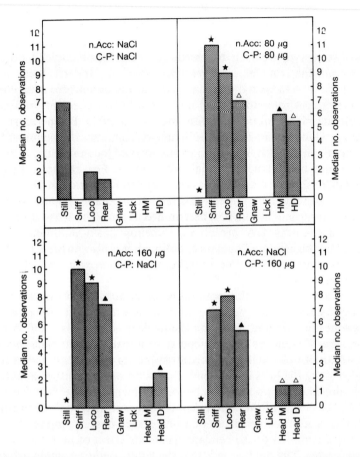

Fig. 2.7. Effects of combined nucleus accumbens (n. Acc) and caudate–putamen (C-P) bilateral microinjections upon components of unconditioned behaviour at the sites depicted in Figs. 2.6. Other details as in legends to Fig. 2.3 and 2.4. Stars refer to significant differences compared to control values $p < 0.01$; filled triangles, $p < 0.02$; open triangles, $p < 0.05$; (Wilcoxon matched pairs). (J. O'Brien, P. Winn, and T. W. Robbins, unpublished results.)

the findings of Fink and Smith (1980) and also Winn and Robbins (1985) that amphetamine hyperactivity depends upon DA projections in the anteroventral head of caudate nucleus as well as the nucleus accumbens. Fink and Smith have suggested that the amphetamine locomotor response depends upon the 'mass-action' of the central DA systems, and of course, are not far from our current speculations about stereotypy.

A further problem has been the lack of strong *oral* (gnawing, licking) responses in response to amphetamine, when these are often (though variably) reported as qualitative changes in the stereotyped pattern. Kelley *et al.* (1988) have recently reported data which importantly bear on this issue. They found that microinjection of 20 μg (in 0.5 μl) of D-amphetamine into a posterior ventrolateral site in the head of the caudate nucleus induced a strong biting and licking response. This restricted site would not normally be reached by injections into the middle of the striatum and these results suggest that there is a degree of topographical organization within the striatum for the *type* of behavioural response observed following amphetamine. A further study has shown that much lower doses than 20 μg into the same sub-region stimulate eating (Kelley and Gauthier 1987) suggesting that the oral response is made more intense (and stereotyped) by enhanced D A activity within that region. This may reflect the disruption of a sequence of behaviour produced by repetitive stimulation of a single element of it, as hypothesized previously, and would appear to contradict a 'Mass Action' account of stereotypy. However, it is possible that such specific effects in restricted areas are inter-mixed with responses (such as locomotion and sniffing) depending upon more diffuse regions of the striatum, and, together, determine the form of the behavioural output following systemic amphetamine.

In summarizing our present position, it seems easiest to conceive the effects of amphetamine activation as occurring in the following sequence. Initially, D A release from the nucleus accumbens and caudate is sufficient to allow the independent, but co-ordinated stimulation of somewhat distinct response elements (such as locomotion, head, and oral movements) permitting quite complex sequences, which may begin to exhibit stereotyped features as the dose increases. The nucleus accumbens may even promote further activity in the DA projection to the head of the caudate. As the effects increase, the progressively greater activation of the caudate occludes the behavioural response arising from the accumbens which is only apparent if the effect of DA-receptor activation in the caudate is blocked, either pharmacologically or by environmental means (see p. 32). It is assumed that the posterior head of the caudate–putamen is largely responsible for the mediation of the intense head, sniffing, and oral movements which gradually dominate the locomotor activation resulting from dopamine release in the ventral anterior striatum. This position clearly depends somewhat on defining the independent neural systems efferent to the striatum which mediate various aspects of the amphetamine response, a topic in which considerable progress has been made.

Striatal efferents mediating the amphetamine response

Many of the behavioural manifestations of amphetamine administration can be found following pharmacological stimulation of non-dopaminergic output pathways such as the substantia nigra, pars reticulata, and globus pallidus (see Fig. 2.2), which then presumably are responsible for the execution of behavioural stereotypy. The work in particular of Scheel-Krüger and colleagues has shown, for example, how local infusions of GABA agonists into substantia nigra, pars reticulata evoke sniffing, licking, and biting in rats, as well as some locomotor changes (e.g. Scheel-Krüger *et al.* 1980; Groves and Tepper 1983). Others have traced the responses yet further. The substantia nigra, pars reticulata projects to the superior colliculus, ventromedial thalamus, and the pontine reticular formation. Each of these routes appears to mediate distinct aspects of amphetamine stereotypy. Thus, electrolytic lesions of the superior colliculus reduce the oral components of stereotypy elicited by apomorphine and amphetamine (Pope *et al.* 1980; Redgrave *et al.* 1980). Manipulations of the ventromedial thalamic nucleus seem not to produce stereotypy, but unilateral alteration of GABA function produces postural deviation (though not active circling; see Leigh *et al.* 1983). Finally, Sirkin and Teitelbaum (1983) have shown that electrolytic lesions of the pontine reticular formation abolish amphetamine- and apomorphine-induced head turns.

A similar picture may be emerging for the output pathways from the nucleus accumbens and the mainly locomotor aspects of the amphetamine response. A combination of neuroanatomical, electrophysiological, and behavioural evidence has shown that the locomotor response to amphetamine and the apomorphine is mediated by projections to the ventral pallidum and thence to a 'mesencephalic locomotor centre' (Mogenson and Nielsen 1984; Swerdlow *et al.* 1984: Swanson *et al.* 1984).

While there is some evidence that stereotypy is a diffuse response following stimulation of many structures efferent to the striatum, these demonstrations indicate some differentiation of its response components. They further support the hypothesis of Lyon and Robbins that progressively increasing activation by stimulant drugs will eventually produce fractionation of complex response sequences and autonomous, repetitive behaviour. This position is also not incompatible with one suggesting the existence of motor 'subsystems' and the possibility that stereotypy reflects the initial co-ordination and then the dissociation of these subsystems (cf. Szechtman *et al.* 1985).

Limbic and cortical influences

The argument we have been pursuing has stressed the initial complexity of stereotyped behaviour and how its final form represents a breakdown in communication between different neuronal systems. This applies particularly to the likely hierarchical levels of control provided by limbic and cortical interactions with the striatum. A general neuroanatomical principle has emerged which links the dorsal striatum to its neocortical inputs and the ventral striatum to its limbic ones, perhaps including the prefrontal cortex (see Fig. 2.2). What types of influence then can these inputs exert over stereotyped behaviour? We can begin to answer this question by reference back to the differences in stereotyped behaviour produced by amphetamine in novel and home-cage environments (Sahakian and Robbins 1975a). First, the drug-treated animals showed no obvious stereotypy in a novel environment, although there was a good deal of apparent stereotyped 'staring'. Clearly, the influence of novelty was in some way inhibitory to stereotypy and was presumably mediated by some area concerned with novelty processing. Whether the interruption occurs via the cortex or limbic system or both is difficult to say. However, it is notable that the hippocampus, which has been linked to functions associated with novelty, projects to the medial nucleus accumbens (Kelley and Domesick 1982) which could influence the functioning of the rest of the striatum via its projection to substantia nigra, pars compacta. This possibility is perhaps greater in the rat, where novelty leads to the replacement of stereotypy by more spatially diverse locomotor activity, a response probably under control of the ventral striatum.

Second, in the home cage one guinea-pig treated with the drug chose in a stereotyped manner to pursue a particular cage-mate, of the several in its home cage. This suggests that experiential factors can contribute to the selection of stereotypy, which could well hinge upon a limbic influence. Such an influence would again be expected to be mediated via the ventral striatum, and some evidence of this is provided by the enhancement of effects of conditioned reinforcement by intra-accumbens amphetamine (Taylor and Robbins 1984). The progressive autonomy of this form of conditioned behaviour may well depend however upon the additional involvement of DA within the caudate–putamen (see Robbins and Everitt 1982).

Finally, the actual guidance of the form of the complex sequence of movements involved in the tracking response by the 'predatory' guinea-pig, including the switching between different directions and the orientation of the gnawing response to a particular location of the fleeing animal's fur probably requires quite detailed sensory feedback and response organization, presumably deriving from the neocortical and perhaps, thalamic inputs to the striatum.

Thus, neocortical and limbic influences are postulated to enable environmental and experiential factors to prevent behaviour overactivated by striatal DA release from becoming too divorced from environmental or historical context. This analysis, of course, is somewhat reminiscent of Kraepelin's notion of an inhibitory forebrain keeping primitive automatisms in check. It would predict that damage to neocortex or limbic structures such as the hippocampus would lead to an exaggeration of stereotyped behaviour produced by amphetamine. Some of our recent evidence broadly confirms this prediction. Figure 2.8 shows the effects of either total decortication or total hippocampectomy upon the stereotyped behaviour produced by

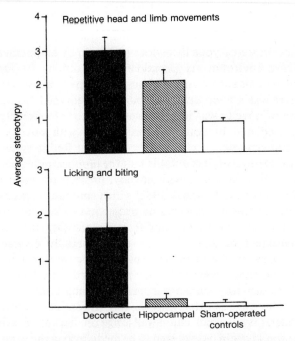

Fig. 2.8. The effect of an acute dose of D-amphetamine (5 mg/kg, intraperitoneal) on repetitive head and limb movements and oral behaviour (licking and biting) in decorticate ($n = 6$), hippocampal ($n = 6$), and sham-operated control rats ($n = 4$). Rats were injected with amphetamine 5 min prior to observation every 5 min in a 30-min period, using a time-sampling procedure. The average stereotypy score for the 30-min period is depicted. Both components of stereotypy were rated on a two-point scale for their duration (1 = discontinuous, 2 = continuous) and a three-point scale for their intensity (1 = none or very weak, 2 = moderate, 3 = intense). The duration and intensity scores were multiplied to provide a stereotypy score for each 5 min interval analysed by analysis of variance. This revealed a significant Group effect for both oral ($F = 3.90$, d$f = 2$, 13, $p < 0.05$) and head and limb components ($F = 8.36$, df, 2, 13, $p < 0.01$). All three groups differed significantly for head and limb movements (top). The decorticates showed significantly more oral components than the other two groups (bottom). (G. Mittleman, unpublished results.)

5 mg/kg D-amphetamine. The lesions had differential effects upon various components of the stereotypy. Thus, hippocampectomy increased the incidence of repetitive head and limb movements, whereas decortication elevated stereotyped oral movements. It appears again that stereotyped behaviour is made up of different response elements, perhaps controlled by different regions of the striatum. In this context it may be relevant that the hippocampus projects primarily to ventral striatum, in fact to the medial

nucleus accumbens, whereas neocortex projects primarily to the dorsal striatum (Fig. 2.2).

The effects of hippocampal lesions are relevant to the results and speculations of Devenport and his colleagues (1981). They provide evidence that, for rats with hippocampal damage, the signalled presentation of reward (food following deprivation) is sufficient to induce behaviour resembling the stereotypy and locomotion produced by amphetamine. This behaviour in fact consisted of 'locomotion along relatively fixed routes, rearing, orienting towards sources of stimuli that were not obvious to the observer, sniffing and head-bobbing'. The behaviour could be blocked by administration of the DA-antagonist, haloperidol. They link these results to the other well-known effects of hippocampal lesions to produce perseverative and 'superstitious' behaviour and postulate that the hippocampus normally promotes behavioural variability by opposing the effects of catecholaminergic activity. This account is allied to the concept that stereotypy can resemble the exaggerated effects of reinforcement (cf. Robbins 1976). It is consistent with the fact that the nucleus accumbens is sensitive to the effects of amphetamine upon responding maintained by conditioned reinforcement (Taylor and Robbins 1984) as this seems to be the most likely locus of interaction of the hippocampus with the ascending DA systems. The experimental findings of Devenport et al. (1981) have also been broadly confirmed by L. Annett (unpublished results) although she found that the DA-antagonist, α-flupenthixol, or catecholamine depletion in the nucleus accumbens blocked the behaviour evoked by reward to the same extent in both sham-operated controls and rats with total hippocampectomies. The question posed by this research is whether the enhanced stereotypy of hippocampal lesioned rats represents effects which are specific to reward or to any conditions conducive to stereotypy, such as the 'stress' of isolation rearing. The hippocampal influence would then be of a generally inhibitory nature rather than one specifically tied to reinforcement processes.

The other major forebrain influence upon behavioural stereotypy is likely to be the prefrontal cortex. Lesions of this region enhance the production of oral dyskinetic movements in both monkeys (Gunne et al. 1982) and in rats (Iversen 1971). Frontal lesions are known to produce perseverative behaviour in man and monkeys, in the latter case including stereotyped pacing. Ridley and Baker (1982) have pointed out these similarities in effects of amphetamine and frontal lesions. This pattern of results again points to an opposing effect of the frontal cortex upon activity in the DA projections ascending to the striatum. The analysis though is complicated by considering the functions of the mesocortical DA projection which of course would also be affected by systemically administered DA-agonists. There were early reports that mesocortical DA-depletion enhanced the behavioural effects of DA-agonists and increased indices of subcortical DA turnover (Carter and

Pycock 1980; Bannon and Roth 1983). However, some of the behavioural results have been difficult to replicate (e.g. Joyce *et al.* 1983).

The mesocortical DA system also seems to be especially sensitive to the effects of stressors such as footshock or isolation (Thierry *et al.* 1976; see Bannon and Roth 1983 for review). If this system is indeed inhibitory to the subcortical DA projections, then it may represent a mechanism for regulating stress and preventing the deleterious behavioural effects of overactivation. Thus 'coping responses' to stress may be correlates of this regulatory action. If then some of the sequelae of activation, such as schedule-induced polydipsia or behaviour evoked by hypothalamic electrical stimulation, are indeed 'coping responses', then their performance might be expected to lead to elevated DA turnover in prefrontal cortex, their prevention presumably having the opposite effect. It seems much less likely from this perspective that amphetamine stereotypy itself has such a function.

Implications and conclusions

One of the main aims of this chapter has been to show that stereotypy is more than a convenient behavioural response for assaying the effects of DA agonists and antagonists. It can be a complex pattern of behaviour, whose analysis at the behavioural, as well as the neural, level can tell us much about brain mechanisms of behaviour, as well as about psychological processes in general. We have considered stereotypy as resulting from a behavioural process of activation, mediated mainly by dopaminergic mechanisms in the striatum. This is held to be essentially the same process that, at a lower intensity, mediates such behavioural phenomena as schedule-induced drinking, tail-pinch-induced behaviour, behaviour evoked by hypothalamic stimulation, displacement behaviour, the behavioural effects of rearing in isolation, and even certain aspects of incentive-motivation or reward. We have outlined a theory (Lyon and Robbins 1975) suggesting that stereotypy is the culmination of a continuous process of psychomotor stimulation and behavioural competition. We have considered, but in the main rejected, hypotheses maintaining that there is some sort of function for amphetamine-induced stereotypy—largely from lack of evidence. This does not rule out the possibility that some of the other expressions of behavioural activation listed above may serve in a coping capacity, but again there is only limited evidence for this view.

By showing how environment and experience can influence stereotyped behaviour, we have pointed to its behavioural and neural complexity. This is significant for two main reasons. First, it provides a model for studying how the basal ganglia interact with other forebrain regions, in particular how these influences normally antagonize the autonomous and stereotyped behaviour that can result from overactivation. This goes somewhat beyond the precepts of early writers on brain function, such as Hughlings Jackson and is of some significance for modern neuropsychological theories concerning action selection, such as that of Norman and Shallice (1980). They, for example, postulate that there is a 'supervisory system' which either resolves conflicts between otherwise automatic actions having similar probabilities of occurrence or is engaged during novel situations to organize new actions (or 'schema'). The elicitation of actions is held to depend on the presence of the appropriate stimuli and upon a general motivational influence which we would broadly equate with activation and the ascending DA system. According to this model, action selection could break down in two main ways, either because of a malfunctioning supervisor or because of excessive activation which overwhelms its modulatory function. The analogies with the prefrontal cortex and basal ganglia are clear and have been previously discussed (see Robbins and Sahakian 1983).

Second, stereotypy induced in animals can be seen as a much more convincing model of human psychopathology, including aspects of schizophrenia, autism, and mania, if its potential complexity is taken into account. To take one example, Frith and Done (1983) have recently described stereotyped sequences of behaviour of schizophrenics in an operant situation disguised as a video game, effects which have recently been confirmed cross-culturally in another sample of schizophrenics in Denmark (Lyon *et al.* 1985). Analogous effects have been seen in rats performing under a similar random schedule of reinforcement distributed over two levers, following treatment with amphetamine (cf. Evenden and Robbins 1983*b*). The qualitative similarity of these effects obviously gives the animal model stronger face validity than say, the apomorphine gnawing response, which has, nevertheless, been widely and successfully used to screen new neuroleptic drugs; indeed the reported correlation between the potency of neuroleptics to antagonize this response and their minimal effective dose clinically is close to 0.9 (Creese *et al.* 1978). Perhaps the more realistic animal model would have even greater success, although it also seems likely that the ability to define exactly how complex patterns of stereotyped behaviour differ from normal will reveal that the pharmacological antagonism of stereotypy may not necessarily also result in a return to objectively-defined normal performance. For example, Robbins (1980) found it difficult to convert the stereotyped operant behaviour back into the normal control pattern of responding, using the neuroleptics α-flupenthixol or clozapine, even at doses which successfully antagonized the stereotyped lever-pressing. This, too, may enable a better understanding of what precisely the drug therapy may be achieving.

The realization that stereotypy can be a complex response, reflecting a disruption of co-ordinated function, not only within the basal ganglia, but also between striatal and other forebrain influences, may also afford some insights into the possible neural sites of dysfunction in conditions such as schizophrenia, as Devenport *et al.* (1981) among others have pointed out. Thus, enhanced stereotypy need not result merely from a primary change in the ascending DA systems; it could also occur, for example, following neuropathology within the prefrontal cortex or hippocampus. This would then perhaps be consistent with the rather limited direct neurochemical evidence that has accrued for the dopamine hypothesis of schizophrenia.

In considering the questions and implications raised in this chapter, we believe that resolving the nature of stimulant stereotypy will require insights from at least three main areas of study, namely neuropsychology, psychopharmacology, and psychopathology, with an integrated approach and what we think would be a mutually profitable outcome.

Acknowledgements

G.M. was supported by a NATO post-doctoral fellowship. P.W. was the Pinsent–Darwin student in Mental Pathology. J.O'B. was supported by a Kenneth Craik Studentship. We thank Dr Jane Taylor for providing Fig. 2.2, I. Cannell for photography, and Drs L. Annett, J. Evenden, and T.E. Robinson for valuable comments.

References

Abelson, J.S. and Woods, J.H. (1980). Effects of apomorphine on elicited and operant pecking in pigeons. *Psychopharmacology* **71**, 237–41.

Annett, L.E., Ridley, R.M., Gamble, S.J., and Baker, H.F. (1983). Behavioural effects of intracerebral amphetamine in the marmoset. *Psychopharmacology* **81**, 18–27.

Antelman, S.M. and Chiodo, L.S. (1983). Amphetamine as a stressor. In *Stimulants: neurochemical, behavioral and clinical perspectives* (ed. I. Creese), pp. 269–99. Raven Press, New York.

Antelman S.M. and Chiodo, L.S. (1984). Stress: its effects on interactions among biogenic amines and role in the induction and treatment of disease. In *Handbook of psychopharmacology* (ed. L.L. Iversen, S.D. Iversen, and S.H. Snyder), Vol. 18. Plenum Press, New York.

Antelman, S.M. and Szechtman, H. (1975). Tail pinch induces eating in sated rats which appears to depend on nigrostriatal dopamine. *Science*, N.Y. **189**, 731–3.

Bannon, M. and Roth, R.H. (1983). Pharmacology of mesocortical dopamine. *Pharmacol. Rev.* **35**, 53–68.

Barrett, J.A. and Stanley, J.A. (1982). Effects of chlorpromazine and D-amphetamine on schedule-controlled and schedule-related behavior of rabbits. *Psychopharmacology* **78**, 197–203.

Berlyne, D. E. (1960). *Conflict, arousal and curiosity.* McGraw-Hill, New York.

Bleuler, E. P. (1950). *Dementia praecox or the group of schizophrenias.* International University Press, New York.

Brett, L. P. and Levine S. (1979). Schedule-induced polydipsia suppresses pituitary–adrenal activity in rats. *J. comp. physiol. Psychol.* **5**, 946–56.

Broadbent, D. E. (1971). *Decision and stress.* Academic Press, London.

Broekkamp, C. P. E., Pijnenberg, A. J. J., and Van Rossum, J. M. (1973). Dopaminergic transmission in relation to mechanisms underlying stereotyped behavior. In *Frontiers in catecholamine research* (ed. E. Usdin and S. H. Snyder), pp. 675–6. Pergamon Press, New York.

Campbell, B. A. and Fibiger, H. C. (1971). Potentiation of amphetamine-induced arousal by starvation. *Nature, London* **233**, 424–5.

Carter, C. J. and Pycock, C. J. (1980). Behavioural and biochemical effects of dopamine and noradrenaline depletion within the medial prefrontal cortex of the rat. *Brain Res.* **192**, 163–76.

Connell, P. H. (1958). *Amphetamine psychosis.* Maudsley Monographs No. 5. Chapman and Hall, London.

Costall, B., Naylor, R. J., and Olley, J. E. (1972). Stereotypy and anti-cataleptic activities of amphetamine after intra-cerebral injection. *Eur. J. Pharmacol.* **18**, 83–94.

Creese, I. and Iversen, S. D. (1975). The pharmacological and anatomical substrates of the amphetamine response in the rat. *Brain Res.* **83**, 419–36.

Creese, I., Burt, D., and Snyder, S. H. (1978). Biochemical actions of neuroleptic drugs. In *Handbook of psychopharmacology* (ed. L. L. Iversen, S. D. Iversen, and S. H. Snyder), Vol. 10, pp. 37–89. Plenum Press, New York.

Devenport, L. D., Devenport, J. A., and Holloway, F. A. (1981). Stereotypy: modulation by the hippocampus. *Science, NY* **212**, 1288–9.

Dooley D. J. and Bowden, D. M. (1983). Differential effects of dopaminergic agonists on food-reinforced operant behavior in the long-tailed macaque (Macaca fascicularis). *Psychopharmacology* **81**, 170–6.

Eichler, A. J., Antelman, S. M., and Black, C. (1980). Amphetamine stereotypy is not a homogeneous phenomenon: sniffing and licking show distinct profiles of sensitization and tolerance. *Psychopharmacology* **68**, 287–90.

Einon, D. F. and Sahakian, B. J. (1979). Environmentally-induced differences in susceptibility of rats to CNS stimulants and CNS depressants: evidence argues against a unitary explanation. *Psychopharmacology* **61**, 299–307.

Ellinwood, E. H. and Kilbey, M. M. (1975). Amphetamine stereotypy: the influence of environmental factors and prepotent behavioral patterns on its topography and development. *Biol. Psychiat.* **10**, 3–16.

Ernst, A. M. and Smelik, P. G. (1966). Site of action of dopamine and apomorphine in compulsive gnawing in the rat. *Experientia* **22**, 837–8.

Evenden, J. L. and Robbins, T. W. (1983a). Dissociable effects of D-amphetamine, chlordiazepoxide and alpha-flupenthixol on choice and rate measures of reinforcement in the rat. *Psychopharmacology* **79**, 180–6.

Evenden, J. L. and Robbins, T. W. (1983b). Increased response switching, perseveration and perseverative switching following D-amphetamine in the rat. *Psychopharmacology* **80**, 67–73.

Fentress, J.C. (1983). Ethological models of hierarchy and patterning of species-specific behavior. In *Handbook of behavioral neurobiology* (ed. E. Satinoff and P. Teitelbaum), Vol. 6, pp. 185–234. Plenum Press, New York.

Fink, J.S. and Smith, G.P. (1980). Relationship between selective denervation of dopamine terminal fields in the anterior forebrain and behavior in response to amphetamine and apomorphine. *Brain Res.* **201**, 107–27.

Fitzgerald, F.L. (1967). Effects of D-amphetamine upon behaviour of young chimpanzees reared under different conditions. In *Proceedings of the 5th International Congress of Neuropsychopharmacology* (ed. H. Brill, J.O. Cole, P. Deniker, H. Hippius, and P.B. Bradley), pp. 1226–7. Excerpta Medica, Amsterdam.

Fog, R. and Pakkenberg, H. (1971). Behavioral effects of D-amphetamine and P-hydroxyamphetamine injections into the corpus striatum of rats. *Exp. Neurol.* **31**, 75–86.

Fray, P.J. Sahakian, B.J. Robbins, T.W., Koob, G.F., and Iversen, S.D. (1980). An observational method for quantifying the behavioural effects of dopaminergic agonists: contrasting effects of D-amphetamine and apomorphine. *Psychopharmacology* **69**, 253–9.

Friedman, S.B. and Ader, R. (1967). Adrenocortical response to novelty and noxious stimuli. *Neuroendocrinology* **2**, 209–12.

Frith, C.D. and Done, D.J. (1983). Stereotyped responding by schizophrenic patients on a two-choice guessing task. *Psychol. Med.* **13**, 779–86.

Fuxe, K. and Ungerstedt, U. (1970). Histochemical, biochemical and functional studies on central monoamine neurones after acute and chronic amphetamine administration. In *Amphetamines and related compounds* (ed. E. Costa and S. Garattini), pp. 257–88. Raven Press, New York.

Groves P.M. and Rebec, G.V. (1976). Biochemistry and behavior: some central actions of amphetamine and certain anti-psychotic drugs. *Ann. Rev. Psychol.* **27**, 91–127.

Groves, P.M. and Tepper, J.M. (1983). Neuronal mechanisms of action of amphetamine. In *Stimulants: neurochemical, behavioral, and clinical perspectives* (ed. I. Creese), pp. 81–129. Raven Press, New York.

Gunne, L.M., Growdon, J., and Glaeser, B. (1982). Oral dyskinesia following rat brain lesions and neuroleptic drug administration. *Psychopharmacology* **77**, 134–9.

Heyman, G.M. (1983). A parametric evaluation of the hedonic and motoric effects of the drugs pimozide and amphetamine. *J. Exp. Anal. Behav.* **40**, 113–22.

Hill, R.T. (1970). Facilitation of conditioned reinforcement as a mechanism of psychomotor stimulation. In *Amphetamines and related compounds* (ed. E. Costa and S. Garattini), pp. 781–95. Raven Press, New York.

Hutt, C. and Hutt, S.J. (1965). Effect of environmental complexity upon stereotyped behaviour in children. *Animal Behav.* **13**, 1–4.

Iversen, S.D. (1971). The effect of surgical lesions to frontal cortex and substantia nigra on amphetamine responses in rats. *Brain Res.* **31**, 295–311.

Jones, G.H., Mittleman, G., and Robbins, T.W. (1989). Attenuation of amphetamine-stereotypy by mesostriatal dopamine depletion enhances plasma corticosterone: implications for stereotypy as a coping response. *Behav. Neural Biol.* **51**, 80–91.

Joyce, E. M. and Iversen, S. D. (1984). Dissociable effects of 6-O HD A lesions of the neostriatum on anorexia, locomotor activity and stereotypy: the role of behavioural competition. *Psychopharmacology* **83**, 363–6.

Joyce, E. M., Stinus, L., and Iversen, S. D. (1983). Effects of injections of 6-O HD A into either nucleus accumbens septi or frontal cortex on spontaneous locomotor activity. *Neuropharmacology* **22**, 1141–5.

Kelley, A. E. and Domesick, V. (1982). The amygdalostriatal projection in the rat—an anatomical study by anterograde and retrograde tracing methods. *Neuroscience* **7**, 615–30.

Kelley, A. E. and Gauthier, A. M. (1987). Differential effects on spontaneous motor behaviour, feeding and oral stereotypy following amphetamine microinjection into anatomically defined subregions of rat striatum. *Society for Neuroscience Abstract* **13**, 31.

Kelley, A. E., Lang, C. G., and Gauthier, A. M. (1988). Induction of oral stereotypy following amphetamine microinjection into a discrete subregion of the striatum. *Psychopharmacology*, **95**, 556–9.

Kelly, P. H. and Moore, K. E. (1976). Mesolimbic dopamine neurons in the rotational model of nigrostriatal function. *Nature, London* **263**, 695–6.

Kelly, P. H., Seviour, P., and Iversen, S. D. (1975). Amphetamine and apomorphine responses in the rat following 6-O HD A lesions of the nucleus accumbens septi and corpus striatum. *Brain Res.* **94**, 507–22.

Kraepelin, E. (1919). *Dementia praecox and paraphrenia*. Livingstone, Edinburgh.

Kramer, J. C., Fischman, V. S., and Littlefield, D. C. (1967). Amphetamine abuse. *J. Am. med. Ass.* **201**, 305–9.

Kuczenski, R. (1983). Biochemical action of amphetamine and other stimulants. In *Stimulants: neurochemical, behavioural and clinical perspectives* (ed. I. Creese), pp. 31–61. Raven Press, New York.

Leigh, P. N., Reavill, C., Jenner, P., and Marsden, C. D. (1983). Basal ganglia outflow pathways and circling behaviour in the rat. *J. neural Transmiss.* **58**, 1–41.

Lyon, M. and Randrup, A. (1972). The dose–response effect of amphetamine upon avoidance behaviour in the rat seen as a function of increasing stereotypy. *Psychopharmacologia, Berlin* **23**, 334–47.

Lyon, M. and Robbins, T. (1975). The action of central nervous system stimulant drugs: a general theory concerning amphetamine effects. In *Current developments in psychopharmacology* (ed. W. Essman and L. Valzelli), Vol. 2, pp. 79–163. Spectrum, New York.

Lyon, N., Mejsholm, B., and Lyon, M. (1986). Stereotyped responding by schizophrenic outpatients: cross-cultural confirmation of perseverative switching in a two choice test. *J. psychiat. Res.* **20**, 137–50.

MacLennan, A. J. and Maier, S. F. (1983). Coping and stress-induced potentiation of stimulant stereotypy in the rat. *Science, NY* **219**, 1091–3.

Meyer-Holzapel, M. (1968). Abnormal behavior in zoo animals. In *Abnormal behaviour in animals* (ed. M. Fox), pp. 476–503. Saunders, London.

Mittleman, G. M. and Valenstein, E. S. (1984). Ingestive behaviour evoked by hypothalamic stimulation and schedule-induced polydipsia are related. *Science, NY* **224**, 415-17.

Mittleman, G. M. and Valenstein, E. S. (1985). Individual differences in non-regulatory ingestive behavior and catecholamine systems. *Brain Res.* **348**, 112-17.

Mittleman, G. M., Castaneda, E., Robinson, T. E., and Valenstein, E. S. (1986). The propensity for non-regulatory ingestive behaviour is related to differences in dopamine systems: behavioural and biochemical evidence. *Behav. Brain Res.* **100**, 213-20.

Mogenson, G. J. and Nielsen, M. (1984). Neuropharmacological evidence to suggest that the nucleus accumbens and subpallidal region contribute to exploratory locomotion. *Behav. neural Biol.* **42**, 52-66.

Moore, K. E. (1978). Amphetamines: biochemical and behavioral actions in animals. In *Handbook of psychopharmacology* (ed. L. L. Iversen, S. D. Iversen, and S. H. Snyder), Vol. 11, pp. 41-98. Plenum Press, New York.

Morley, J. E. and Levine, A. S. (1980). Stress-induced eating is mediated by endogenous opioids. *Science, NY* **209**, 1259-61.

Nauta, W. J. H. and Domesick, V. (1984). Afferent and efferent relations of the basal ganglia. In *Functions of the basal ganglia*, CIBA Foundation Symposium 107, pp. 23-41. Pitman, London.

Nieto, J., Makhlouf, C., and Rodriguez, R. (1979). D-Amphetamine effects on behaviour produced by periodic food deliveries in the rat. *Pharmacol. Biochem. Behav.* **11**, 423-30.

Norman, D. A. and Shallice, T. (1980). *Attention to action: willed and automatic control of behavior.* Center for Information Processing Technical Report No. 99. University of California San Diego.

Pellegrino, L. J. and Cushman, A. J. (1967). *A stereotaxic atlas of the rat brain.* Appleton-Century-Crofts, New York.

Phillips, A. G. and Fibiger, H. C. (1976). Long term deficits in stimulation-bound behaviour and self-stimulation after 6-hydroxydopamine administration in the rat. *Behav. Biol.* **16**, 127-43.

Pijnenberg, A. J. J., Honig, W. M. M., van der Heyden, J. A. M., and van Rossum, J. M. (1976). Effects of chemical stimulation of the mesolimbic dopamine system upon locomotor activity. *Eur. J. Pharmacol.* **35**, 45-58.

Pope, S. G., Dean, P., and Redgrave, P. (1980). Dissociation of D-amphetamine-induced locomotor activity and stereotyped behaviour by lesions of the superior colliculus. *Psychopharmacology* **70**, 297-302.

Randrup, A. and Munkvad, I. (1970). Biochemical, anatomical and psychological investigations of stereotyped behaviour induced by amphetamine. In *Amphetamines and related compounds* (ed. E. Costa and S. Garattini), pp. 695-713. Raven Press, New York.

Ranje, Ch. and Ungerstedt, U. (1974). Chronic amphetamine treatment: vast individual differences in performance of a learned response. *Eur. J. Pharmacol.* **29**, 307-11.

Rebec, G. V. and Segal, D. S. (1978). Dose-dependent biphasic alterations in the spontaneous activity of neurons in the rat neostriatum produced by D-amphetamine and methylphenidate. *Brain Res.* **150**, 353–66.

Redgrave, P. Dean, P., Donohoe, T.P., and Pope, S.G. (1980). Superior colliculi lesion selectively attenuates apomorphine-induced oral behaviour; a possible role for the nigro-tectal pathway. *Brain Res.* **196**, 541–6.

Ridley, R.M. and Baker, H.F. (1982). Stereotypy in monkeys and humans. *Psychol. Med.* **12**, 61–72.

Robbins, T.W. (1976). Relationship between reward-enhancing and stereotypical effects of psychomotor stimulant drugs. *Nature, London* **264**, 57–9.

Robbins, T.W. (1980). Stereotypy of a learned response after apomorphine. *Br. J. Pharmacol.* **69**, 275–6P.

Robbins, T.W. (1984). Cortical noradrenaline, attention and arousal. *Psychol. Med.* **14**, 13–21.

Robbins, T.W. and Everitt, B.J. (1982). Functional studies of the central catecholamines. *Int. Rev. Neurobiol.* **23**, 303–65.

Robbins, T.W. and Koob, G.F. (1980). Selective disruption of displacement behaviour by lesions of the mesolimbic dopamine system. *Nature, London* **285**, 409–12.

Robbins, T.W. and Sahakian, B.J. (1981). Behavioural and neurochemical determinants of drug-induced stereotypy. In *Metabolic disorders of the nervous system* (ed. F.C. Rose) pp. 244–91. Pitman, London.

Robbins, T.W. and Sahakian, B.J. (1983). Behavioral effects of psychomotor stimulant drugs; clinical and neuropsychological implications. In *Stimulants: neurochemical, behavioral and clinical perspectives* (ed. I. Creese), pp. 301–38. Raven Press, New York.

Robbins, T.W., Watson, B.A., Gaskin, M., and Ennis, C. (1983). Contrasting interactions of pipradrol, D-amphetamine, cocaine, cocaine analogues, apomorphine and other drugs with conditioned reinforcement. *Psychopharmacology* **80**, 113–19.

Rowland, N. and Marques, D. (1980). Stress-induced eating: misrepresentation? *Appetite* **1**, 225–8.

Rowland, N., Marques, D., and Fisher, A. (1980). Comparison of the effects of brain dopamine-depleting lesions upon oral behavior elicited by tail-pinch and electrical brain stimulation. *Physiol. Behav.* **24**, 273–81.

Rylander, G. (1971). Stereotype behavior in man following amphetamine abuse. In *The correlation of adverse effects in man with observations in animals* (ed, S.B.deC. Baker), pp. 29–31. Excerpta Medica, Amsterdam.

Sahakian, B.J. and Robbins, T.W. (1975*a*). The effects of test environment and rearing condition on amphetamine-induced stereotypy in the guinea pig. *Psychopharmacologia, Berlin* **45**, 115–17.

Sahakian, B.J. and Robbins, T.W. (1975*b*). Potentiation of locomotor activity and modification of stereotypy by starvation in apomorphine treated rats. *Neuropharmacology* **14**, 251–7.

Sahakian, B.J. and Robbins, T.W. (1977). Isolation-rearing enhances tail-pinch induced oral behaviour in rats. *Physiol. Behav.* **18**, 53–8.

Sahakian, B.J., Robbins, T.W., Morgan, M.J., and Iversen, S.D. (1975). The effects of psychomotor stimulants on stereotypy and locomotor activity in socially deprived and control rats. *Brain Res.* **84**, 195–205.

Scheel-Krüger, J., Arnt, J., Magelund, G., Olianas, M., Przewlocka, B., and Christensen, A. V. (1980). Behavioural functions of GABA in basal ganglia and limbic system. *Brain Res. Bull.* **5**, 261–7.

Schwartz, B. (1982). Development of complex, stereotyped behavior in the pigeon. *J. Exp. Anal. Behav.* **33**, 153–66.

Segal, D. S. (1975). Behavioral characterisation of D- and L-amphetamine: neurochemical implications. *Science, NY* **190**, 475–7.

Segal, D. S. and Schuckit, M. A. (1983). Animal models of stimulant-induced psychosis. In *Stimulants: neurochemical, behavioral and clinical perspectives* (ed. I. Creese), pp. 131–67. Raven Press, New York.

Sirkin, D. W. and Teitelbaum, P. (1983). The pontine reticular formation is part of the output pathway for amphetamine and apomorphine-induced lateral head movements: evidence from experimental lesions in the rat. *Brain Res.* **260**, 291–6.

Staton, D. M. and Solomon, P. R. (1984). Microanalysis of D-amphetamine into the nucleus accumbens and caudate-putamen. *Physiol. Psychol.* **12**, 159–62.

Swanson, L. W., Mogenson, G. J. Gerfen, C. R., and Robinson, P. (1984). Evidence for a projection from the lateral preoptic area and substantia innominata to the mesencephalic locomotor region. *Brain Res.* **295**, 161–78.

Swerdlow, N. R., Swanson, L. W., and Koob, G. F. (1984). Electrolytic lesion of the substantia innominata and lateral preoptic area attenuate the 'supersensitive' locomotor response to apomorphine resulting from denervation of the nucleus accumbens. *Brain Res.* **306**, 141–8.

Swenson, R. M. and Vogel, W. H. (1983). Plasma catecholamine and corticosterone as well as brain catecholamine changes during coping in rats exposed to stressful foot-shock. *Pharmacol. Biochem. Behav.* **18**, 689–93.

Szechtman, H. Ornstein, K. Teitelbaum, P., and Golani, I. (1985). The morphogenesis of stereotyped behavior induced by the dopamine receptor agonist apomorphine in the laboratory rat. *Neuroscience* **14**, 783–98.

Taylor, J. R. and Robbins, T. W. (1984). Enhanced behavioural control by conditioned reinforcers following microinjections of D-amphetamine into the nucleus accumbens. *Psychopharmacology* **84**, 405–12.

Teitelbaum, P. and Derks, P. (1958). The effect of amphetamine on forced drinking in the rat. *J. comp. physiol. Psychol.* **51**, 801–10.

Thierry, A. M., Tassin, J. P., Blanc, G., and Glowinski, J. (1976). Selective activation of the mesocortical DA system by stress. *Nature London* **263**, 242–4.

Valenstein, E. S. (1976). Stereotyped behavior and stress. In *Psychopathology of human adaptation* (ed. G. Serban and J. W. Mason), pp. 113–24. Plenum Press, New York.

Van der Kooy, D. and Phillips, A. G. (1979). Involvement of the trigeminal motor system in brain stem self-stimulation and stimulation-induced behavior. *Brain Behav. Evol.* **16**, 293–314.

Wallace, M., Singer, G., Finlay, J., and Gibson, G. (1983). The effect of 6-OHDA lesions of the nucleus accumbens septi on schedule-induced drinking, wheel-running and corticosterone levels in the rat. *Pharmacol. Biochem. Behav.* **18**, 129–36.

Winn, P. and Robbins, T.W. (1985). Comparative effects of infusions of 6-hydroxydopamine into nucleus accumbens and anterolateral hypothalamus on the response to dopamine agonists, body weight, locomotor activity and measures of exploration in the rat. *Neuropharmacology* **24**, 25–32.

Wise, R. (1981). Brain dopamine and reward. In *Theory in psychopharmacology* (ed. S. J. Cooper), Vol. 1. pp. 103–22. Academic Press, London.

Yerkes, R.M. and Dodson, J.P. (1908). The relation of strength of stimulus to rapidity of habit formation. *J. comp. neurol. Psychol.* **18**, 459–82.

3

Aspects of stereotyped and non-stereotyped behaviour in relation to dopamine receptor subtypes

JOHN L. WADDINGTON, ANTHONY G. MOLLOY,
KATHY M. O'BOYLE, and MARK T. PUGH

Introduction

Historical perspective

The rise of interest in stereotyped behaviour since the 1960s has occurred in close temporal contiguity with recognition of the important role for the neurotransmitter dopamine in motor function, and identification of the action of various drugs to influence dopaminergic activity. This relationship is often perceived as being of such intimacy that, at least in certain disciplines, stereotypy is in common usage equated automatically with dopaminergic function and drug action on that function. We are reminded in this volume that stereotypy is a broad, long-standing neuropsychological concept with general applicability to behaviour and cognition. It is often overlooked that, in animals, the induction of stereotyped motor behaviour by apomorphine, the involvement of striatal function in its manifestation, and its sensitivity to antagonism by neuroleptic drugs had all been recognized by 1960. At the time of each of these individual studies, it was not yet known that apomorphine was a direct dopamine receptor agonist, that the striatum was a major terminal field of ascending dopaminergic neurones, or that neuroleptics were potent dopamine receptor antagonists (Neumeyer *et al.* 1981).

However, the strength of the relationship between drug-induced stereotyped motor behaviour and the function of forebrain dopaminergic neurones cannot be ignored. It is beyond the scope of this chapter to discuss the now voluminous experimental evidence in this area. Reviews over the past decade have carefully discussed the general evolution of this relationship, the nature, pharmacology, and assessment of dopamine-mediated stereotypies, and the extent to which differing or overlapping terminal regions of nigrostriatal, mesolimbic, and mesocortical dopamine neurones might subserve distinct elements of stereotyped behaviour (Randrup and Munkvad 1974; Iversen 1977; Seeman 1980; Robbins and Sahakian 1981; Joyce 1983; Rebec and Bashore 1984).

The range of drugs inducing repetitious and inappropriate patterns of motor behaviour which show invariant form is wide, but these diverse compounds have a common action to increase or mimic dopaminergic neurotransmission with varying degrees of selectivity. Since the identification of the prototype inducers of such stereotyped motor behaviour, the direct dopamine receptor agonist apomorphine and the indirect dopamine-releasing agent amphetamine, a substantial number of dopaminergic drugs have been shown to share this property; the range of such agents has recently been reviewed (Seeman 1980; Robbins and Sahakian 1981; Bradbury *et al.* 1984). The stimulation of dopamine receptor sites induced by these direct or indirect agonist actions then initiates a series of physiological events which are poorly understood (Scheel-Krüger and Arnt 1985) but ultimately result in the manifestation of stereotyped motor behaviour.

The purpose of this article is to re-examine this classical drug-induced stereotypy in rodents, in the light of evidence that dopamine receptors appear to exist as a number of subtypes. By analogy with cholinergic and adrenergic systems, where receptor heterogeneity is well established and has important physiological consequences, the general question is whether dopamine receptor subtypes can also be differentiated functionally; more specifically, can stereotyped behaviour(s) be equated with drug action at any particular class of dopamine receptor site? It may seem strange that such a fundamental question should need to be posed about a system of receptor multiplicity. However, while cholinergic and adrenergic receptor subtyping evolved from distinct functional/physiological responses to drugs, receptor subtyping in relation to dopaminergic neurotransmission evolved substantially from neurochemical and direct radioligand-receptor binding techniques. The extent of confusion over the nature of dopamine receptor heterogeneity, to be discussed below, stems to a considerable extent from excessive reliance on the significance of the binding of drugs to synaptic membrane preparations, in the absence of clear physiological distinctions. By proceeding in this inverse manner, a system for the subclassification of dopamine receptors has evolved and achieved widespread acceptance; however, its behavioural correlates are not yet clear.

The subclassification of brain dopamine receptors

Proposals for receptor subclassification historically stem from pharmacological inconsistencies, usually anomalous physiological responses to putative agonist and antagonist drugs. Only a few authors who have reviewed the area (e.g. Costall and Naylor 1981) have acknowledged that the first systematic discussion of the possibility of dopamine receptor multiplicity originates with Klawans (1973). His proposals stemmed from just such considerations—primarily in relation to behavioural phenomena in clinical populations that appeared anomalous in the absence of receptor heterogeneity. A more specific scheme subsequently proposed by Costall and Naylor (1975) had its basis in the selective ability of certain neuroleptics to antagonize oral dyskinesias induced in the guinea-pig by intrastriatal dopamine. Such blockade was designated to occur at 'DA-2' receptors, with blockade of associated hyperactivity being designated to occur at 'DA-1' receptors. Cools and Van Rossum (1976) proposed a scheme of 'DA$_e$' and 'DA$_i$' receptors mediating electrophysiological excitation and inhibition, respectively. These subtypes were distinguished by anatomical, as well as neurophysiological criteria. Based on complex topographical studies of specific motor responses to local intracerebral injections into the monkey and cat striatum, some behavioural distinctions were also drawn.

Each of the above schemes for dopamine receptor subclassification has yet to achieve widespread acceptance in relation to dopaminergic function. While they importantly draw attention to anomalies in particular areas of dopaminergic behaviour, the small numbers of drugs specified as showing any selectivity of action within each scheme has limited the possibility of investigating the generality of these proposals.

The scheme for dopamine receptor subclassification that is most widely accepted evolved from rather different considerations. In the early-1970s, the ability of dopamine and dopamine agonist drugs to stimulate the activity of the enzyme adenylate cyclase in dopamine-rich areas of the brain was identified. As this stimulation was shown to be sensitive to antagonism by neuroleptics, these processes were offered as a neurochemical index of dopamine receptor function (Kebabian *et al.* 1972; Iversen 1975). However, a number of anomalies became apparent in relation to behavioural correlates. For some neuroleptics, such as the butyrophenone haloperidol and the diphenylbutylpiperidine pimozide, there was a substantial discrepancy between their high *in vivo* potency as dopamine antagonists and their low potency to inhibit the dopaminergic stimulation of adenylate cyclase. These anomalies became more exaggerated with the identification of the ergot derivatives, such as bromocriptine, and the substituted benzamides, such as sulpiride, as dopaminergic agonists and antagonists, respectively; both groups of agents had negligible actions on the activity of adenylate cyclase. It was from such considerations that Spano *et al.* (1978) and Kebabian (1978) speculated that dopamine receptors might exist in at least two forms, distinguished by their association or non-association with adenylate cyclase.

The application of radioligand-receptor binding techniques to dopaminergic systems produced a number of results that were at variance with those derived from drug effects on adenylate cyclase activity. Radioligands such as the butyrophenones ³H-haloperidol and ³H-spiperone appeared to bind to a population of sites showing many of the characteristics of dopamine receptors. Significantly, they were potently displaced by the dopaminergic ergots, by other butyrophenones and diphenylbutylpiperidines, and by the substituted benzamides, in addition to those drugs influencing the activity of dopamine-sensitive adenylate cyclase. Thus, these *in vitro* binding indices of dopamine receptor interactions appeared much more in concordance with the *in vivo* pharmacological activity of dopamine agonist and antagonist drugs, and appeared unrelated to those derived from effects on adenylate cyclase (Seeman 1977).

These two lines of evidence led Kebabian and Calne (1979) to formally propose a classification scheme for dopamine receptors that has become the basis for most of the subsequent work on dopamine receptor multiplicity: D-1 receptors were defined as those coupled to the stimulation of adenylate cyclase activity, the prototype receptor system being the dopaminergic stimulation of parathyroid hormone release; D-2 receptors were defined as those not coupled to adenylate cyclase and labelled by ³H-butyrophenone (and subsequently other) ligands, the prototype receptor system being the dopaminergic inhibition of pituitary prolactin secretion. Inspection of Kebabian and Calne's original scheme reveals two points that are of particular importance for the receptor basis of dopaminergic stereotyped behaviour. First, while it would be wrong to state that the D-1:D-2 scheme is solely determined from neurochemical considerations, typical dopaminergic behaviours are not a fundamental element of their classification; writing subsequently, Kebabian revealed that the hypothesis had its origins in the observation that the dopamine agonist lergotrile inhibited prolactin secretion yet blocked the dopamine-induced stimulation of striatal adenylate cyclase activity (Kebabian *et al.* 1983). Second, the scheme arose in the absence of any drugs known to act selectively as D-1 antagonists.

Since the introduction of radioligand binding techniques in the middle-1970s there has been a literature explosion. In the dopaminergic field this has clearly outstripped efforts to identify the physiological role of the various 'binding sites' identified, without which the designation 'receptor' is unwarranted. This has had two paradoxical consequences. Some workers have proposed further subdivision within the D-1:D-2 scheme, culminating in a 'four dopamine receptor' hypothesis derived essentially from *in vitro* binding considerations (Seeman 1980; Sokoloff *et al.* 1980). This in itself has led to two substrategies; a search for newer drugs with yet greater selectivity to discriminate between these various new binding sites, and greater potential to probe their physiological/behavioural relevance (Martres *et al.* 1984), or attempts to rationalize the four putative 'receptors' within the scheme originally proposed. The results of this latter approach have achieved more widespread acceptance, with D-3 being proposed as a subspecies of

D-1, and D-4 (in the sense of Seeman 1980) proposed as a subspecies of D-2. The intricacies of *in vitro* binding which have led to this rationalization are available in several articles and reviews (Creese *et al.* 1983; Leff and Creese 1983; Seeman *et al.* 1985). Needless to say, behavioural data are not prominent in these arguments.

Alternatively, the second of these paradoxical consequences has been to seek regression to a unitary dopamine receptor hypothesis. Laduron (1981, 1983) has argued that the 'D-1 receptor' is simply an enzyme, and that there is no evidence that changes in the activity of adenylate cyclase have any relationship with the other known pharmacological actions of dopamine agonists and antagonists. He took the extreme position that the D-2 site is the unitary receptor mediating all of the known central actions of dopamine and dopaminergic drugs.

This article will discuss the evidence that stereotyped behaviour in rodents may or may not be associated with drug action at one particular subtype of dopamine receptor. The system of receptor classification adopted for this purpose will be the rationalized D-1:D-2 scheme outlined above with one minor modification; evidence has emerged that, while D-2 receptors are not linked to the stimulation of adenylate cyclase activity, some can inhibit the activity of this enzyme (Creese *et al.* 1983; Stoof and Kebabian 1984).

Some procedural issues: pharmacological tools and behavioural assessment

A first requirement for probing the role(s) of multiple dopamine receptors in stereotyped motor behaviour is clearly a range of agonist and antagonist drugs known to act selectively at differing subtypes. The prototype stereotypy-inducing agents, apomorphine and amphetamine, have little to distinguish their actions at D-1 and D-2 receptors; apomorphine is a potent D-2 agonist and a weaker partial agonist at the D-1 receptor, while amphetamine releases dopamine itself to act ubiquitously on all dopamine receptors. The dopaminergic ergot agonists such as bromocriptine and lergotrile are potent D-2 agonists with weaker antagonist or partial agonist activity at the D-1 receptor (Fuxe and Calne 1979; Kebabian and Calne 1979; Seeman 1980). Similarly, among the classical antagonists of stereotypy the phenothiazine and thioxanthene neuroleptics, such as chlorpromazine and flupenthixol, act non-selectively to block both D-1 and D-2 receptors. The butyrophenones and related neuroleptics, including haloperidol and pimozide, show some (but not absolute) selectivity to block D-2 receptors. Substituted benzamide neuroleptics such as sulpiride and metoclopramide are much more selective as D-2 antagonists but have considerably reduced potency (Kebabian and Calne 1979; Jenner and Marsden 1979; Seeman 1980).

Thus, within the ranks of conventional pharmacological agents, there is a paucity of compounds that are both potent and selective as agonists or antagonists at dopamine receptor subtypes, and drugs acting with any degree of selectivity at D-1 receptors are conspicuous by their absence. Fortunately, these concepts of dopamine receptor multiplicity have been a stimulus for medicinal chemists either to look for new compounds with such actions or, in more than one case, to re-evaluate previously discarded agents. Some of the experimental compounds that will be discussed at length below are indicated in Table 3.1. The indices of their selectivity are their relative potencies to displace the *in vitro* binding of the D-1 ligand ^{3}H-piflutixol, or the D-2 ligand ^{3}H-spiperone. Given IC_{50} values represent the concentration of the experimental drug which will displace 50 per cent of the specifically-bound ligand under the specified conditions; thus low numbers indicate high affinity for the designated receptor. The use of these ligands, including complexities in their displacement by agonist drugs that are as yet functionally obscure, have been described in detail (Seeman 1980; Hyttel 1982; Creese *et al.* 1983; O'Boyle and Waddington 1984*a*).

Table 3.1 Affinities of some investigational agents for D-1 and D-2 dopamine receptors

| | $IC_{50}(nM)$ | | D-1 |
| | ^{3}H-piflutixol | ^{3}H-spiperone | |
Drug	(D-1)	(D-2)	D-2
D-1 agonists			
R-SK&F 38393	810	33 300	0.024
S-SK&F 38393	>100 000	>50 000	—
D-1 antagonists			
SCH 23390	1.0	1 565	0.0006
R-SK&F 83566	1.9	2 710	0.0007
S-SK&F 83566	561	11 400	0.049
D-2 agonists			
RU 24213	> 50 000	377	>133
D-2 antagonists			
Metoclopramide	>100 000	330	>303
Sulpiride	>100 000	273	>366
Ro 22–2586	18 300	84	217
Non-selective antagonists			
cis(Z)-Flupenthixol	1.1	2.4	0.48

Data from O'Boyle and Waddington (1984*a*, *b* and unpublished) and Pugh *et al.* (1985).

A second requirement for probing the contributions of dopamine receptor subtypes to stereotypy is a clear definition of stereotyped behaviour and a consistent procedure for its assessment. Most of the early work on dopamine agonist-induced motor stereotypy relied on the use of simple rating scales to assess a series of transitions between supposedly mutually exclusive categories of behaviour; these transitions were thought to reflect the increasing activation of a unitary dopaminergic process. It is now widely recognized that many of the assumptions underlying such procedures are likely to be invalid; such scales do not invariably constitute an ordinal scale of measurement and do not in fact reflect the progressive stimulation of a homogeneous dopaminergic system. Furthermore, they are insensitive to many of the individual behaviours constituting a typical syndrome of stereo-typed motor behaviour. Several articles and reviews have discussed these points in detail (Ungerstedt and Ljungberg 1977; Fray *et al.* 1980; Robbins and Sahakian 1981; Rebec and Bashore 1984). Stereotypy syndromes in rodents can consist of a variety of behaviours, including sniffing, rearing, locomotion, licking, gnawing, and other head and limb movements. There is no *a priori* reason to assume that all components of dopaminergic stereotypy involve any common subtype of receptor. Therefore, any study of dopamine receptor multiplicity in relation to stereotypy syndromes must include not only selective agonist and antagonist drugs, but also some means for assessing the individual sensitivities of the range of behaviours encountered to such pharmacological manipulations.

In addition to stereotypy rating scales, there are numerous alternative or adjunctive procedures for assessment of component behaviours by direct visual observation. One is the use of a behavioural check-list, to specify the presence or absence of a range of typical individual behaviours at a given assessment point (Fray *et al.* 1980). This approach has recently been extended by the use of data collection and analysis by computer and an extended range of behavioural categories (Lewis *et al.* 1985). As a new refine-ment, the complex system of Eshkol–Wachman Movement Notation has been successfully applied to the assessment of stereotyped behaviour (Szechtman *et al.* 1985). We have adopted the concurrent use of both a behavioural check-list (Fray *et al.* 1980) and an extended stereotypy rating scale (Robbins and Sahakian 1981) to allow us to distinguish the elements of behaviour present and make a coarse global estimation of the stereotyped nature of the syndrome to which they contribute (Molloy and Waddington 1984, 1985*a*; Pugh *et al.* 1985).

Stereotypy and D-2 dopamine receptors

Indirect correlational analyses

Following the introduction of ³H-butyrophenone ligands for what is now termed the D-2 receptor, behavioural correlates of drug interaction with this site were sought. The affinities for the D-2 receptor of a wide range of neuroleptic drugs were found to be highly correlated with their potencies to block stereotyped behaviour induced by a single dose of apomorphine or amphetamine (Creese *et al*. 1976; Leysen *et al*. 1978). In these studies the measure of antagonism of stereotypy was simply the dose of neuroleptic which inhibited the 'syndrome' (on an all-or-none basis) in 50 per cent of animals. Similarly, Seeman (1980) reported that the affinities for the D-2 receptor of a range of direct dopaminergic agonists were correlated with the minimum doses at which they induced stereotypy. These doses were those required to produce a consistent 'motor response' sustained for a least 30 min.

As previously discussed, there is no such general relationship between either the stereotypy-inducing or stereotypy-blocking potencies of dopaminergic agonists/antagonists and their affinities for D-1 receptors. Such indirect data have been conventionally interpreted as indicating that D-2 rather than D-1 receptors may be the more important for the initiation and expression of dopaminergic motor stereotypy. However, correlational analyses cannot prove a cause-and-effect relationship, and any distinct relationships between D-2 affinity and changes in specific behaviours do not appear to have been examined.

Blockade of apomorphine-induced stereotypy by selective D-2 antagonists

An important role for D-2 rather than D-1 receptors in stereotyped behaviour would also be indicated if responses to the essentially non-selective agonist apomorphine were to be blocked by selective D-2 antagonists. The substituted benzamide sulpiride is now widely accepted as such a selective D-2 antagonist, albeit of low affinity and potency (at least on peripheral administration). Reviews indicate that sulpiride, and some related benzamides, have been shown by certain authors to antagonize apomorphine stereotypy at high doses, but that the literature is not consistent on this point (Jenner and Marsden 1979; Worms 1982). Sulpiride has alternatively been reported to antagonize locomotion but to have little or no effect on the classical licking or gnawing induced by apomorphine (Ljungberg and Ungerstedt 1978; Jenner and Marsden 1979; Table 3.2). It is often not clear whether 'apomorphine-induced locomotion' is activity that distributes stereotyped behaviours over a range of locations, or is itself stereotyped in nature by way of invariance and/or repetition of route (Ljungberg and Ungerstedt 1978; cf. Schiorring 1979). The general significance of such distinctions is not clear in relation to the heterogeneity of dopamine receptors. Studies with sulpiride are also confounded by its low *in vivo* potency and debate as to the extent of its penetration into the brain and into distinct brain regions (Dross and Hopf 1979).

Metoclopramide, a related benzamide, shows similar characteristics as a selective D-2 antagonist in *in vitro* binding assays and neurochemical studies,

Table 3.2 Antagonism of apomorphine-induced stereotypy and of associated sniffing and locomotion by non-selective and selective D-2 antagonists

Drug	Dose (mg/kg)	Stereotypy score	Prevalence of behaviours	
			Sniffing	Locomotion
Apomorphine	0.5	3.2 ± 0.4	7/7	4/7
+ *cis*(Z)-flupenthixol	0.1	1.3 ± 0.5*	4/6	2/6
	0.5	0.1 ± 0.1**	1/7**	1/7
+ metoclopramide	1.0	1.2 ± 0.3*	7/8	3/8
	5.0	0 ± 0**	2/7 **	0/7 *
Apomorphine	0.5	3.1 ± 0.1	8/8	7/8
+ sulpiride	50	2.0 ± 0.5	8/10	4/10
	100	1.0 ± 0.2**	7/9	2/9*

Data from Molloy and Waddington (1985*a* and unpublished), as means ± SEM.
*$p < 0.05$.
**$p < 0.01$.

but has greater *in vivo* potency on peripheral administration. Some authors have maintained that the benzamides do not exhibit any intrinsic pharmacological differences (Worms 1982), while others have proposed that metoclopramide may have a preferential action on apomorphine-induced biting/gnawing (Ljungberg and Ungerstedt 1978; Jenner and Marsden 1979). The proposal that sulpiride and metoclopramide may be doubly dissociated by their respective actions on apomorphine-induced locomotion and gnawing is in contrast to the similarity of their moderate affinity for D-2 receptors and their negligible affinity for D-1 receptors. Whether these differences have their basis in pharmacodynamic, pharmacokinetic, or procedural factors is unknown. In our hands, metoclopramide dose-dependently antagonizes the overall stereotypy syndrome induced by apomorphine, and use of the behavioural check-list reveals that this arises from antagonism of both the stereotyped sniffing and locomotion which contribute to the overall response (Table 3.2); there was little rearing, licking, or gnawing induced by the dose of apomorphine used. It should be noted that these actions of the selective D-2 antagonist metoclopramide were qualitatively indistinguishable from those of the non-selective D-1 and D-2 antagonist *cis*(Z)-flupenthixol (Table 3.2), though this thioxanthene neuroleptic has greater potency (and greater affinity for D-2 receptors; Table 3.1).

A newer experimental substituted benzamide derivative, YM-09151-2, is a highly potent and highly selective D-2 antagonist (Grewe *et al.* 1982; Fleminger *et al.* 1983). It has been shown to be a potent antagonist of apomorphine-induced stereotyped behaviour when assessed using a rating scale sensitive predominantly to the sniffing and gnawing components of the syndrome (Fleminger *et al.* 1983). These authors also found a significant correlation between the potencies of a series of mostly substituted benzamide neuroleptics to inhibit apomorphine stereotypy and their affinities for the D-2 receptor, but not with their affinities for the D-1 receptor. Similar to our own findings with metoclopramide, the effects of YM-09151-2 on stereotyped behaviour were qualitatively indistinguishable from those of the non-selective dopamine receptor antagonist *cis*(Z)-flupenthixol.

In summary, these results complement the earlier studies investigating correlations between antistereotypic potency and affinities for D-1 and D-2 receptors. They further indicate an important role for D-2 receptors in dopamine agonist-induced stereotyped behaviour. However, the apparent absence of any functional role for D-1 receptors in these processes is indicated only indirectly by both the correlational analyses and the 'subtraction' strategy (i.e. comparing the actions of a selective D-2 antagonist with those of a non-selective antagonist of both D-1 and D-2 receptors).

Induction of stereotyped behaviour by selective D-2 agonists

A third line of evidence for an important role for D-2 receptors in stereotyped behaviour would be its induction by selective D-2 agonist drugs. As noted previously, the dopaminergic ergots, of which bromocriptine is the most well known, are potent D-2 agonists; however, some may also have weak partial agonist or weak antagonist activity at the D-1 receptor. They induce forms of stereotyped behaviour, but these actions do not always completely mimic those of apomorphine. Ergot-induced stereotypies may sometimes be less compulsive and perhaps less continuous than typical apomorphine-induced behaviours. These responses can be blocked by haloperidol and, less consistently, by sulpiride. Dopaminergic ergots have a complex pharmacology, which also includes: (1) a mode of interaction with D-2 receptors that is different from that of apomorphine and of dopamine itself; (2) sensitivity to manipulations of presynaptic dopaminergic function; and (3) highly potent interactions with several non-dopaminergic receptors, as previously reviewed (Fuxe and Calne 1979; Seeman 1980; Rosenfeld and Makman 1981). For these reasons, it is difficult to relate unequivocally their behavioural actions to a particular receptor subtype.

We have preferred to use the N-diphenylethylamine derivative RU 24213 as a selective D-2 agonist (Euvrard *et al.* 1980; Pugh *et al.* 1985; Table 3.1) in our behavioural studies. This agent dose-dependently induces stereotyped behaviour characterized by sniffing and locomotion; there were no consistent rearing or licking/biting responses (Pugh *et al.* 1985; Table 3.3). This profile is similar to that induced by apomorphine, at least at the dose utilized in Table 3.2. To confirm the involvement of D-2 receptors in these

Table 3.3 Induction of stereotyped behaviours by the selective D-2 agonist RU 24213 and their antagonism by a selective D-2 antagonist

Drug	Dose (mg/kg)	Stereotypy score	Prevalence of behaviours	
			Sniffing	Locomotion
Vehicle	—	0.4 ± 0.2	0/5	0/5
RU 24213	0.5	$1.8 \pm 0.2*$	5/5*	2/5
	3.0	$2.0 \pm 0.0**$	4/5*	2/5
	15.0	$3.0 \pm 0.0**$	5/5*	4/5*
RU 24213	15.0	3.0 ± 0.2	8/8	6/8
+ Ro 22–2586	0.04	2.6 ± 0.2	7/8	6/8
	0.2	$0.8 \pm 0.2**$	2/8**	0/8*

Data from Pugh *et al.* (1985), as means ± SEM.
*$p < 0.05$.
**$p < 0.01$.

responses to RU 24213, we investigated their sensitivity to blockade by a new selective D-2 antagonist Ro 22–2586, the active 4aR, 8aR enantiomer of the pyrrolo-(2,3-g)-isoquinoline neuroleptic piquindone (Ro 22–1319; Olson *et al.* 1981; Davidson *et al.* 1983; O'Boyle and Waddington 1984*b*). Stereotyped behaviour induced by RU 24213 was potently blocked by Ro 22–2586 in a dose-dependent manner, and both the sniffing and locomotor components of the syndrome were sensitive to antagonism (Table 3.3). Among other putative agents, the pyrazole partial ergoline LY 141865 (or its resolved active *trans*-(–)-4aR enantiomer LY 171555; Titus *et al.* 1983) appears to be a selective D-2 agonist (Tsuruta *et al.* 1981). However, while it appears selective, it has low potency (Frey *et al.* 1982). Behaviourally, it can induce some form of 'locomotor activity' in electronic activity monitors that are sensitive to antagonism by haloperidol (Titus *et al.* 1983). We have found it to be selective but to have a low potency to displace the striatal binding of ^{3}H-spiperone, and not to be a potent inducer of compulsive stereotyped behaviours. The napthoxazine (+)-PHNO is a potent D-2 receptor agonist, whose actions at the D-1 receptor appear minimal but have yet to be thoroughly evaluated (Martin *et al.* 1984). It potently induces stereotyped behaviour, when defined as the occurrence of biting, licking, or gnawing on an all-or-none basis, and this response is sensitive to antagonism by haloperidol. For both LY 141865 and (+)-PHNO, the syndromes they induce and the sensitivity of their constituent behaviours to selective antagonists remain to be characterized in detail.

While these studies with putative selective D-2 agonists are not conclusive, the results are consistent with the indirect correlational analyses, and the effects of selective D-2 antagonists on apomorphine stereotypy. Thus, there is clearly some general weight of evidence that drug action on D-2 receptors is crucially associated with the induction and antagonism of stereotyped behaviour. However, only the role of D-2 receptors has been investigated directly; any role for D-1 receptors appears still to be excluded only on the basis of indirect analyses.

Non-induction of stereotyped behaviour by selective D-1 agonists

Clearly, evidence for the involvement of D-2 receptors in stereotyped behaviour would be considerably strengthened by more direct evidence that appeared to exclude a role for D-1 receptors. The 1-phenyl-1H-3-benzazepine derivative, SK&F 38393, has remained, until very recently, the only agent with any selectivity of action on brain D-1 receptors, where it exerts partial agonist activity (Setler *et al.* 1978; Stoof and Kebabian 1981; Waddington *et al.* 1982; Sibley *et al.* 1982).

In the whole animal, SK&F 38393 fails to induce stereotyped behaviour, even when given at high doses (Setler *et al.* 1978; Waddington *et al.* 1982). In further studies with SK&F 38393, using a behavioural check-list as well as a stereotypy rating scale, we noted some activation of behaviours in the well-habituated animal; however, as will be discussed in detail below, they were not exhibited in a stereotyped fashion (Molloy and Waddington 1984, 1985*a*). These behaviours were allocated low (borderline) scores on the stereotypy rating scale to distinguish them from vehicle-injected animals (Table 3.5), but were readily distinguishable from typical stereotyped responses to apomorphine and RU 24213. SK&F 38393 is a chiral compound whose *R*- and *S*-enantiomers have been resolved (Kaiser *et al.* 1982); both D-1 agonist activity (Kaiser *et al.* 1982; O'Boyle and Waddington 1984*a*) and its non-stereotyped behavioural actions (Molloy and Waddington 1984, 1985*a*) reside predominantly in its *R*-enantiomer.

The failure of this centrally active, selective D-1 agonist to induce stereo-typed behaviour appears to add considerable weight to the other lines of evidence indicating the importance of D-2 receptors. Very similar arguments relate not just to the induction and antagonism of stereotyped behaviour, but extend also to the other central nervous system effects of dopaminergic manipulations, including behavioural actions such as catalepsy and inhibition of conditioned avoidance, the regulation of emesis, neurochemical and neuroendocrine effects, and the clinical antipsychotic activity of neuroleptics. The totality of the above lines of evidence, indicating that D-2 receptors mediate at the very least the vast majority of the physiological actions of dopamine and of related drugs in the brain, achieved widespread acceptance (Seeman 1980; Laduron 1981; Creese *et al.* 1983). Thus, any functional role for the D-1 receptor was described as 'unknown'

(Creese *et al.* 1983), or else the D-1 receptor was relegated to a 'site' that still remains in search of a function (Laduron 1983).

In other transmitter systems where receptor subtypes have been postulated, selective antagonists which define distinct physiological responses have been an essential part of their characterization. Despite all of the above evidence, indicating the prepotent functional role of D-2 receptors, the potentially conclusive studies of the effects of a selective D-1 antagonist have remained conspicuous by their absence.

Impact of new drugs which selectively influence D-1 receptors

The effects of selective D-1 antagonists on stereotyped behaviours

In 1983, Hyttel noted an abstract by Iorio *et al.* (1981) which described some atypical properties of the 7-chlorophenyl-1H-3-benzazepine derivative SCH 23390. Using radioligand binding and neurochemical indices, he was able to show that SCH 23390 appeared to be the first representative of that so far elusive group of compounds, selective D-1 antagonists (Hyttel 1983). These results were elaborated by Iorio *et al.* (1983) and subsequently extended in several laboratories (Cross *et al.* 1983; O'Boyle and Waddington 1984*a*; Christensen *et al.* 1984; Hyttel 1984). They have confirmed the status of SCH 23390 as the first potent and selective antagonist of brain D-1 dopamine receptors. The essential question was whether studies with SCH 23390 would confirm the prepotent role of D-2 receptors in stereotyped (and other dopamine-mediated) behaviours.

From the very outset, studies of the effects of SCH 23390 on stereotyped behaviour produced unexpected results. Iorio *et al.* (1981, 1983) initially reported that SCH 23390 blocked the induction by apomorphine of biting, licking, or gnawing. This was subsequently extended to blockade of apomorphine-induced sniffing and locomotion (Molloy and Waddington 1984, 1985*a*; Table 3.4), and amphetamine- and methylphenidate-induced gnawing (Christensen *et al.* 1984). Similar results were noted by Mailman *et al.* (1984). Such data clearly threw into some confusion the earlier, apparently consistent series of arguments which indicated the exclusivity of the role of D-2 receptors in mediating stereotyped behaviour. A possible way out of the dilemma is presented by the nature of the agonists which induced SCH 23390-sensitive stereotypy; apomorphine is a non-selective dopamine receptor agonist, while amphetamine and methylphenidate both act indirectly on release and uptake mechanisms to enhance non-selectively dopaminergic transmission. Perhaps their resultant effects on D-1 as well as on D-2 receptors render their behavioural actions sensitive to SCH 23390 in some as yet unappreciated way. This would be resolved by studying the

Table 3.4 Antagonism of apomorphine- and RU 24213-induced stereotyped behaviours by selective D-1 antagonists

Drug	Dose (mg/kg)	Stereotypy score	Prevalence of behaviours	
			Sniffing	Locomotion
Apomorphine	0.5	3.2 ± 0.4	7/7	4/7
+ SCH 23390	0.1	0 ± 0**	2/6*	0/6*
Apomorphine	0.5	3.2 ± 0.2	8/8	5/8
+ S-SK&F 83566	0.2	3.0 ± 0.0	3/3	3/3
+ R-SK&F 83566	0.04	1.4 ± 0.2**	6/10	2/10
+ R-SK&F 83566	0.2	0.7 ± 0.3**	3/9*	0/9*
RU 24213	15	3.0 ± 0.2	8/8	6/8
+ SCH 23390	0.04	1.4 ± 0.3**	6/8	4/8
	0.2	1.1 ± 0.3**	2/8*	1/8*
RU 24213	15	2.8 ± 0.1	10/10	10/10
+ S-SK&F 83566	0.2	2.6 ± 0.3	7/7	6/7
+ R-SK&F 83566	0.04	1.3 ± 0.2**	9/9	4/9*
	0.2	0.6 ± 0.3**	5/9*	0/9**

Data from Molloy and Waddington (1985a–c), as mean ± SEM.
*$p < 0.05$.
**$p < 0.01$.

effects of SCH 23390 on stereotypy induced by a selective D-2 agonist such as RU 24213.

We have found SCH 23390 to be a potent antagonist of stereotyped sniffing and locomotion induced by RU 24213 (Pugh *et al.* 1985; Table 3.4). In fact, SCH 23390 was both qualitatively and quantitatively similar to the selective D-2 antagonist Ro 22–2586 in blocking RU 24213-induced stereotypy (Tables 3.3 and 3.4). Thus, the same conceptual problem remains. A further possible explanation might be found by reconsidering the weak residual D-2 antagonist activity of SCH 23390. Though the low affinity of SCH 23390 for the D-2 receptor is orders of magnitude less than its very high affinity for D-1 receptors, this might be functionally relevant if it occurred at some unappreciated but critical subspecies of D-2 receptor, or if some pharmacokinetic idiosyncrasy such as selective regional penetration was operating. It has been possible to investigate further the mechanism(s) of this paradoxical blockade of both apomorphine- and RU 24213-induced stereotyped behaviour using a newer selective D-1 antagonist, the 7-bromo-1-phenyl-1H-3-benzazepine SK&F 83566.

The benzazepine D-1 antagonists are also chiral compounds, existing as true enantiomeric pairs, and we have been able to study the receptor and behavioural pharmacology of the resolved *R*- and *S*-enantiomers of SK&F 83566. The *R*-enantiomer shows high stereoselective affinity for D-1 receptors, comparable with that of SCH 23390, while its *S*-antipode is less active by orders of magnitude; conversely, these enantiomers display only very weak affinity for D-2 receptors and this residual activity shows negligible stereoselectivity (O'Boyle and Waddington 1984*b*; Table 3.1). Thus, if any action of SK&F 83566 to block stereotypy has its basis in weak residual D-2 antagonist activity, this effect should exhibit little or no enantioselectivity. Conversely, if SK&F 83566 were to antagonize stereotypy in an enantioselective manner, this would be consistent with a basis in D-1 receptor blockade.

We have found that *R*-SK&F 83566 but not *S*-SK&F 83566 blocks stereotyped behaviour induced by either apomorphine or RU 24213, and that this effect is manifest on both the sniffing and locomotor components of the syndrome (Molloy and Waddington 1985*b*, *c*; Table 3.4). This criterion of enantioselectivity is strong (but not conclusive) evidence that it is indeed blockade of D-1 receptors which underlays antagonism of stereotypy by SCH 23390 and SK&F 83566. Therefore, the apparent paradox between the weight of evidence indicating an exclusive role for D-2 receptors in stereotypy, and the blockade of stereotypy by D-1 antagonists, clearly remains. The paradox is not exclusive to stereotyped behaviour; it extends to other dopaminergic behavioural effects thought to be mediated through D-2 receptors, such as catalepsy and inhibition of conditioned avoidance (Iorio *et al.* 1983; Christensen *et al.* 1984; Arnt 1985).

Are these agents really selective?

Such results clearly pose problems for assumptions about the pharmacology of these agents and/or concepts of the functional roles of D-1 and D-2 receptors. The interpretation of these behavioural studies rests on the extent to which drugs such as SCH 23390, RU 24213, and Ro 22-2586 can be considered to act selectively at D-1 and D-2 receptors *in vivo*. In this regard, there are three principal questions which need to be asked.

1. Do these drugs show adequate *in vitro* selectivity for D-1 and D-2 receptors? In terms of current criteria for distinguishing drug action at these receptor subtypes (Kebabian and Calne 1979; Seeman 1980; Creese *et al.* 1983; Stoof and Kebabian 1984), SCH 23390 potently inhibits the stimulation of striatal adenylate cyclase activity induced by dopamine (the definition of a D-1 antagonist) and potently displaces the binding of ^{3}H-piflutixol to D-1 receptors; it fails to influence prolactin secretion and is only a very weak

displacer of ^{3}H-spiperone binding, the two prototype indices of D-2 activity (Iorio *et al.* 1983; Hyttel 1983; O'Boyle and Waddington 1984*a*; Christensen *et al.* 1984; Table 3.1). Conversely, RU 24213 and Ro 22-2586 negligibly influence the activity of dopamine-stimulated adenylate cyclase and only very weakly displace the binding of ^{3}H-piflutixol; however, they appropriately influence prolactin secretion and potently displace the binding of ^{3}H-spiperone (Euvrard *et al.* 1980; Olson *et al.* 1981; Davidson *et al.* 1983; Pugh *et al.* 1985; Table 3.1). Thus, according to prevailing definitions and nomenclature, the compounds used in this study appear to exert substantial selectivity of action *in vitro* at the designated D-1 and D-2 subtypes of the dopamine receptor.

2. Might these drugs have active metabolites with non-selective actions? The ability to elevate or inhibit prolactin secretion *in vivo* is a property shared by all known D-2 antagonists and agonists, respectively, and is one of the criteria defining activity at the D-2 receptor (Kebabian and Calne 1979; Seeman 1980; Creese *et al.* 1983; Stoof and Kebabian 1984). SCH 23390, under a variety of conditions which include doses considerably higher than those influencing behaviour, reliably fails to elevate prolactin secretion (Iorio *et al.* 1983; Christensen *et al.* 1984). This indicates that SCH 23390 itself has negligible D-2 antagonist activity and that no active metabolites with functionally significant D-2 antagonist activity are formed *in vivo*. Also, D-2 but not D-1 agonists induce emesis in dogs; their emetic potency is highly correlated with their affinity for D-2 receptors (Seeman 1980), as is anti-emetic potency of dopaminergic antagonists. SCH 23390 fails to antagonize apomorphine-induced emesis even at high doses (Iorio *et al.* 1983; Christensen *et al.* 1984), again indicating that the compound has negligible D-2 antagonist activity and that no active metabolite with functionally significant D-2 antagonist activity is formed *in vivo*. Selective antagonism at peripheral DA-1 but not DA-2 dopamine receptors is similarly retained *in vivo* (Hilditch *et al.* 1984). Likewise, RU 24213 potently inhibits prolactin secretion *in vivo* (Euvrard *et al.* 1980), as well as inducing stereotyped behaviour, confirming that D-2 agonist activity is indeed preserved.

3. Might non-dopaminergic actions of these drugs contribute to these unexpected results? Consistent with its failure to elevate prolactin secretion, the weak affinity of SCH 23390 for brain D-2 receptors is 500–1000-fold less than its very high affinity for D-1 receptors (Hyttel 1983; Cross *et al.* 1983; O'Boyle and Waddington 1984*a*). In both ligand binding and pharmacological studies, SCH 23390 similarly has little affinity for many non-dopaminergic receptors such as those for noradrenalin, histamine, acetylcholine, and the benzodiazepines (Hyttel 1983; Cross *et al.* 1983; Christensen *et al.* 1984). However, it has been consistently found that SCH 23390 has a modest affinity for 5-HT receptors, although this is some 35-fold less

than its affinity for D-1 receptors (Hyttel 1983; Cross *et al.* 1983); it can act as a modest 5-HT antagonist *In vitro* (Hicks *et al.* 1984). When given at doses which markedly antagonized stereotyped behaviour induced by RU 24213, SCH 23390 had no effect on the classical serotonergic behavioural syndrome induced by the 5-HT agonist 5-methoxy-N, N-dimethyltryptamine (Pugh *et al.* 1985). This indicates that at these low doses SCH 23390 was exerting little functional serotonergic antagonist action. Even potent 5-HT antagonists have inconsistent effects on dopamine agonist-induced stereotyped behaviour, and fail to exert the specific blockade of these responses associated with dopamine antagonists (Robbins and Sahakian 1981).

Thus, the available evidence indicates that the 'paradoxical' antagonism by the D-1 antagonist SCH 23390 of stereotypy induced by both apomorphine and the D-2 agonist RU 24213 is not readily explained in terms of a non-selective metabolite or by an action on any known non-dopaminergic system. SCH 23390, like Ro 22–2586, dose-dependently antagonized both the sniffing and locomotor components of RU 24213-induced stereotypy at a low dose (40 μg/kg), which was below a previously reported ED50 for the induction of catalepsy (Christensen *et al.* 1984). This, together with the failure of even a fivefold higher dose of SCH 23390 to antagonize the serotonergic behavioural syndrome, further indicated that the present effect of SCH 23390 is not a non-specific or general sedative effect to depress behaviour.

Are D-1 agonists behaviourally active?

An effect of D-1 receptor antagonists on the manifestation of stereotyped behaviour would be more credible were D-1 agonists also active behaviourally. As noted above, SK&F 38393, the only compound readily available, had been considered to be essentially inert in the whole animal; its effects in animals with 6-hydroxydopamine lesions or given long-term neuroleptic treatment (Setler *et al.* 1978; Waddington *et al.* 1982) were of unknown significance in view of resultant changes in dopamine receptor characteristics and in the absence of selective antagonists such as SCH 23390. It is well established that SK&F 38393 fails to induce stereotypy, but most studies had addressed this issue alone without seeking other perhaps more subtle effects.

When SK&F 38393 is given to well-habituated animals, in whom the baseline of spontaneous behaviours is very low, a number of behavioural responses are evident which can be quantified using a rapid sampling behavioural check-list procedure. Episodes of prominent grooming behaviour are most obvious, together with episodes of sniffing. These behaviours are discontinuous and non-stereotyped in nature, and cannot be appropriately quantified using a stereotypy rating scale. They are stereoselectively induced

Table 3.5 Induction of non-stereotyped grooming behaviour by
R-SK&F 38393 and apomorphine, and the influence of selective D-1 and
D-2 antagonists

Drug	Dose (mg/kg)	Stereotypy score	Prevalence of grooming
Vehicle	—	0.1 ± 0.1	1/13
R-SK&F 38393	20	1.7 ± 0.1	17/26
+ metoclopramide	1.0	1.4 ± 0.3	6/8
	5.0	1.3 ± 0.3	5/8
+ SCH 23390	0.1	0.1 ± 0.1*	2/8*
	0.5	0.1 ± 0.1*	0/8*
Apomorphine	0.5	3.2 ± 0.4	0/7
+ metoclopramide	1.0	1.2 ± 0.3*	5/8*
	5.0	0 ± 0**	1/7
Apomorphine	0.5	3.1 ± 0.1	0/8
+ sulpiride	50	2.0 ± 0.5	5/10*
	100	1.0 ± 0.2**	4/9

Data from Molloy and Waddington (1984, 1985a, and unpublished), as means ± SEM.
*$p < 0.05$.
**$p < 0.01$.

by the R- but not the S-enantiomer of SK&F 38393, paralleling the enantioselectivity of their D-1 agonist activity and distinct from the lack of enantioselectivity of their weak residual affinity for D-2 receptors. Grooming and
sniffing induced by SK&F 38393 is blocked by SCH 23390 (Molloy and
Waddington 1984, 1985a; Table 3.5). This behavioural profile is consistent
with a basis in D-1 receptor stimulation.

Episodes of non-stereotyped rearing and locomotion can also be induced
by this D-1 agonist, but appear to have a more complex basis. They are less
reliably induced than grooming and sniffing, are selectively more prevalent
in aged than in young animals, and are sensitive to antagonism by both SCH
23390 and metoclopramide (Molloy and Waddington 1984, 1985a; Molloy
et al. 1986). Similarly, locomotion and climbing induced by intra-accumbal
injections of SK&F 38393 have previously been noted to be antagonized by
sulpiride (Freedman et al. 1979; Costall et al. 1984). Rosengarten et al.
(1983) have described apparently non-stereotyped perioral movements after
acute challenge with SK&F 38393 and these were sensitive to antagonism by
a non-selective D-1 blocker. We have also noted such movements but find
this response also to be most evident in aged animals (Molloy et al. 1986),

where the D-1:D-2 ratio is perturbed by selective loss of D-2 receptors (O'Boyle and Waddington 1984c).

We have been able to induce grooming in rats with apomorphine when they are pre-treated with metoclopramide or sulpiride (Molloy and Waddington 1985a; Table 3.5). Such pre-treatment appears to 'unmask' the D-1 agonist component of apomorphine by blocking competing D-2 agonist effects such as stereotypy. Interestingly, these apparent 'unmasking' effects of the substituted benzamides had unusual dose dependencies. In a complex manner, they were evident at moderate doses but somewhat diminished at a higher dose (Table 3.5). No grooming was seen with RU 24213 with or without pre-treatment with a selective D-2 antagonist, consistent with it having no *in vivo* D-1 agonist component that could be 'unmasked' in this way.

The above evidence suggests that behavioural responses attributable to D-1 agonist action can be observed under particular experimental conditions. However, they are fragmented and non-stereotyped in nature, and are not prominent under conventional circumstances. Certainly, the profound behavioural effects of selective D-1 antagonists in the whole animal have not been matched to date by similarly profound, inverse effects of D-1 agonists. Nevertheless, such effects of D-1 agonists do suggest that D-1 receptors can subserve a behavioural role, and results from 6-hydroxydopamine lesion models such as rotational behaviour (circling/turning) support this general view (Arnt and Hyttel 1984; Herrera-Marschitz and Ungerstedt 1985; Arnt 1985). This issue would be clarified further were highly potent and selective D-1 agonists to become available. Rejection of D-1-mediated functions (Laduron 1981, 1983) appears to have been premature, and the above data on D-1 agonist effects provide some indirect support for the principle of behavioural effects of D-1 antagonists.

Conclusions and caveats

Anomalies relating to a primary role for D-2 receptors

The above data, on the effects of D-1 antagonists on D-2 agonist-induced stereotyped behaviour, should prompt us to review critically the evidence that appeared to suggest an exclusive role for D-2 mechanisms. If we do so, certain anomalies are evident. For example, dopamine agonist-induced stereotypy is not a homogeneous phenomenon. It is clear that differing drugs with apparently similar D-2 agonist activities induce qualitatively distinct patterns of stereotyped behaviour. While D-2 agonist activity appears essential for stereotyped behaviour to be initiated, certainly some other property is able to influence both the intensity of stereotypy and its qualitative expression. The extent to which this might relate to actions on differing substates or subpopulations of D-2 receptor, to pharmacokinetically or pharmacodynamically determined differences in regional actions, to additional non-dopaminergic actions, or, perhaps, to various additional effects on D-1 receptors remains unclear.

While D-2 antagonists have a general (but not absolute) action to block D-2 agonist-induced stereotypy, D-1 antagonists share this action.

Is there a mechanism for D-1 antagonist effects on stereotypy?

One explanation could be that SCH 23390 and SK&F 83566 are genuinely antagonizing stereotypy responses to drugs such as apomorphine and RU 24213 through blockade of tonic activity in ascending forebrain D-1 dopaminergic systems. This would imply that D-1 dopaminergic activity was able to influence processes stimulated by D-2 dopaminergic activity, i.e. that D-1 and D-2 dopaminergic systems do not invariably function independently. Such a possibility had not been previously considered prior to the recent introduction of the first selective D-1 antagonists, but has been proposed recently (Molloy and Waddington 1984, 1985a; Christensen et al. 1984; Arnt 1985). Behavioural studies in the whole animal are, of course, neither intended to nor able to indicate directly any synaptic basis for any such interaction. However, some possibilities which can be tested suggest themselves.

First, SCH 23390 might interact with D-1 receptors which are able to influence directly the characteristics of D-2 receptors possibly located in the same membrane, perhaps to alter their affinity for D-2 agents. However, our preliminary *in vitro* binding data, while not conclusive, are not consistent with such an effect (O'Boyle et al. 1986). Second, SCH 23390 might block D-1 receptors in dopaminergic systems which exert an important modulatory influence on those processes which are initiated by D-2 stimulation. Such interactions between D-1 and D-2 mechanisms would not have been previously indicated because of the lack of availability of selective D-1 antagonists, until the very recent introduction of SCH 23390. In general terms, it is possible that by blocking tonic dopaminergic activity at forebrain D-1 receptors SCH 23390 is able to influence behavioural effects that are initiated by drugs acting selectively on D-2 receptors.

These 'paradoxical' actions of SCH 23390 are not confined to antagonism of stereotyped behaviour, as the typical D-2 antagonist response of inhibition of conditioned avoidance responding is also mimicked by SCH 23390 (Iorio et al. 1983). Similarly, SCH 23390 can attenuate efflux responses to the D-2 agonist LY 141865 in functional rat striatal slice preparations held in perfusion chambers (Plantje et al. 1984); this is also important additional evidence that such paradoxical effects of SCH 23390 do not have their basis

In formation of a non-selective antagonist metabolite. It is striking that SCH 23390 appears to be a 'selective' D-1 antagonist not only in isolated, non-functional synaptic membrane preparations, as used in *in vitro* ligand binding assays; it also appears 'selective' when the criterion involves an *in vivo* physiological system that contains only D-2 receptors, such as regulation of emesis by the chemoreceptive trigger zone and of prolactin secretion by the pituitary (Creese *et al.* 1983). Similarly, SCH 23390 appears 'selective' in the rotational model where tonic D-1 dopaminergic activity in the hemisphere initiating the response is removed by a 6-hydroxydopamine lesion (Arnt and Hyttel 1984; Herrera-Marschitz and Ungerstedt 1985). However, when the test procedure is one that contains functional D-1 and D-2 receptors in the intact forebrain, such as in behavioural studies using whole animals, or uses striatal slice preparations where local functional integrity of D-1 and D-2 systems is preserved (Plantje *et al.* 1984), SCH 23390 appears to exert 'paradoxical' antagonism of D-2 agonist responses. Some potential neural substrates for such interactions have been discussed by Stoof and Kebabian (1981, 1984), Saller and Salama (1985), and Scheel-Krüger and Arnt (1985).

It seems that D-2 receptor stimulation may be required for initiating stereotyped behaviour in the whole animal. However, evidence suggests that tonic dopaminergic activity at D-1 receptors exerts an important modulatory influence over these processes (Pugh *et al.* 1985). Also, any putative neural mechanism for such interactions would have to account for complex results seen following prolonged denervation or sustained abolition of tonic dopaminergic activity (Arnt 1987). Neuropsychologically, more information is required on the extent to which processes governing selection of a stereotyped mode of behaviour might be dissociated from factors influencing the intensity and qualitative expression of stereotypy. Psychopharmacologically, potent and selective D-1 agonist and antagonist drugs are required from chemical classes other than the benzazepines to clarify the generality of the complex results derived from their exclusive use. For a further account of developments in this rapidly expanding field, see Waddington and O'Boyle (1989).

Acknowledgements

Studies carried out in the authors' laboratory were supported by the Medical Research Council of Ireland and the Royal College of Surgeons in Ireland. They were greatly aided by generous gifts of investigational drugs by Lundbeck, Roche, Roussel-UCLAF, Schering, and Smith, Kline, and French.

References

Arnt, J. (1987). Behavioural studies of dopamine receptors: evidence for regional selectivity and receptor multiplicity. In *Structure and function of dopamine receptors* (ed. I. Creese and C. Fraser) pp. 199-231. Alan R. Liss, New York.

Arnt, J. and Hyttel, J. (1984). Differential inhibition by dopamine D-1 and D-2 antagonists of circling behaviour induced by dopamine agonists in rats with unilateral 6-hydroxydopamine lesions. *Eur. J. Pharmacol.* **102**, 349-54.

Bradbury, A. J., Cannon, J. G., Costall, B., and Naylor, R. J. (1984). A comparison of dopamine agonist action to inhibit locomotor activity and to induce stereotyped behaviour in the mouse. *Eur. J. Pharmacol.* **105**, 33-47.

Christensen, A. V., Arnt, J., Hyttel, J., Larsen, J-J., and Svendsen, O. (1984). Pharmacological effects of a specific dopamine D-1 antagonist SCH 23390 in comparison with neuroleptics. *Life Sci.* **34**, 1529-40.

Cools, A. R. and Van Rossum, J. M. (1976). Excitation-mediating and inhibition-mediating dopamine receptors: a new concept towards a better understanding of electrophysiological, biochemical, pharmacological, functional and clinical data. *Psychopharmacology* **45**, 243-54.

Costall, B. and Naylor, R. J. (1975). Neuroleptic antagonism of dyskinetic phenomena. *Eur. J. Pharmacol.* **33**, 301-12.

Costall, B. and Naylor, R. J. (1981). The hypotheses of different dopamine receptor mechanisms. *Life Sci.* **28**, 215-29.

Costall, B., Eniojukan, J., and Naylor, R. J. (1984). D-1 and D-2 dopamine agonist-antagonist action in the nucleus accumbens to modify mouse spontaneous climbing behaviour. *Br. J. Pharmacol.* **81**, 115P.

Creese, I., Burt, D. R., and Snyder, S. H. (1976). Dopamine receptor binding predicts clinical and pharmacological potencies of antischizophrenic drugs. *Science* **192**, 481-3.

Creese, I., Sibley, D. R., Hamblin, M. W., and Leff, S. E. (1983). The classification of dopamine receptors: relationship to radioligand binding. *Ann. Rev. Neurosci.* **6**, 43-71.

Cross, A. J., Mashal, R. D., Johnson, J. A., and Owen, F. (1983). Preferential inhibition of ligand binding to calf striatal dopamine D-1 receptors by SCH 23390. *Neuropharmacology* **22**, 1327-9.

Davidson, A. B., Boff, E., MacNeil, D. A., Wenger, J., and Cook, L. (1983). Pharmacological effects of Ro 22-1319: a new antipsychotic agent. *Psychopharmacology* **79**, 32-9.

Dross, K. and Hopf, A. (1979). Studies on the distribution of ^{14}C-sulpiride and its metabolites in the rat and guinea pig. *Pharmacopsychiatry* **12**, 438-44.

Euvrard, C., Ferland, L., Di Paulo, T., Beaulieu, M., Labrie, F., Oberlander, C., Raynaud, J. P., and Boissier, J. R. (1980). Activity of two new potent dopaminergic agonists at the striatal and anterior pituitary levels. *Neuropharmacology* **19**, 379-86.

Fleminger, S., Van de Waterbeemd, H., Rupniak, N. M. J., Reavill, C., Testa, B., Jenner, P., and Marsden, C. D. (1983). Potent lipophilic substituted benzamide drugs are not selective D-1 dopamine receptor antagonists in the rat. *J. Pharm. Pharmacol.* **35**, 363–8.

Fray, P. J., Sahakian, B. J., Robbins, T. W., Koob, G. F., and Iversen, S. D. (1980). An observational method for quantifying the behavioural effects of dopamine agonists: contrasting effects of d-amphetamine and apomorphine. *Psychopharmacology* **69**, 253–9.

Freedman, S. B., Wait, C. P., and Woodruff, G. N. (1979). Effects of dopamine receptor agonists and antagonists in the rat nucleus accumbens. *Br. J. Pharmacol.* **67**, 430P–431P.

Frey, E. A., Cote, T. E., Grewe, C. W., and Kebabian, J. W. (1982). ^{3}H-spiroperidol identifies a D-2 dopamine receptor inhibiting adenylate cyclase activity in the intermediate lobe of the rat pituitary gland. *Endocrinology* **110**, 1897–904.

Fuxe, K. and Calne, D. B. (1979). *Dopaminergic ergot derivatives and motor function.* Pergamon Press, Oxford.

Grewe, C. W., Frey, E. A., Cote, T. E., and Kebabian, J. W. (1982). YM-09151-2: a potent antagonist for a peripheral D-2 dopamine receptor. *Eur. J. Pharmacol.* **81**, 149–52.

Herrera-Marschitz, M. and Ungerstedt, U. (1985). Effect of the dopamine D-1 antagonist SCH 23390 on rotational behaviour induced by apomorphine and pergolide in 6-hydroxy-dopamine denervated rats. *Eur. J. Pharmacol.* **109**, 349–54.

Hicks, P. E., Shoemaker, H., and Langer, S. Z. (1984). 5-HT receptor antagonist properties of SCH 23390 in vascular smooth muscle and brain. *Eur. J. Pharmacol.* **105**, 339–42.

Hilditch, A., Drew, G. M., and Naylor, R. J. (1984). SCH 23390 is a very potent and selective antagonist at vascular dopamine receptors. *Eur. J. Pharmacol.* **97**, 333–4.

Hyttel, J. (1982). Preferential labelling of adenylate cyclase-coupled dopamine receptors with thioxanthene neuroleptics. *Adv. Biosci.* **37**, 147–52.

Hyttel, J. (1983). SCH 23390: the first selective dopamine D-1 antagonist. *Eur. J. Pharmacol.* **91**, 153–4.

Hyttel, J. (1984). Functional evidence for selective dopamine D-1 receptor blockade by SCH 23390. *Neuropharmacology* **23**, 1395–401.

Iorio, L. C., Houser, V., Korduba, C. A., Leitz, F., and Barnett, A. (1981). SCH 23390, a benzazepine with atypical effects on dopaminergic systems. *Pharmacologist* **23**, 137.

Iorio, L. C., Barnett, A., Leitz, F. H., Houser, V. P., and Korduba, C. A. (1983). SCH 23390, a potential benzazepine antipsychotic with unique interactions on dopaminergic systems. *J. Pharmacol. exp. Ther.* **226**, 462–8.

Iversen, L. L. (1975). Dopamine receptors in the brain. *Science* **188**, 1084–9.

Iversen, S. D. (1977). Neural substrates mediating amphetamine responses. *Adv. behav. Biol.* **21**, 31–45.

Jenner, P. and Marsden, C. D. (1979). The substituted benzamides: a novel class of dopamine antagonists. *Life Sci.* **25**, 479–86.

Joyce, J. N. (1983). Multiple dopamine receptors and behaviour. *Neurosci. Biobehav. Rev.* **7**, 227–56.

Kaiser, C., Dandridge, P.A., Garvey, E., Hahn, R.A., Sarau, H.M., Setler, P.E., Bass, L.S., and Clardy, J. (1982). Absolute stereochemistry and dopaminergic activity of enantiomers of 2,3,4,5-tetrahydro-7,8-dihydroxy-1-phenyl-1H-3-benzazepine. *J. Med. Chem.* **25**, 697-703.

Kebabian, J.W. (1978). Multiple classes of dopamine receptors in mammalian central nervous system: the involvement of dopamine-sensitive adenyl cyclase. *Life Sci.* **23**, 479-84.

Kebabian, J.W. and Calne, D.B. (1979). Multiple receptors for dopamine. *Nature* **277**, 93-6.

Kebabian, J.W., Petzold, G.L., and Greengard, P. (1972). Dopamine-sensitive adenylate cyclase in caudate nucleus of rat brain, and its similarity to the "dopamine receptor". *Proc. nat. Acad. Sci., USA* **69**, 2145-9.

Kebabian, J.W., Beaulieu, M., Cote, T.E., Eskay, R.L., Frey, E.A., Goldman, M.E., Grewe, C.W., Munemura, M., Stoof, J.C., and Tsuruta, K. (1983). The D-2 dopamine receptor in the intermediate lobe of the rat pituitary gland: physiology, pharmacology and biochemistry. In *Dopamine receptors* (ed. C. Kaiser and J.W. Kebabian), pp. 33-52. American Chemical Society, Washington, DC.

Klawans, H.L. (1973). *The pharmacology of extrapyramidal movement disorders.* Karger, Basel.

Laduron, P. (1981). Dopamine receptor: a unique site with multiple postsynaptic localisation. In *Apomorphine and other dopaminomimetics* (ed. G.L. Gessa and G.U. Corsini), Vol. 1, pp. 95-103. Raven Press, New York.

Laduron, P. (1983). Dopamine-sensitive adenylate cyclase as a receptor site. In *Dopamine receptors* (ed. C. Kaiser and J.W. Kebabian), pp. 22-31. American Chemical Society, Washington, DC.

Leff, S.E. and Creese, I. (1983). Dopamine receptors re-explained. *Trends pharmacol. Sci.* **4**, 463-7.

Lewis, M.H., Baumeister, A.A., McCorkle, D.L., and Mailman, R.B. (1985). A computer-supported method for analysing behavioural observations: studies with stereotypy. *Psychopharmacology* **85**, 204-9.

Leysen, J.E., Niemegeers, C.J.E., Tollenaere, J.P., and Laduron, P.M. (1978). Serotonergic component of neuroleptic receptors. *Nature* **272**, 168-71.

Ljungberg, T. and Ungerstedt, U. (1978). Classification of neuroleptic drugs according to their ability to inhibit apomorphine-induced locomotion and gnawing: evidence for two different mechanisms of action. *Psychopharmacology* **56**, 239-47.

Mailman, R.B., Schulz, D.W., Lewis, M.H., Staples, L., Rollema, H., and DeHaven, D.L. (1984). SCH 23390: a selective D-1 dopamine antagonist with potent D-2 behavioural actions. *Eur. J. Pharmacol.* **101**, 159-60.

Martin, G.E., Williams, M., Pettibone, D.J., Yarbrough, G.G., Clineschmidt, B.V., and Jones, J.H. (1984). Pharmacologic profile of a novel potent direct-acting dopamine agonist, (+)-4-propyl-9-hydroxynaphthoxazine ((+)-PHNO). *J. Pharmacol. exp. Ther.* **230**, 569-76.

Martres, M.P., Sokoloff, P., Delandre, M., Schwartz, J.C., Protais, P., and Costentin, J. (1984). Selection of dopamine antagonists discriminating various behavioural responses and radioligand binding sites. *Naunyn-Schmiedeberg's Arch. Pharmacol.* **325**, 102–15.

Molloy, A. G. and Waddington, J. L. (1984). Dopaminergic behaviour stereospecifically promoted by D-1 agonist *R*-SK&F 38393 and selectively blocked by the D-1 antagonist SCH 23390. *Psychopharmacology* **82**, 409–10.

Molloy, A. G. and Waddington, J. L. (1985a). Sniffing, rearing and locomotor responses to the D-1 dopamine agonist *R*-SK&F 38393 and to apomorphine: differential interactions with the selective D-1 and D-2 antagonists SCH 23390 and metoclopramide. *Eur. J. Pharmacol.* **108**, 305–8.

Molloy, A. G. and Waddington, J. L. (1985b). Mechanism of paradoxical blockade of D-2 agonist-induced stereotypy by the enantiomers of the D-1 antagonist SK&F 83566. *Br. J. Pharmacol.* **85**, 242P.

Molloy, A. G. and Waddington, J. L. (1985c). Stereoselective blockade of behavioural responses to the dopamine agonist apomorphine by the enantiomers of the selective D-1 antagonist SK&F 83566. *Irish J. med. Sci.* **154**, 332–3.

Molloy, A. G., O'Boyle, K. M., and Waddington, J. L. (1986). The D-1 dopamine receptor and ageing: behavioural and neurochemical studies. In *The Neurobiology of dopamine systems* (ed. W. Winlow and R. Markstein) pp. 104–7. Manchester University Press.

Neumeyer, J. L., Lal, S., and Baldessarini, R. J. (1981). Historical highlights of the chemistry, pharmacology, and early clinical uses of apomorphine. In *Apomorphine and other dopaminomimetics* (ed. G. L. Gessa and G. U. Corsini), Vol. 1, pp. 1–17. Raven Press, New York.

O'Boyle, K. M. and Waddington, J. L. (1984a). Selective and stereospecific interactions of *R*-SK&F 38393 with ^{3}H-piflutixol but not ^{3}H-spiperone binding to striatal D-1 and D-2 dopamine receptors: comparisons with SCH 23390. *Eur. J. Pharmacol.* **98**, 433–6.

O'Boyle, K. M. and Waddington, J. L. (1984b). Identification of the enantiomers of SK&F 83566 as specific and stereoselective antagonists at the striatal D-1 dopamine receptor: comparisons with the D-2 enantioselectivity of Ro 22-1319. *Eur. J. Pharmacol.* **106**, 219–20.

O'Boyle, K. M. and Waddington, J. L. (1984c). Loss of rat striatal dopamine receptors with ageing is selective for D-2 but not D-1 sites: association with increased non-specific binding of the D-1 ligand ^{3}H-piflutixol. *Eur. J. Pharmacol.* **105**, 171–4.

O'Boyle, K. M., Molloy, A. G., and Waddington, J. L. (1986). Benzazepine derivatives: nature of the selective and stereospecific interactions of SK&F 38393 and SCH 23390 with brain D-1 receptors. In *Dopamine systems and their regulation* (ed. G. N. Woodruff) pp. 385–6. Macmillan Press, London.

Olson, G. L., Cheung, H-C., Morgan, K. D., Blount, J. F., Todaro, L., Berger, L., Davidson, A. B., and Boff, E. (1981). A dopamine receptor model and its application in the design of a new class of rigid pyrrolo (2,3-g)isoquinoline antipsychotics. *J. Med. Chem.* **24**, 1026–34.

Plantje, J. F., Daus, F. J., Hansen, H. A., and Stoof, J. C. (1984). SCH 23390 blocks D-1 and D-2 dopamine receptors in rat neostriatum in vitro. *Naunyn-Schmiederberg's Arch. Pharmacol.* **327**, 180–2.

Pugh, M.T., O'Boyle, K.M., Molloy, A.G., and Waddington, J.L. (1985). Effects of the putative D-1 antagonist SCH 23390 on stereotyped behaviour induced by the D-2 agonist RU 24213. *Psychopharmacology* **87**, 308–12.

Randrup, A. and Munkvad, I. (1974). Pharmacology and physiology of stereotyped behaviour. *J. Psychiat. Res.* **11**, 1–10.

Rebec, G.V. and Bashore, T.R. (1984). Critical issues in assessing the behavioural effects of amphetamine. *Neurosci. Biobehav. Rev.* **8**, 153–9.

Robbins, T.W. and Sahakian, B.J. (1981). Behavioural and neurochemical determinants of drug-induced stereotypy. In *Metabolic disorders of the nervous system* (ed. F.C. Rose), pp. 244–91. Pitman Books, London.

Rosenfeld, M.R. and Makman, M.H. (1981). The interaction of lisuride, an ergot derivative, with serotonergic and dopaminergic receptors in rabbit brain. *J. Pharmacol. exp. Ther.* **216**, 526–31.

Rosengarten, H., Schweitzer, J.W., and Friedhoff, A.J. (1983). Induction of oral dyskinesias in naive rats by D-1 stimulation. *Life Sci.* **33**, 2479–82.

Saller, C.F. and Salama, A.I. (1985). Dopamine receptor subtypes: in vivo biochemical evidence for functional interaction. *Eur. J. Pharmacol.* **109**, 297–300.

Scheel-Krüger, J. and Arnt, J. (1985). New aspects on the role of dopamine, acetylcholine and GABA in the development of tardive dyskinesia. In *Dyskinesia: research and treatment* (ed. D.E. Casey, T.N. Chase, A.V. Christensen, and J. Gerlach), pp. 46–57. Springer-Verlag, Berlin.

Schiørring, E. (1979). An open field study of stereotyped locomotor activity in amphetamine-treated rats. *Psychopharmacology* **66**, 281–9.

Seeman, P. (1977). Antischizophrenic drugs: membrane receptor sites of action. *Biochem. Pharmacol.* **26**, 1741–8.

Seeman, P. (1980). Brain dopamine receptors. *Pharmacol. Rev.* **32**, 229–313.

Seeman, P., Ulpian, C., Grigoriadis, D., Pri-Bar, I., and Buchman, O. (1985). Conversion of dopamine D-1 receptors from high to low affinity for dopamine. *Biochem. Pharmacol.* **34**, 151–4.

Setler, P.E., Sarau, H.M., Zirkle, C.L., and Saunders, H.L. (1978). The central effects of a novel dopamine agonist. *Eur. J. Pharmacol.* **50**, 419–30.

Sibley, D.R., Leff, S.E., and Creese, I. (1982). Interactions of novel dopaminergic ligands with D-1 and D-2 dopamine receptors. *Life Sci.* **31**, 637–45.

Sokoloff, P., Martres, M.P., and Schwartz, J.C. (1980). Three classes of dopamine receptor (D-2, D-3, D-4) identified by binding studies with ^{3}H-apomorphine and ^{3}H-domperidone. *Naunyn-Schmiedeberg's Arch. Pharmacol.* **315**, 89–102.

Spano, P.F., Govoni, S., and Trabucchi, M. (1978). Studies on the pharmacological properties of dopamine receptors in various areas of the central nervous system. *Adv. Biochem. Psychopharmacol.* **19**, 155–65.

Stoof, J.C. and Kebabian, J.W. (1981). Opposing roles of D-1 and D-2 dopamine receptors in efflux of cyclic AMP from rat neostriatum. *Nature* **294**, 366–8.

Stoof, J.C. and Kebabian, J.W. (1984). Two dopamine receptors: biochemistry, physiology and pharmacology. *Life Sci.* **35**, 2281–96.

Szechtman, H., Ornstein, K., Teitelbaum, P., and Golani, I. (1985). The morphogenesis of stereotyped behaviour induced by the dopamine receptor agonist apomorphine in the laboratory rat. *Neuroscience* **14**, 783–98.

Titus, R.D., Kornfeld, E.C., Jones, N.D., Clemens, J.A., Smalstig, E.B., Fuller, R.W., Hahn, R.A., Hynes, M.D., Mason, N.R., Wong, D.T., and Foreman, M.M. (1983). Resolution and absolute configuration of an ergoline-related dopamine agonist, trans-4, 4a, 5, 6, 7, 8, 8a, 9-octahydro-5-propyl-1H (or 2H)-pyrazolo (3, 4-g) quinoline. *J. Med. Chem.* **26**, 1112–16.

Tsuruta, K., Frey, E.A., Grewe, C.W., Cote, T.E., Eskay, R.L., and Kebabian, J.W. (1981). Evidence that L Y 141865 specifically stimulates the D-2 dopamine receptor. *Nature* **292**, 463–5.

Ungerstedt, U. and Ljungberg, T. (1977). Behavioural patterns related to dopamine neurotransmission: effect of acute and chronic antipsychotic drugs. *Adv. Biochem. Psychopharmacol.* **16**, 193–9.

Waddington, J.L. and O'Boyle, K.M. (1989). Drugs acting on brain dopamine receptors: a conceptual re-evaluation five years after the first selective D-1 antagonist. *Pharmacol. Ther.* **43**, 1–52.

Waddington, J.L., Cross, A.J., Gamble, S.J., and Bourne, R.C. (1982). Functional heterogeneity of multiple dopamine receptors during six months treatment with distinct classes of neuroleptic drugs. *Adv. Biosci.* **37**, 143–6.

Worms, P. (1982). Behavioural pharmacology of the benzamides as compared to standard neuroleptics. In *The benzamides: pharmacology, neurobiology and clinical aspects* (ed. J. Rotrosen and M. Stanley), pp. 7–16. Raven Press, New York.

4

Neural basis of drug-induced yawning

COLIN T. DOURISH and STEVEN J. COOPER

Introduction

In a study of human yawning Robert Provine (1986) remarked that yawning is a prominent stereotyped action pattern and releasing stimulus which 'does not deserve its current status as a minor behavioural curiosity'. Indeed, 'yawning may have the dubious distinction of being the least understood, common, human behaviour'. In contrast, a large body of experimental data has been collected during the past 30 years on drug-induced yawning in animals (particularly rodents). In this chapter we consider the neural basis of drug-induced yawning in rodents and discuss the relevance of this pharmacological phenomenon to 'spontaneous' yawning in animals and man.

We propose that yawning may be controlled by a complex interaction of catecholaminergic, serotonergic, and peptidergic neuronal mechanisms. A model is put forward to explain how yawning may be caused largely by peptidergic and cholinergic excitation and dopaminergic inhibition. Furthermore, we present evidence which suggests that, in animals and man, yawning may be a marker of recovery from acute stress and that these responses may be closely associated with an inhibition of brain dopamine metabolism.

Historical perspective: peptide hormones

Drug-induced yawning and stretching were first reported in the 1950s by W. Ferrari and colleagues working at the University of Cagliari in Italy (Ferrari *et al.* 1955; Ferrari 1958; early studies are reviewed by Ferrari *et al.* 1963 and Gessa *et al.* 1967). Ferrari injected dogs intracisternally with adrenocorticotropic hormone (ACTH) and after about an hour observed recurrent yawning and stretching (see Fig. 4.1). The behaviour persisted for 24 to 72 hours depending on the dose of ACTH given (Ferrari *et al.* 1963). The syndrome appeared to be centrally mediated as intra-arterial injections of large doses of ACTH did not produced yawning and stretching (Ferrari *et al.* 1963). After this initial discovery a large number of other peptides were

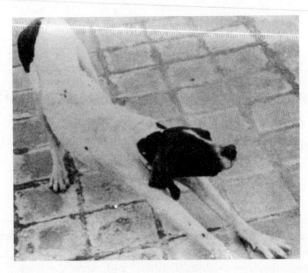

Fig. 4.1. Stretching induced by intracisternal injection of ACTH in the dog. (From Ferrari *et al.* 1963, with permission of the authors and publisher.)

tested for their ability to provoke the yawning syndrome, but of these only α-melanocyte stimulating hormone (α-MSH), β-lipotropic hormone (β-LPH) (Ferrari *et al.* 1963), and, more recently, oxytocin (Argiolas *et al.* 1985) produced a positive result. In subsequent studies, intraventricular or intracisternal injection of ACTH and α-MSH were found to elicit the syndrome in a wide variety of other species including cats, rabbits, monkeys, guinea-pigs, mice, and rats. Interestingly, in dogs and cats stretching was the dominant response, whereas in monkeys, rabbits, and rats yawning was more frequently observed (Gessa *et al.* 1967). In rats, excessive grooming is also an important feature of the ACTH-induced syndrome. Peptide-induced grooming is discussed in detail by Isaacson and Gispen in Chapter 5 of this volume.

In an effort to identify the site of action of ACTH in producing the yawning–stretching syndrome, Gessa *et al.* (1967) examined the effects of intracerebral injection of the hormone into various brain regions in cats. These experiments revealed two principal sites of action of ACTH in the brain which were the hypothalamic areas lining the third ventricle and the caudate nucleus. A hypothalamic site of action was not unexpected as another feature of the yawning–stretching syndrome is sexual arousal and there is considerable evidence that hypothalamic mechanisms are important in the control of sexual behaviour (Sandler and Gessa 1975). (A detailed consideration of the sexual arousal component of the syndrome is beyond the scope of this chapter. For further discussion of this subject the reader is referred to reviews by Bertolini *et al*. 1975 and Bertolini and Gessa 1981.) The most intense stretching and yawning was observed upon injection of ACTH into the anterior and ventromedial hypothalamic nuclei. Potent effects were also observed in the posterior and lateral hypothalamic nuclei and in the caudate nucleus (Gessa *et al*. 1967). Weak responses were produced by application of ACTH to the putamen, globus pallidus, and substantia nigra. This early observation that the hypothalamus and the caudate nucleus play an important role in the mediation of stretching and yawning induced by ACTH is consistent with recent experiments showing that these regions are crucially involved in the control of yawning induced by dopamine agonists (see below for further discussion).

During the 10 years subsequent to the 1967 review of Gessa and colleagues little or no work was published on the neuropharmacology of yawning. However in the mid-1970s interest in the yawning syndrome was rekindled by the discovery that certain pharmacological manipulations of either cholinergic or dopaminergic neurotransmitter systems could elicit yawning (Baraldi and Bertolini 1974; Urba-Holmgren *et al*. 1977; Mogilnicka and Klimek 1977). These seminal findings provoked a considerable research effort on the yawning syndrome and a consideration of the results of these studies and their theoretical implications forms the basis of the remainder of this chapter.

Acetylcholine

Yawning induced by cholinergic agents

In 1977 Holmgren and his colleagues observed that small doses of pilocarpine (a cholinergic agonist) or physostigmine (which inhibits acetylcholine metabolism) produced yawning in infant rats. Each yawn was preceded by salivation, licking of the forepaws and cleaning movements of the snout, chewing movements, or forelimb stretching (Urba-Holmgren *et al*. 1977). The yawn consisted of a slow wide opening of the mouth with marked protrusion of the tongue and had a maximum frequency of 8–10 responses in 15 min and a duration of 3–4 seconds.

The response appeared to be centrally mediated since the peripheral cholinergic agonist neostigmine methylsulphate did not induce yawning. Furthermore, the yawning seemed to involve muscarinic receptors as the response was inhibited by the muscarinic antagonist scopolamine and was not produced by nicotine (Urba-Holmgren *et al*. 1977). Furthermore, the nicotinic receptor blocker mecamylamine had no effect on yawning induced by pilocarpine or physostigmine (Ushijima *et al*. 1984a).

Yawning induced by cholinergic agonists is critically dependent on the age of the animal during testing. Thus, physostigmine-induced yawning is highest in early postnatal days and tends to decline from the seventh day onward (Holmgren and Urba-Holmgren 1980). (It should be noted that this developmental sequence contrasts with that of yawning induced by dopaminergic drugs which does not appear until 11–15 days of age and is maximal in adults.) There has been disagreement is subsequent studies as to whether pilocarpine significantly increases yawning in adult rats. Yamada and colleagues (Yamada and Furukawa 1980; Ushijima *et al*. 1984a, 1985) have reported that pilocarpine induces a peak yawning response in adult rats at a dose of 4.0 mg/kg. However, Salamone *et al*. (1986) disagree and suggest that Ushijima *et al*. (1984a, 1985) may have recorded an exaggerated yawning response by scoring 'gaping' responses as yawns.

Gaping is a rapid opening and closing of the mouth which is wide enough to see the teeth. In contrast, yawning has been defined as a gradual opening of the mouth, followed by a retention of the open position, frequently accompanied by a lifting back of the head, and usually finished with a closure of the mouth more rapid than the orginal opening (Salamone *et al*. 1986). Since Ushijima *et al*. (1984a) recorded yawns as total number of mouth openings, it is possible that gaping responses may have been scored as yawns in their study.

Ushijima *et al*. (1984a, 1985) have suggested that spontaneous physiological yawning and yawning induced by physostigmine are very similar in appearance. Both responses are reported to be characterized by a slow wide opening of the mouth (3.6 s in duration) with the head moving mainly upward (Ushijima *et al*. 1985). Thus, they have speculated that physiological yawning may be mediated by endogenous acetycholine.

Responses associated with yawning induced by cholinergics

Some attention has also been paid to two other components of the cholinergic yawning syndrome, i.e. tongue protrusion and chewing mouth movements. It has been proposed that tongue protrusion (in contrast to yawning) may be mediated by nicotinic receptors since this response is inhibited by the nicotinic antagonist mecamylamine (Ushijima *et al*. 1984a, 1985). Chewing mouth movements (described as teeth chattering by some authors) have been observed after pilocarpine and physostigmine; like yawning, these responses are attenuated by scopolamine but unaffected by the peripheral muscarinic antagonist methyl scopolamine (Ushijima *et al*. 1984a; Salamone *et al*. 1986). The frequency of chewing is considerably higher than that of yawning with as many as 40 responses per minute being observed at some doses (Salamone *et al*. 1986). The chewing response has been proposed by Salamone and colleagues (1986) as a reliable index of central muscarinic agonist activity in rats.

Chewing mouth movements have also been observed in rats treated acutely and chronically with certain neuroleptic drugs including haloperidol and sulpiride (Rupniak *et al*. 1983*a*). This response was decreased by anticholinergics and increased by cholinergic agonists (Rupniak *et al*. 1983*a*, 1985). It has been suggested that this chewing response may be an acute dystonic reaction (Rupniak *et al*. 1983*a*, 1985).

Yawning and associated behaviours elicited by cholinergic agonists are sensitive to dopaminergic drug treatments. For example, the dopamine antagonists spiroperidol and fluphenazine potentiated yawning induced by physostigmine (Holmgren and Urba-Holmgren 1980; Yamada and Furukawa 1980). Thus, a dopaminergic–cholinergic link has been implicated in the control of yawning (see pp. 105–8).

Dopamine

Early studies

In recent years, the role of dopamine in yawning has been the subject of more attention than that of any other neurotransmitter. This is due in part to the fact that yawning and related behaviours have been used to examine the functional role of certain dopamine receptor subtypes in the CNS which were identified by receptor binding and neurochemical studies (see Carlsson 1975; Seeman 1980; Stoof and Kebabian 1984 for further details of the biochemistry and pharmacology of multiple dopamine receptors). Therefore, a correspondingly large section of this chapter is devoted to a consideration of the role of dopaminergic mechanisms in yawning.

The first reports of yawning induced by dopaminergic agents came from Baraldi and colleagues (Baraldi and Bertolini 1974; Baraldi and Benassi-Benelli 1975) who observed that apomorphine and amantadine produced yawning and penile erections in male rats. Subsequently, Mogilnicka and Klimek (1977) discovered that a large number of dopamine agonists, including piribedil, nomifensine, and L-dopa, when given in small doses produced yawning, stretching, chewing, and penile erection in rats. The list of dopamine agonists which have since been reported to produce the yawning syndrome is extensive and the rank order of potency of some of these compounds is shown in Table 4.1.

Yawning induced by dopamine agonists appears to be mediated by an action on dopamine receptors as it is prevented by pre-treatment with small doses of dopamine antagonists (Mogilnicka and Klimek 1977; Protais *et al*. 1983; Gower *et al*. 1984). The yawning syndrome contrasts with the well-known effects of high-dose dopamine agonist treatment (consisting of hyperactivity and stereotyped sniffing, rearing, headbobbing, and oral movements) which are mediated by stimulation of postsynaptic dopamine

Table 4.1 Rank order of potency of various dopamine agonists for inducing yawning in rats

Drug	Minimum dose required to elicit yawning in the rat*	Reference
n-propyl-nor apomorphine	0.5 μg/kg SC	Gower *et al*. (1984)
N,N-dipropyl A-5,6-DTN	2.0 μg/kg SC	Gower *et al*. (1984)
B-HT 920	10.0 μg/kg IP	Ferrari (1985)
Apomorphine	10.0 μg/kg SC	Urba-Holmgren *et al*. (1982)
Lisuride	12.5 μg/kg IP	Baggio and Ferrari (1983)
Pergolide	40.0 μg/kg SC	Gower *et al*. (1984)
CQ 32084	60.0 μg/kg SC	Protais *et al*. (1983)
Lergotrile	0.2 mg/kg SC	Protais *et al*. (1983)
TL-99	0.25 mg/kg SC	Gower *et al*. (1984)
(±)-3-PPP	0.5 mg/kg SC	Gower *et al*. (1984)
Nomifensine	0.5 mg/kg SC	Mogilnicka and Klimek (1977)
Piribedil	1.25 mg/kg SC	Dourish *et al*. (1985)
Bromocriptine	1.3 mg/kg SC	Protais *et al*. (1983)
L-dopa	13.5 mg/kg SC	Protais *et al*. (1983)

*SC, subcutaneous; IP, intraperitoneal.

receptors located in striatum and nucleus accumbens (Ernst 1967; Kelly *et al*. 1975).

Is yawning mediated by dopamine autoreceptors?

Mogilnicka and Klimek (1977) suggested that yawning was mediated via the activation of presynaptic inhibitory dopamine receptors caused by low-dose dopamine agonist treatment. These presynaptic receptors (named auto-receptors by Carlsson 1975), located on the cell bodies, dendrites, axons, and presynaptic terminals of dopamine neurones (see Fig. 4.2), are considerably more sensitive to dopamine and dopamine agonists than postsynaptic dopamine receptors and are, therefore, activated by very small drug doses. Stimulation of dopamine autoreceptors was shown by Carlsson (1975) to inhibit both the synthesis and release of dopamine and consequently to functionally decrease brain dopaminergic neurotransmission. Numerous subsequent studies have supported the autoreceptor explanation advanced by Mogilnicka and Klimek (1977) and some authors have proposed that yawning behaviour may be a useful index of brain dopamine autoreceptor activation (Gower *et al*. 1984; Stahle and Ungerstedt 1984; Dourish and Cooper 1985). Indeed, there is a good correlation between the potencies of

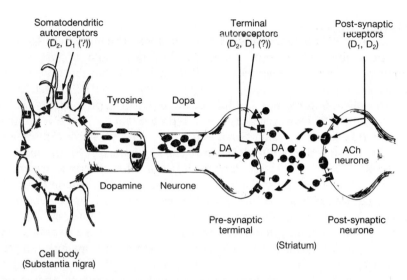

Tyrosine Dopa

Somatodendritic
autoreceptors
(D_2, D_1 (?))

Terminal
autoreceptors
(D_2, D_1 (?))

Post-synaptic
receptors
(D_1, D_2)

DA DA ACh
neurone

Dopamine Neurone

DA

Cell body
(Substantia nigra)

Pre-synaptic
terminal

Post-synaptic
neurone

(Striatum)

Fig. 4.2. Schematic representation of a nigrostriatal dopamine neurone illustrating the location of pre- and postsynaptic dopamine receptors. Abbreviations: DA, dopamine; ACh, acetylcholine.

drugs in producing yawning and their potencies in biochemical tests thought to identify dopamine autoreceptor activity (Gower *et al*. 1984). In addition, yawning is elicited by certain novel dopamine agonists, including (±)-3-PPP, TL-99, and B-HT 920 which are claimed to act selectively on dopamine autoreceptors (Gower *et al*. 1984; Mogilnicka *et al*. 1984; Ferrari 1985). Another novel drug (+)-AJ 76 which is thought to be a selective dopamine autoreceptor antagonist (Svensson *et al*. 1986) blocks yawning induced by apomorphine (Dourish *et al*. 1988).

Dopamine depletion produced by bilateral 6-hydroxydopamine (6-OHDA) lesions of the striatum or the substantia nigra prevents yawning induced by a low dose of apomorphine (Dourish and Hutson 1985; Stoessl *et al*. 1987). Similarly, apomorphine-induced yawning is prevented by chronic haloperidol treatment which potentiates stereotyped sniffing and oral behaviour induced by a high dose of the drug (Ushijima *et al*. 1984*b*). These findings support mediation of yawning by dopamine autoreceptors since it is well established that postsynaptic dopamine receptors become supersensitive to dopamine agonists after treatments with neuroleptics or denervation by 6-OHDA (Ungerstedt 1971; Rupniak *et al*. 1983*b*).

However, some recent findings have cast doubt on whether the receptors which mediate yawning induced by dopamine agonists are autoreceptors. The racemic form of 3-PPP has been resolved into two stereoisomers which have different pharmacological properties. (+)-3-PPP is a 'classical' dopamine agonist which stimulates dopamine autoreceptors at low doses and postsynaptic dopamine receptors at high doses. In contrast, ( ) 3 PPP is a dopamine autoreceptor agonist at low doses and a postsynaptic dopamine antagonist at high dose (Clark *et al*. 1985). If yawning reflects activation of dopamine autoreceptors then clearly (−)3-PPP which is an agonist only at autoreceptors should be more potent in producing yawning than (+)-3-PPP. However, it has been reported that (−)-3-PPP is either inactive (Gower *et al*. 1984; Serra *et al*. 1986) or less active (Stahle and Ungerstedt 1984) than (+)-3-PPP in producing yawning. Furthermore, it has been claimed that catecholamine depletion after reserpine treatment induces yawning and potentiates apomorphine-induced yawning (Yamada and Furukawa 1980; Serra *et al*. 1986). However, there is disagreement in the literature regarding this finding since Mogilnicka and Klimek (1977) have reported that reserpine attenuates dopamine agonist-induced yawning. Our view of these data is that yawning involves activation of a dopamine receptor population which is more sensitive to dopamine agonists than postsynaptic dopamine receptors which mediate hypermotility, stereotypy, and so on. Further research is needed to resolve the controversy regarding the pre- or postsynaptic location of this receptor population. (See pp. 101–2 for further discussion.)

Mediation of yawning by D-2 dopamine receptors

Dopamine receptors have been classified as D-1 or D-2 subtypes on the basis of adenylate cyclase stimulation and ligand binding studies (Kebabian and Calne 1979; Seeman 1980). Selective agonists and antagonists at these receptors have been synthesized (see review by Stoof and Kebabian 1984). It appears that yawning is mediated by D-2 receptors as D-2 agonists elicit yawning whereas the D-1 agonist SKF 38393 does not (Gower *et al*. 1984). Furthermore, the selective D-2 antagonist sulpiride is a potent blocker of dopamine agonist-induced yawning (Baggio and Ferrari 1983; Gower *et al*. 1984), whereas the D-1 antagonist SCH 23390 has no effect on the response (unpublished data of Serra *et al*. cited in Serra *et al*. 1986). It is also of interest that a high dose of apomorphine (1 mg/kg), which produces stereotypy in normal rats, elicits sedation and sleep in rats pre-treated with SCH 23390 (Gessa *et al*. 1985). This suggests that blockade of excitatory D-1 receptors by SCH 23390 reveals the existence of a D-2 receptor population which mediates sleep and related behaviour. Interestingly, Urba-Holmgren *et al*. (1982) have reported that very high doses of apomorphine (5–10 mg/kg) produce yawning which has a very long latency of 90–120 min. Yawning is only apparent in these animals, following recovery from intense stereotyped sniffing, locomotion etc., when brain levels of apomorphine have declined. Thus, it has been suggested that yawning appears when a certain critical level of apomorphine in the brain is attained. Above this level yawning is inhibited (Urba-Holmgren *et al*. 1982). Similarly, it has been noted that treatments with high doses of neuroleptics can cause the appearance of yawning in rats treated with a high dose of apomorphine (Protais *et al*. 1983). Presumably, blockade of hyperactivity, stereotyped sniffing, headbobbing, etc. allows the expression of yawning in animals given a large dose of apomorphine. Systemic administration of high doses of haloperidol alone does not produce yawning. However, injection of the drug in microgram amounts into the septal area produces yawning and penile erections in rats (Nickolson and Berendsen, unpublished data cited in Nickolson and Berendsen 1980). This suggests that the expression of septally-mediated yawning after peripheral haloperidol may be blocked by various effects of the drug at other brain sites.

Responses associated with yawning induced by dopamine agonists

Yawning induced by dopamine agonists is generally accompanied by tongue protrusion, chewing, and stretching (as is yawning induced by cholinergic agents: see p. 105).

Tongue protrusion induced by dopamine agonists is probably mediated by an indirect action on nicotinic receptors since it is most effectively blocked by the nicotinic antagonist mecamylamine (Ushijima *et al*. 1985). Chewing almost invariably precedes and succeeds yawning induced by peripheral or central dopamine agonists and is blocked by treatments (i.e. neuroleptics, scopolamine, 6-OHDA lesions) which also prevent yawning (Yamada and Furukawa 1980; Dourish *et al*. 1985; Dourish and Hutson 1985).

The principal distinction between the profiles of yawning induced by dopaminergic and cholinergic agonists is that the dopaminergic syndrome includes a sexual arousal component (i.e. penile grooming, erection, ejaculation) whereas the cholinergic syndrome does not (Gower *et al*. 1984; Holmgren *et al*. 1985). There appears to be an important association between yawning and sexual arousal elicited by dopamine agonists and, interestingly, both responses are abolished by striatal 6-OHDA lesions or haloperidol pre-treatment (Gower *et al*. 1984; Dourish *et al*. 1985; Dourish and Hutson 1985). Recently, Holmgren *et al*. (1985) have bred a Sprague–Dawley derived rat strain which exhibits a high incidence of spontaneous yawning behaviour. Observation of these animals after saline or dopamine agonist treatments suggests that yawning and penile erection are regulated by a common dopaminergic mechanism (for further discussion of dopamine autoreceptor modulation of sexual behaviour see Gessa *et al*. 1980; Napoli-Farris *et al*. 1984).

Sexual arousal is also associated with peptide-induced yawning (see above). Recent lesion studies have enabled the differentiation of the yawning and sexual arousal components of the syndrome induced by dopamine agonists and peptide hormones (see p. 108).

Sex hormones appear to modulate yawning. Thus, yawning induced by apomorphine is less intense in female than in male rats (Berendsen and Nickolson 1981). Further, castration of male but not female rats reduces yawning. Testosterone treatment counteracts this effect and increases yawning in both intact and ovariectomized female rats (Berendesen and Nickolson 1981). Therefore, Berendsen and Nickolson (1981) have proposed that apomorphine-induced yawning is under androgenic influence and that oestrogens play little or no part.

Brain pathways involved in dopamine agonist-induced yawning

There is strong evidence that yawning induced by dopamine agonists is a phenomenon which is mediated centrally. First, yawning induced by systemic agonist administration is abolished by central dopamine receptor antagonists such as haloperidol and pimozide (Mogilnicka and Klimek 1977; Protais *et al.* 1983) whereas the peripheral dopamine antagonist domperidone has no effect on the response (Gower *et al.* 1984; Stahle and Ungerstedt 1984). Second, intracerebral injections of dopamine agonists elicit yawning in rats (Dourish *et al.* 1985; Dourish *et al.* 1986; Melis *et al.* 1987; see Fig. 4.3).

Bilateral application of piribedil or apomorphine to the caudate nucleus produces yawning, chewing, stretching, and sexual arousal, a syndrome which is identical to that observed after systemic administration of these

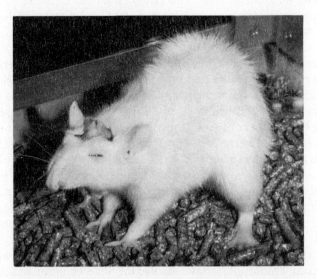

Fig. 4.3. Yawning induced by bilateral instrastriatal injection of apomorphine in the rat.

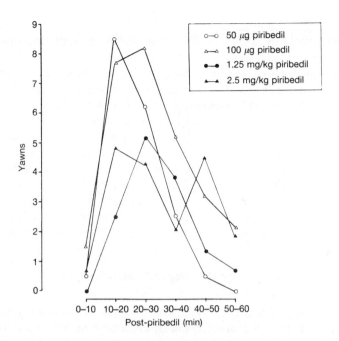

Fig. 4.4. Time course of yawning induced by piribedil injected bilaterally into the striatum or systemically injected subcutaneously. Doses are given in micrograms bilaterally or milligrams per kilogram. Data are mean number of yawns per 10-min period (From Dourish *et al.* (1985)).

drugs (Dourish *et al.* 1985). Systemic administration of a low dose of the dopamine antagonist haloperidol prevents yawning induced by intrastriatal piribedil. Yawning was induced by intrastriatal application of piribedil at doses which were 25 times lower than those required to elicit the response by systemic injection (see Fig. 4.4). Furthermore, the intrastriatal response had a shorter latency to onset and a longer duration than that produced by systemic administration of piribedil. This strongly suggests that the behaviour is centrally mediated.

These experiments also provide clues to the location of the central site of action of dopamine agonists (and possibly other compounds) in producing yawning. Apomorphine-induced yawning appears to be dependent on the integrity of dopaminergic innervation of the striatum, since the response to a small dose of the drug given systemically, is abolished by bilateral 6-OHDA lesions of the striatum (Dourish and Hutson 1985) or the substantia nigra (Stoessl *et al.* 1987). Striatal involvement in yawning is also supported by observations that the caudate nucleus is one of the most effective brain sites for producing yawning in response to piribedil and apomorphine (Dourish *et al.* 1985, 1986) or ACTH (Gessa *et al.* 1967). In addition, yawning is elicited by injections of dopamine agonists or ACTH into other dopamine-rich brain regions (i.e. putamen, globus pallidus, substantia nigra, nucleus accumbens) with dense neuronal projections to and/or from the caudate nucleus (Gessa *et al.* 1967; Dourish *et al.* 1985, 1986).

Yawning is also elicited by injection of small doses of apomorphine into the paraventricular nucleus of the hypothalamus (PVN) (Melis *et al.* 1987). Indeed yawning can be induced by PVN injections of doses of apomorphine that are 1000-fold lower than the doses of the drug required to induce yawning by intrastriatal injection. Injection of peptide hormones (ACTH, oxytocin) into various regions of the hypothalamus also induces yawning (Melis *et al.* 1986; see pp. 105–8). Thus, there may be independent striatal and hypothalamic dopaminergic mechanisms involved in the mediation of yawning (see pp. 105–8).

Environmental influences on the temporal characteristics of apomorphine-induced yawning

In a recent study (Cooper, de Mars, and Dourish, unpublished results) we examined the temporal characteristics of apomorphine-induced yawning in rats tested under either novel or familiar conditions. The frequency and duration of yawning, stretching, penile grooming, face and body grooming, resting, chewing, rearing, and locomotion were determined from videotape recordings of behaviour. The results are illustrated in Fig. 4.5 which shows the time of occurrence of each yawn in individual rats during a 60-min test. The numbers at the right of each figure give the total number of yawns for each rat. On occasions yawns occurred so closely together that it was not possible to represent each response separately on the chosen time scale. Under both experimental conditions yawns occurred in bursts.

In animals tested in familiar conditions there were few episodes of yawning after vehicle injection (range 0–4 responses). These animals exhibited locomotion and rearing during the first 10 min of the test but were generally inactive thereafter. When injected with 0.025 mg/kg apomorphine, yawning was evident early in the test (0–20 min) and late in the test (40–60 min). At higher drug doses most yawning occurred within 20–25 minutes of injection. After the yawning episodes these animals became inactive, like controls.

In animals tested in a novel environment, yawning occurred in all animals after vehicle injection (indeed two animals attained high scores, 24 and 48 responses). In the novel situation the animals also showed high levels of grooming and were very active during the first 30 min of the test. Yawning and inactivity occurred late in the test. Thus, these animals showed a sequence of behaviour consisting of activity/exploration succeeded by

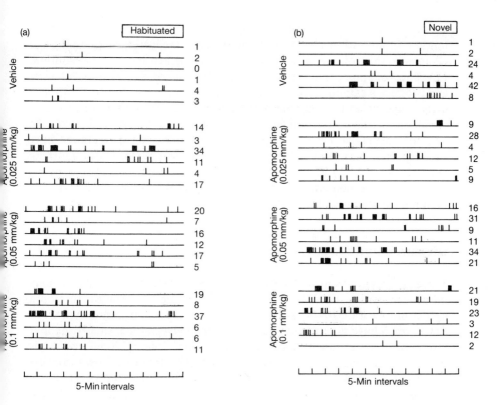

Fig. 4.5. (a) Frequency of yawning in individual rats during a 60-min test after injection of vehicle or various doses of apomorphine in a familiar environment. Drug doses are expressed in milligrams per kilogram subcutaneous (Cooper, de Mars, and Dourish, unpublished results). (b) Frequency of yawning in individual rats during a 60-min test after injection of vehicle or apomorphine in a novel environment. Details are as described for (a).

yawning and resting. Apomorphine-treated animals tested in novel conditions showed a great deal of yawning. With increasing drug dosage, the onset of yawning seemed to occur earlier in the test. Thus, apomorphine considerably reduced the 'hyperactivity' phase exhibited by vehicle-treated animals exposed to novelty and attenuated novelty-induced excessive grooming.

Our interpretation of these data is that low doses of apomorphine attenuate responses produced by novelty (i.e. increased rearing, locomotion, and grooming) and increase yawning and associated behaviour. This suggests that yawning is associated with a decreasing level of arousal (or stress). We propose that novelty may be associated with increased dopamine release causing activation of postsynaptic dopamine receptors. The resulting behavioural responses of this 'arousal' or 'stress' state are increased grooming (see Chapter 5, this volume, by Isaacson and Gispen), rearing, and locomotion. Low doses of apomorphine attenuate novelty-induced behavioural responses and produce a calming effect which results in yawning and resting. Interestingly, it has recently been reported that low doses of apomorphine have an anxiolytic action in an animal model of anxiety (Hjorth *et al*. 1986). In addition, beneficial effects of low-dose dopamine agonist treatment have been reported in patients suffering from mania (Post 1976). The diminishing arousal and anxiolytic effects of apomorphine may be mediated by an agonist action at dopamine autoreceptors (Carlsson 1975) or at postsynaptic inhibitory dopamine receptors (Cools and Van Rossum 1976).

Serotonin and noradrenalin

There is evidence that both serotonergic and noradrenergic neurones may influence yawning. Urba-Holmgren *et al*. (1979) reported that the serotonin uptake inhibitor Lu 10–171 potentiates yawning induced by physostigmine at doses which have no effect on behaviour when given alone, suggesting that serotonin exerts a positive modulating effect on yawning. Similarly, it has been observed that the serotonin antagonist methysergide supresses yawning induced by α-MSH or piribedil (Yamada and Furukawa 1981). Since serotonergic neurones may tonically inhibit nigrostriatal and mesolimbic dopamine neurones, Yamada and Furukawa (1981) have suggested that methysergide could decrease piribedil-induced yawning by causing disinhibition of dopaminergic neurones. The consequent increase in dopamine release produced by methysergide would prevent yawning.

In cats and monkeys (but not rats) the serotonin agonists LSD and N,N-dimethyltryptamine elicit yawning which can be blocked by methysergide (Jacobs *et al*. 1977; Trulson and Jacobs 1979; Marini 1981). Thus, data on the whole tend to support a facilitatory role of serotonin in yawning. In contrast, noradrenalin appears to have an inhibitory influence on peptide-induced yawning. Thus, yawning induced by ACTH in rats is potentiated by the α_2-adrenoceptor antagonist yohimbine but blocked by the α_2-agonist clonidine (Poggioli *et al*. 1984, 1985).

Interactions of α_2-adrenoceptor agonists and antagonists with apomorphine-induced yawning are not so straightforward. Thus, Gower *et al*. (1986) report that the α_2-antagonists piperoxan and idazoxan and the α_2-agonist clonidine all inhibit apomorphine-induced yawning. Although there seems to be some doubt regarding the exact nature of the dopaminergic–noradrenergic link in yawning, the identity of the adrenoceptor population involved has been clearly established as being of the α_2 subtype, as the α_1-antagonists prazosin and phenoxybenzamine have no effect on apomorphine-induced yawning (Gower *et al.* 1986).

Interaction of brain dopaminergic, cholinergic, and peptidergic neurones in the mediation of yawning: an hypothesis and a model

It is clear from the preceding pages that yawning behaviour is influenced by a number of interacting neurotransmitter systems. Major influences are exerted by brain dopaminergic, cholinergic, and peptidergic neurones and in this section we propose a hypothesis which explains how these various neurotransmitter mechanisms may interact to control yawning and associated behaviours.

There is strong evidence for the involvement of dopaminergic inhibition and cholinergic excitation in yawning. Thus, yawning induced by dopaminergic drugs is probably caused by activation of dopamine autoreceptors (or inhibitory postsynaptic dopamine receptors) which reduces dopamine synthesis and release. In contrast, yawning induced by cholinergic agents appears to be due to increased release of acetylcholine and stimulation of postsynaptic muscarinic receptors (see pp. 93–4).

In cross-blocking studies, it has been shown that dopamine agonist-induced yawning is attenuated or abolished by treatment with muscarinic receptor antagonists (Yamada and Furukawa 1980, 1981; Holmgren and Urba-Holmgren 1980). In contrast, dopamine antagonists potentiate yawning induced by physostigmine (Yamada and Furukawa 1980; Holmgren and Urba-Holmgren 1980). Therefore, these authors have proposed that yawning is produced by the release of cholinergic neurones from tonic dopaminergic inhibition. This disinhibition may be caused by activation of dopamine autoreceptors at presynaptic neuronal sites induced by low doses of dopamine agonists (see Fig. 4.2). Thus, the same functional effect (i.e. increased yawning) is produced by stimulation of postsynaptic cholinergic receptors or presynaptic (inhibitory) dopamine receptors. Blockade of postsynaptic dopamine receptors by a dopamine antagonist would also activate cholinergic neurones and this probably accounts for the potentiation of physostigmine-induced yawning by neuroleptics (Yamada and Furukawa 1980).

It seems that the striatum may be the central locus for this dopaminergic–cholinergic neuronal interface. The striatum in the rat receives innervation from approximately 3500 dopaminergic neurones located in the zona compacta of the substantia nigra (Andén *et al.* 1964, 1966). The terminals of these dopamine neurones make synaptic connections with striatal interneurones (which represent the majority of striatal

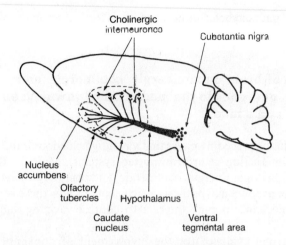

Fig. 4.6. Schematic representation of a dopaminergic–cholinergic neuronal interaction which may mediate yawning.

neurones) and neurones which innervate the substantia nigra and globus pallidus. Acetylcholine is a major striatal transmitter and most of it is located in interneurones (Hassler 1978). The dopaminergic nigrostriatal neurones make synaptic contact with these cholinergic neurones (Hattori *et al.* 1976) and inhibit their firing (Roth and Bunney 1976; Trabucchi *et al.* 1975; see Fig. 4.6). In contrast, there is no apparent dopaminergic–cholinergic link in other major dopamine terminal regions such as nucleus accumbens and olfactory tubercles (Ladinsky *et al.* 1975).

In yawning experiments, it has been shown that the striatum is very sensitive to dopamine agonist treatments and that 6-OHDA lesions of the striatum or substantia nigra abolish yawning induced by a small dose of apomorphine (Dourish *et al.* 1985; Dourish and Hutson 1986; Stoessl *et al.* 1987). Furthermore, yawning induced by intrastriatal injection of piribedil is abolished by blockade of either dopamine autoreceptors (with low-dose haloperidol) or postsynaptic muscarinic receptors (with scopolamine) (Dourish *et al.* 1985). At this point, our yawning model comprises striatal cholinergic excitation and dopaminergic inhibition. We noted earlier that the peptide hormones ACTH, α-MSH, β-LPH and oxytocin are potent yawning inducers. Therefore, the question arises as to how peptidergic mechanisms interact with neuronal dopamine and acetylcholine to control yawning.

There is evidence that ACTH and α-MSH injection can activate cholinergic neurones (Torda and Wolff 1952; Marx 1975). Accordingly, yawning induced by ACTH and α-MSH is paralleled by a twofold elevation of

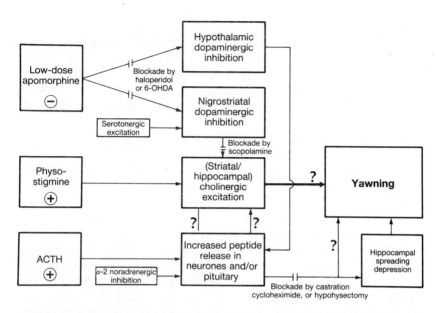

Fig. 4.7. Schematic diagram illustrating control of yawning behaviour by interacting excitatory cholinergic, peptidergic, and serotonergic neurotransmitter systems and inhibitory dopaminergic and noradrenergic mechanisms.

acetycholine turnover in hippocampus (Wood *et al.* 1978). This is consistent with evidence that peptide-induced yawning is suppressed by cholinergic antagonists and neuroleptics (Ferrari *et al.* 1963; Yamada and Furukawa 1981). These data suggest that yawning is associated with cholinergic and peptidergic excitation and dopaminergic inhibition (see Fig. 4.7).

Indeed it is known that α-MSH-producing cells in the pituitary are under the inhibitory control of dopaminergic neurones originating from the arcuate nucleus of the hypothalamus (Tilders and Smelik 1977). Therefore, it is possible that inhibition of dopamine release (caused by low-dose dopamine agonist treatment) may indirectly result in release of newly synthesized peptides (ACTH, α-MSH, β-LPH, oxytoxin) from the pituitary or from peptidergic neurones (Serra *et al.* 1983*a*).

The importance of the pituitary in mediating yawning is illustrated by the observation that hypophysectomy prevents yawning induced by apomorphine (Serra *et al.* 1983*a*). Similarly, apomorphine-induced yawning is prevented by treatment with the protein synthesis inhibitor cycloheximide (Serra *et al.* 1983*b*).

The observation of Wood *et al.* (1978) that ACTH and α-MSH specifically increased acetylcholine turnover in the hippocampus indicates that this brain region may be of importance in the control of yawning. This idea is supported by evidence from lesion studies in which it has been demonstrated that partial ablation of the hippocampus potentiates ACTH-induced yawning whereas total hippocampectomy abolishes the response (Colbern *et al.* 1977). This study also implicated the amygdala and the mammillary bodies in the control of yawning since lesions in these areas modified the response to ACTH.

Interestingly, lesion studies have also enabled the differentiation of the yawning and sexual arousal components of the ACTH-induced syndrome. Thus, pre-optic lesions, destroying structures which take up labelled testosterone, abolished penile grooming and erection but did not affect yawning (Bertolini *et al.* 1975).

The model we propose to explain the neural control of yawning is illustrated in Fig. 4.7. It is clear that there are cholinergic, peptidergic, serotonergic (all excitatory), dopaminergic, and noradrenergic (both inhibitory) inputs to the system. At this point it is unclear whether the final step in the pathway is peptidergic or cholinergic (hence the reciprocal connections with question marks in Fig. 4.7). However, it is noteworthy that all of these influences may precede a mechanism illustrated on the bottom right portion of Fig. 4.7. Cortical spreading depression was shown to produce yawning and sexual arousal by Huston (1971). In a subsequent study, Jakobartl and Huston (1977) observed that intracranial injection of ACTH produced spreading depression and that the hippocampus was more sensitive to the peptide than the cortex. Thus, it is possible that yawning and related behaviour elicited by ACTH could be secondary to hippocampal spreading depression.

Conclusions

In this chapter we have described how drug-induced yawning is mediated by the interaction of various brain neurotransmitter systems. Dopaminergic, peptidergic, and cholinergic neurones appear to be primarily responsible for the control of yawning. At the pharmacological level yawning and sexual arousal appears to be useful as a model for identifying drugs with agonist activity at inhibitory dopamine receptors (Gower *et al.* 1984). Similarly, chewing mouth movements have been proposed as a useful index of agonist action at central muscarinic receptors (Salamone *et al.* 1986).

In behavioural terms, the evidence suggests that in most cases pharmacologically-induced yawning bears a close resemblance to spontaneous, physiological yawning. Thus, the posture of rats yawning in response to physostigmine or apomorphine is very similar to that of spontaneous physiological yawning in rats (Ushijima *et al.* 1985). Furthermore, apomorphine-induced yawns in rats occur in clusters (Szechtman 1984; Cooper, de Mars, and Dourish, unpublished results; Fig. 4.5) which is consistent with anecdotal reports that yawning in humans occurs in bursts (Barbizet 1958).

The only comprehensive study to date on physiological yawning in animals was carried out by Anias *et al.* (1984) who produced a 'high yawning frequency' line of Sprague–Dawley rats through selective breeding. They found a clear circadian pattern in spontaneous yawning with the highest frequency being evident during the last hour of the light period. Interestingly, this coincides with the time of the lowest daily dopamine turnover rate (Cahill and Ehret 1981) which suggests some form of dopaminergic control of spontaneous yawning.

Spontaneous, physiological yawning is a behaviour categorized by ethologists as a 'stereotyped action pattern' (see Provine 1986 and references therein). In humans, yawns can be released by observing yawns, thinking about yawning, or even reading about yawning (Provine 1986). There have been a number of speculations concerning the function of yawning. One proposal is that yawning is useful for 'stretching the face'. By causing contraction of the facial muscles, yawning forces blood through cerebral vessels to the brain which may have an alerting effect (Heusner 1946; Barbizet 1958). Similarly, it has been suggested that yawning may increase blood oxygen levels during the deep air inspiration which accompanies the response (Bartlett *et al.* 1971). However, a study by Provine (1986) has cast doubt on the respiratory hypothesis since there was no correlation between yawn duration and interyawn interval (i.e. infrequent yawners did not compensate by producing yawns of longer duration).

Yawning is also of clinical interest since it has been reported to be associated with a number of disorders including epilepsy, epidemic encephalitis and Huntington's chorea (Heusner 1946), hysteria and brainstem lesions (Barbizet 1958) and adrenoleucodystrophy (which interestingly is accompanied by high blood ACTH levels; Kataoka *et al.* 1980). Yawning is also reported to be associated with opiate withdrawal in man (Himmelsbach 1939). In contrast, it has been reported that apomorphine-induced yawning in rats is reduced by the opiate antagonist naloxone (Szechtman 1984). However, it appears that the effects of naloxone on yawning may not be opiate-receptor-mediated (Berendsen and Gower 1986).

It seems likely that yawning may have an important social function both in apes (Hadidian 1980) and in humans (Barbizet 1958). In man, yawning is often regarded as an expression of indifference and/or boredom although social etiquette demands that the yawn is hidden by putting one's hand over one's mouth.

We believe that yawning and stretching may signal the termination of stressful experience or of sustained concentration. Experimental evidence is lacking, but there are anecdotal observations which suggest that yawning and stretching may be behavioural features of recovery from at least certain forms of stress. For example, one of us (SJC) sat amongst a large class of students in Northern Ireland who were being addressed by a visiting research worker. He wanted them to answer direct questions about the impact of the 'Troubles' (i.e. the period from 1969 to the present day during which there has been widespread violence) on their personal lives, and on those of their families and friends. The effect of his talk on the behaviour of the students was startling. Under normal circumstances, like students anywhere, his audience would have shown periodic fidgeting, whispering, looking-about, coughing, and so on. On this occasion, however, the entire class sat motionless, and expressionless, when it became clear that they were being asked about widespread fears and anxieties, and about injuries and deaths which may have befallen members of their families, their friends, and neighbours. There was a palpable feeling of tension throughout the lecture room. As the speaker came to an end of his talk and signalled this by some closing comments, the behaviour of the class changed remarkably. They relaxed their body postures, they turned to classmates and looked at each other, they smiled, and most strikingly, there was a widespread outbreak of yawning and stretching. These changes were closely synchronized throughout the class. It was difficult to discount the impression that the yawning and stretching occurred as part of a more complex change in the students' behaviour, which was initiated by the end of a distressing experience. Formal observations of the behaviour of people, alone or in large groups, during and following the imposition of stress would be extremely interesting. We suggest that the occurrence of yawning and stretching, in people, may form part of a range of behavioural responses indicative of recovery from stressful events. The animal data which we discuss (see pp. 105–8) imply that in people, too, yawning and stretching may follow from neurochemical changes in the brain, which include an inhibition of central dopaminergic activity. In rats it is clear that spontaneous yawning can be significantly altered by environmental manipulation. In animals and man changes in brain dopamine metabolism and yawning frequency may be closely associated with recovery from acute stress.

During the past decade experiments on drug-induced yawning in animals have facilitated that construction of a model of the neuronal circuitry which subserves yawning. Furthermore, yawning in animals has proved to be a useful pharmacological tool for studying neurotransmitter receptors and receptor subtypes. The challenge remains to discover the physiological trigger for yawning and to fully understand the behavioural and social significance of the response.

References

Andén, N.E., Carlsson, A., Dahlström, A., Fuxe, K., Hillarp, N.A., and Larsson, K. (1964). Demonstration and mapping out of nigro-neostriatal dopamine neurones. *Life Sci.* **3**, 523–30.

Andén, N.E., Dahlström, A., Fuxe, K., and Larsson, K. (1966). Functional role of the nigro-neostriatal dopamine neurones. *Acta pharmacol. toxicol.* **24**, 263–74.

Anias, J., Holmgren, B., Urba-Holgren, R.U., and Eguibar, J.R. (1984). Circadian variation of yawning behaviour. *Acta neurobiolog. exp.* **44**, 179–86.

Argiolas, A., Melis, M.R., and Gessa, G.L. (1985). Intraventricular oxytoxin induces yawning and penile erection in rats. *Eur. J. Pharmacol.* **117**, 395–6.

Baggio, G. and Ferrari, F. (1983). The role of dopaminergic receptors in the behavioural effects induced by lisuride in male rats. *Psychopharmacology* **80**, 38–42.

Baraldi, M. and Benassi-Benelli, A. (1975). Apomorphine-induced penile erection in adult rats. *Riv. Farmacol. Terapia* **6**, 771–2.

Baraldi, M. and Bertolini, A. (1974). Penile erections induced by amantadine in male rats. *Life Sci.* **14**, 1231–5.

Barbizet, J. (1958). Yawning. *J. Neurol. Neurosurg. Psychiat.* **21**, 203–9.

Bartlett, R.H., Gazzaniga, A.B., and Geraghty, T. (1971). The yawn maneuver: prevention and treatment of postoperative pulmonary complications. *Surg. Forum* **21**, 196–8.

Berendsen, H.H.G. and Gower, A.J. (1986). Opiate–androgen interactions in drug-induced yawning and penile erections in rats. *Neuroendocrinology* **42**, 185–90.

Berendsen, H.H.G. and Nickolson, V.J. (1986). Androgenic influences on apomorphine-induced yawning in rats. *Behav. neural Bio.* **33**, 123–8.

Bertolini, A. and Gessa, G.L. (1981). Behavioural effects of ACTH and MSH peptides. *J. endocrinol. Invest.* **4**, 241–51.

Bertolini, A., Gessa, G.L., and Ferrari, W. (1975). Penile erection and ejaculation: a central effect of ACTH-like peptides in mammals. In *Sexual behaviour: pharmacology and biochemistry* (ed. M. Sandler and G.L. Gessa), pp. 247–57. Raven Press, New York.

Cahill, A.L. and Ehret, C.F. (1981). Circadian variations in the activity of tyrosine hydroxylase, tyrosine amino transferase and tryptophan hydroxylase: relationship to catecholamine metabolism. *J. Neurochem.* **37**, 1109–15.

Carlsson, A. (1975). Receptor-mediated control of dopamine metabolism. In *Pre- and postsynaptic receptors* (ed. E. Usdin and W.E. Bunney), pp. 49–63. Marcel Dekker, New York.

Clark, D., Hjorth, S., and Carlsson, A. (1985). Dopamine-receptor agonists— mechanisms underlying autoreceptor selectivity. 1. Review of the evidence. *J. neural Transmission* **62**, 1–52.

Colbern D., Isaacson, R.L., Bohus, B., and Gispen, W.H. (1977). Limbic-midbrain lesions and ACTH-induced excessive grooming. *Life Sci.* **21**, 393–404.

Cools, A.R. and Van Rossum, J.M. (1976). Excitation-mediating and inhibition mediating dopamine receptors: a new concept towards a better understanding of data. *Psychopharmacologia* **45**, 243–54.

Dourish, C.T. and Cooper, S.J. (1985). Behavioural evidence for the existence of dopamine autoreceptors. *Trends pharmacol. Sci.* 6, 17–18.

Dourish, C.T. and Hutson, P.H. (1985). Bilateral lesions of the striatum induced with 6-hydroxydopamine abolish apomorphine-induced yawning in rats. *Neuropharmacology* 24, 1051–5.

Dourish, C.T., Cooper, S.J., and Philips, S.R. (1985). Yawning elicited by systemic and intrastriatal injection of piribedil and apomorphine in the rat. *Psychopharmacology* 86, 175–181.

Dourish, C.T., Cooper, S.J., and Hutson, P.H. (1986). Involvement of the striatum in dopamine agonist-induced yawning. In *The neurobiology of dopamine systems* (ed. W. Winlow and R. Markstein), pp. 463–6. Manchester University Press, Manchester.

Dourish, C.T., Herbert, E.N., and Iversen, S.D. (1988). Blockade of apomorphine-induced yawning in rats by the selective dopamine autoreceptor antagonist (+)-AJ 76. *Br. J. Pharmacol.* 95, 498P.

Ernst, A.M. (1967). Mode of action of apomorphine and d-amphetamine on gnawing compulsion in rats. *Psychopharmacologia* 10, 316–23.

Ferrari, F. (1985). Sexual excitement and stretching and yawning induced by B-HT 920. *Pharmacol. Res. Commun.* 17, 557–64.

Ferrari, W. (1958). Behavioural changes in animals after intracisternal injection with adrenocorticotrophic hormone and melanocyte-stimulating hormone. *Nature* 181, 925–6.

Ferrari, W., Floris, E., and Paulesu, F. (1955). Su di una particolare imponente sinomatologia prodotta nel cane dall'ACTH iniettato nella cisterna magna. *Boll. Soc. Ital. Biol. Sper.* 31, 862–4.

Ferrari, W., Gessa, G.L., and Vargiu, L. (1963). Behavioural effects induced by intracisternally injected ACTH and MSH. *Ann. NY Acad. Sci.* 104, 330–43.

Gessa, G.L., Pisano, N., Vargiu, L., Crabai, F., and Ferrari, W. (1967). Stretching and yawning movements after intracerebral injection of ACTH. *Rev. Can. Biologie* 26, 229–36.

Gessa, G.L., Benassi-Benelli, A., Falaschi, P., and Ferrari, F. (1980). Role of dopamine in erection and ejaculation mechanisms. *Proc. Austral. Acad. Sci.* 1980, 619–21.

Gessa, G.L., Porceddu M.L., Collu M., Mereu G., Serra, M., Ongini, E., and Biggio, G. (1985). Sedation and sleep induced by high doses of apomorphine after blockade of D-1 receptors by SCH 23390. *Eur. J. Pharmacol.* 109, 269–74.

Gower, A.J., Berendsen, H.H.E., Princen, M.M., and Broekkamp, C.L.E. (1984). The yawning–penile erection syndrome as a model for putative dopamine autoreceptor activity. *Eur. J. Pharmacol.* 103, 81–90.

Gower, A.J., Berendsen, H.H.G., and Broekkamp, C.L.E. (1986). Antagonism of drug-induced yawning and penile erections in rats. *Eur. J. Pharmacol.* 122, 239–44.

Hadidian, J. (1980). Yawning in an Old World monkey, *Macaca nigra* (Primates: Cercopithecidae). *Behaviour* 75, 133–47.

Hassler, R. (1978). Striatal control of locomotion, intentional actions and of integrating and perceptive activity. *J. neurol. Sci.* 36, 187–224.

Hattori, T., Singh, U.K., and McGeer, P.L. (1976). Immunohistochemical localization of choline acetyltransferase containing neostriatal neurones and their relationship with dopaminergic synapses. *Brain Res.* **102**, 164–73.

Heusner, A.P. (1946). Yawning and associated phenomena. *Physiol. Rev.* **26**, 156–68.

Himmelsbach, C.K. (1939). Studies of certain addiction characteristics of (a) dihydromorphine ('para morphan'), (b) didhydrodesoxy morphine — D('desomorphine'), (c) dihydrodesoxycodeine —D('desocodeine') and (d) methyldihydromorphinone ('metopon'). *J. Pharmacol. exp. Ther.* **67**, 239–49.

Hjorth, S., Engel, J.A., and Carlsson, A. (1986). Anticonflict effects of low doses of the dopamine agonist apomorphine in the rat. *Pharmacol. Biochem. Behav.* **24**, 237–40.

Holmgren, B. and Urba-Holmgren, R. (1980). Interaction of cholinergic and dopaminergic influences on yawning behaviour. *Acta neurobiol. exp.* **40**, 633–42.

Holmgren, B., Urba-Holmgren, R., Trucios N., Zermeno M., and Eguibar, J.R. (1985). Association of spontaneous and dopaminergic-induced yawning and penile erections in the rat. *Pharmacol. Biochem. Behav.* **22**, 31–5.

Huston, J.P. (1971). Yawning and penile erection induced in rats by cortical spreading depression. *Nature* **232**, 274–5.

Jacobs, B.L., Trulson, M.E., and Stern, W.C. (1977). Behavioural effects of LSD in cats: Proposal of an animal behaviour model for studying the actions of hallucinogenic drugs. *Brain Res.* **132**, 301–14.

Jakobartl, L. and Huston, J.P. (1977). Spreading depression in hippocampus and neocortex of rats induced by $ACTH_{1-24}$. *Neurosci. Lett.* **5**, 189–92.

Kataoka, A., Koriyama, T., Arimura, K., Enatsu, M., Igata, A., and Tokito, S. (1980). Adrenoleukodystrophy and yawning. *J. Autonom. nerv. syst.* **17**, 24–5.

Kebabian, J.W. and Calne, D.B. (1979). Multiple receptors for dopamine. *Nature* **277**, 93–6.

Kelly, P.H, Seviour, P.W, and Iversen, S.D. (1975). Amphetamine and apomorphine responses in the rat following 6-OHDA lesions of the nucleus accumbens septi and corpus striatum. *Brain Res.* **94**, 507–22.

Ladinsky, H., Consolo, S., Bianchi, S., Samanin, R., and Ghezzi, D. (1975). Cholinergic–dopaminergic interaction in the striatum: The effect of 6-hydroxydopamine or pimozide treatment on the increased striatal acetylcholine levels induced by apomorphine, piribedil and d-amphetamine. *Brain Res.* **84**, 221–6.

Marx, J.L. (1975). Learning and behaviour II: The hypothalamic peptides. *Science* **190**, 544–5.

Marini, J.L. (1981). Serotonergic and dopaminergic effects on yawning in the cat. *Pharmacol. Biochem. Behav.* **15**, 711–15.

Melis, M.R., Argiolas, A., and Gessa, G.L. (1986). Oxytocin-induced penile erection and yawning: site of action in the brain. *Brain Res.* **398**, 259–65.

Melis, M.R., Argiolas, A., and Gessa, G.L. (1987). Apomorphine-induced penile erection and yawning: site of action in the brain. *Brain Res.* **415**, 98–104.

Mogilnicka, E. and Klimek, V. (1977). Drugs affecting dopamine neurones and yawning behaviour. *Pharmacol. Biochem. Behav.* **7**, 303–5.

Mogilnicka, E., Boissard, C.G., and Delini-Stula, A. (1984). Effects of apomorphine, TL-99 and 3-PPP on yawning in rats. *Neuropharmacology* **23**, 19–22.

Napoli-Farris, L., Fratta, W., and Gessa, G.L. (1984). Stimulation of dopamine autoreceptors elicits 'premature ejaculation' in rats. *Pharmacol. Biochem. Behav.* **20**, 69–72.

Nickolson, V.J., and Berendsen, H.H.G. (1980). Effects of potential neuroleptic peptide des-tyrosine¹-γ-endorphin and haloperidol on apomorphine-induced behavioural syndromes in rats and mice. *Life Sci.* **27**, 1377–85.

Poggioli, R., Vergoni, A.V., Guarini, S., and Bertolini, A. (1984). Influence of clonidine on the ACTH-induced behavioural syndrome *Eur. J. Pharmacol.* **101**, 299–302.

Poggioli, R., Vergoni, A.V., and Bertolini, A. (1985). Influence of yohimbine on the ACTH-induced behavioural syndrome in rats. *Pharmacol. Res. Commun.* **17**, 671–8.

Post, R.M. (1976). Low doses of piribedil improves mania patients. *Lancet* i, 203–4.

Protais, P., Dubuc, I., and Costentin, J. (1983). Pharmacological characteristics of dopamine receptors involved in the dual effect of dopamine agonists on yawning behaviour in rats. *Eur. J. Pharmacol.* **94**, 271–80.

Provine, R.R. (1986). Yawning as a stereotyped action pattern and releasing stimulus. *Ethology* **72**, 109–122.

Roth, R.H, and Bunney, B.S. (1976). Interaction of cholinergic neurones with other chemically defined neuronal systems in the CNS. In *Biology of cholinergic function* (ed. A.M. Goldberg and I. Hanin), pp. 379–94. Raven Press, New York.

Rupniak, N.M.J., Jenner, P., and Marsden, C.D. (1983a). Cholinergic manipulation of perioral behaviour induced by chronic neuroleptic administration to rats. *Psychopharmacology* **79**, 226–30.

Rupniak, N.M.J., Jenner, P., and Marsden, C.D. (1983b). Long-term neuroleptic treatment and the status of the dopamine hypothesis of schizophrenia. In *Theory in psychopharmacology*, Vol. 2 (ed. S.J. Cooper), pp. 195–237. Academic Press, London.

Rupniak, N.M.J., Jenner, P., and Marsden, C.D. (1985). Pharmacological characterization of spontaneous or drug-associated purposeless chewing movements in rats. *Psychopharmacology* **85**, 71–9.

Salamone, J.D., Lalies, M.D., Channell, S.L., and Iversen, S.D. (1986). Behavioural and pharmacological characterization of the mouth movements induced by muscarinic agonists in the rat. *Psychopharmacology* **88**, 467–71.

Sandler, M. and Gessa, G.L. (1975). *Sexual behaviour: pharmacology and biochemistry*. Raven Press, New York.

Seeman P. (1980). Brain dopamine receptors. *Pharmacol. Rev.* **32**, 229–313.

Serra, G., Collu, M., Loddo, S., Celasco, G., and Gessa, G.L. (1983a). Hypophysectomy prevents yawning and penile erection but not hypomotility induced by apomorphine. *Pharmacol. Biochem. Behav.* **19**, 917–20.

Serra, G., Collu, M., and Gessa, G.L. (1986). Dopamine receptors mediating yawning: are they autoreceptors? *Eur. J. Pharmacol.* **120**, 187–192.

Serra, G., Fratta, W., Collu, M., Napoli-Farris, L., and Gessa, G.L. (1983b).

Cycloheximide prevents apomorphine-induced yawning, penile erection and genital grooming in rats. *Eur. J. Pharmacol.* **86**, 279–84.

Stahle, L. and Ungerstedt, U. (1984). Assessment of dopamine autoreceptor agonist properties of apomorphine, (+)-3-PPP and (–)-3-PPP by recording of yawning behaviour in rats. *Eur. J. Pharmacol.* **98**, 307–10.

Stoessl, A.J., Dourish, C.T., and Iversen, S.D. (1987). Apomorphine-induced yawning in rats is abolished by bilateral 6-hydroxydopamine lesions of the substantia nigra. *Psychopharmacology* **93**, 336—42.

Stoof, J.C. and Kebabian, J.W. (1984). Two dopamine receptors: biochemistry, physiology and pharmacology. *Life Sci.* **35**, 2281–96.

Svensson, K., Johansson, A.M., Magnusson, T., and Carlsson, A. (1986). (+)-AJ 76 and (+)-UH 232: central stimulants acting as preferential dopamine autoreceptor antagonists. *Naunyn Schmiedeberg's Arch. Pharmacol.* **334**, 234–45.

Szechtman, H. (1984) Timing of yawns induced by a small dose of apomorphine and its alteration by naloxone. *Prog. Neuropsychopharmacol. biol. Psychiat.* **8**, 743–6.

Tilders, F. and Smelik, P. (1977). Direct neural control of MSH secretion in mammals: The involvement of dopaminergic tuberohypophyseal neurones. In Melanocyte-stimulating hormone: control chemistry and effects (ed. F.J.H. Tilders *et al.*), pp. 80–93. Karger, Basel.

Torda, C. and Wolff, H.G. (1952). Effect of pituitary hormones, cortisone and adrenalectomy on some aspects of neuromuscular function and acetylcholine synthesis. *Am. J. Physiol.* **169**, 140–9.

Trabucchi, M., Cheney, G.L., Racagni, G., and Costa, E. (1975). In vivo inhibition of striatal acetylcholine turnover by L-dopa, apomorphine and (+)-amphetamine. *Brain Res.* **85**, 130–4.

Trulson, M.E. and Jacobs, B.L. (1979). Effects of 5-methoxy-N, N-dimethyltryptamine on behaviour and raphe unit activity in freely moving cats. *Eur. J. Pharmacol.* **54**, 43–50.

Ungerstedt, U. (1971). Post-synaptic supersensitivity after 6-hydroxydopamine-induced degeneration of the nigro-striatal dopamine system. *Acta physiol. scand.* **83** (Suppl. 367), 69–93.

Urba-Holmgren, R., Gonzalez, R.M., and Holmgren, B. (1977). Is yawning a cholinergic response? *Nature* **267**, 261–2.

Urba-Holmgren, R., Holmgren, B., Rodriguez, R., and Gonzalez, R.M. (1979). Serotonergic modulation of yawning. *Pharmacol. Biochem. Behav.* **11**, 371–2.

Urba-Holmgren, R., Holmgren, B., and Anias, J. (1982) Pre- and post-synaptic dopaminergic receptors involved in apomorphine-induced yawning. *Acta neurobiol. exp.* **42**, 115–25.

Ushijima, I., Yamada, K., Inoue, T., Tokunaya, T., Furukawa, T, and Noda, Y. (1984*a*). Muscarinic and nicotinic effects on yawning and tongue protruding in the rat. *Pharmacol. Biochem. Behav.* **21**, 297–300.

Ushijima, I., Noda, Y., Mizuki, Y., and Yamada, K. (1984*b*). Modification of apomorphine-, physostigmine- and pilocarpine-induced yawning after long-term treatment with neuroleptic or cholinergic agents. *Arch. int. Pharmacodyn. Ther.* **271**, 180–8.

Ushijima, I., Mizuki, Y., Imaizumi, J., Yamada, M., Noda, Y., Yamada, K., and Furukawa, T. (1985). Characteristics of yawning behaviour induced by apomor phine, physostigmine and pilocarpine. *Arch. int. Pharmacodyn. Ther.* **273**, 196–201.

Wood, P. L., Malthe-Sorenssen, D., Cheney, D. L., and Costa, E. (1978). Increase of hippocampal acetylcholine turnover and the stretching–yawning syndrome elicited by alpha-MSH and ACTH. *Life Sci.* **22**, 673–8.

Yamada, K. and Furukawa, T. (1980). Direct evidence for involvement of dopaminergic inhibition and cholinergic activation in yawning. *Psychopharmacology* **67**, 39–43.

Yamada, K. and Furukawa, T. (1981). The yawning elicited by α-melanocyte-stimulating hormone involves serotonergic–dopaminergic–cholinergic neurone link in rats. *Naunyn-Schmiedeberg's Arch. Pharmacol.* **316**, 155–60.

5

Neuropeptides and the issue of stereotypy in behaviour

ROBERT L. ISAACSON and WILLEM H. GISPEN

Introduction

When reviewing our research on excessive grooming elicited by the direct administration of neuropeptides or their fragments into the cerebral ventricles or into the brain, itself, in the context of behavioural stereotypy, we were forced to think about the nature and the significance of stereotypy itself. This, in turn, led us to a further step: the consideration of the adaptive significance of the mechanisms underlying excessive grooming—those neural systems that assist members of a species to survive and prosper in their environment.

Stereotypy is not simply the reproduction of identical motor responses. This definition is clearly insufficient, even though such behaviour does occur in animals after the administration of large doses of certain drugs, especially dopaminergic agonists. As Douglas emphasized some years ago (1967) and as reinforced by Gaffan and his associates (1984a,b), responses should be considered in terms of their consequences, their outcomes, and what they accomplish. Accordingly, behaviours, even though varied, that all lead to the same, less-than-optimal results or consequences should be regarded as stereotyped. Therefore, we will regard stereotypy as a reduction in an individual's usual abilities *to change* ongoing behavioural patterns or strategies subsequent to changes in environmental events so as to produce optimal consequences. Stereotypies can be a consequence of dysfunctions of perceptual, cognitive, or motor abilities, but their net effect is a failure to reach appropriate goals, to maximize rewards, or to minimize misfortunes. In the end, it is a reduced competence of an individual to deal with a changing environment due to a perseveration of cognitive, attention, motor, or strategic aspects of behaviour. As a consequence of this approach, it is clear that stereotypy should not be thought as a single phenomenon.

Examples of stereotyped acts

Since stereotypy is a form of incompetence in dealing with the environment as reflected in inappropriate responding, a common but extreme example would be the behavioural stereotypy, exemplified by uninterruptable, repetitive movements induced by drugs. For example, after dopaminergic stimulation in rodents, there are often movements of the mouth and head, postural deviations, gnawing, and other acts, that are resistant to disruption by extreme environmental changes, including those of an intense nature—the discharge of a gun, loud clicks, hand claps, light flashes, and so forth. In a real sense they resemble the behaviour of animals exhibiting aspects of chemically or environmentally induced motor seizures. After the administration of a sufficient systemic dose of picrotoxin, for example, animals exhibits a narrowly defined *set* of behavioural actions that occur in a specific sequence. These include body postural deviations, stretches (both unilateral and bilateral), twitches, vibrations, jumping, running movements of the four limbs—even when the animal is on its side (Thomas and Isaacson, unpublished observations). One of the earliest signs of seizure onset is the occurrence of repetitive retractions of the lower jaws that continue for 1–3 min before being replaced by 'absence' periods. In these, the animals show few movements but are not in touch with events in their environment. They seem to be counterparts of human epileptic absence attacks.

A similar progression of stereotyped response occurs when gamma aminobutyric acid (GABA) antagonists are injected into the region of the superior colliculus, the major behavioural consequence being explosive running bouts or 'fits' (Spruijt 1985). Temporal lobe epilepsy in humans produces a variety of seizure states in which the patient is unresponsive to environmental changes while engaging in one of a limited set of acts (Delgado-Escuéta and Walsh 1983). Over a short time period, the particular behaviour to be exhibited is not predictable, but a prediction that one of the limited set of behaviours will occur is nearly certain of fulfilment. In essence, then, the seizure-induced action is stereotyped because of its long- but not short-term predictability, its resistance to interruption, but primarily because of its maladaptive consequences. Clearly, drug-induced repetitive acts and seizure-related behaviours are less than ideal adjustments to environmental events. Animals exhibiting extreme forms of stereotypy do not appear to be aware of changes in the environment; they certainly do not respond to them and it is unlikely that they are even 'aware' of them.

Neuropeptide-induced behaviours: excessive grooming

In our work with animals, in which excessive grooming has been induced by neuropeptide administration (Gispen and Isaacson 1981, 1986), the behaviour of our experimental subjects is described as more-or-less repetitive and as highly predictable over an extended time period. On the basis of a high predictability, *per se*, it might be thought to be a form of stereotyped behaviour. However, this lack of variability results in part from the nature of the isolated testing situation that was designed to produce only limited types of responding. After the neuropeptide treatment, the animals are placed in small compartments, alone, under low levels of illumination, and with background 'white noise' often present to mask extraneous sounds. An animal administered saline usually spends most of time asleep after some early periods of locomotion and some short-duration grooming bouts occurring in the first 20–40 min. When active neuropeptides are injected into the ventricular system, excessive grooming occurs instead of sleep. Both the periods of sleep and the grooming can be easily interrupted by environmental events and appear to be reasonable activities in the barren testing environment.

The nature of excessive grooming

When about a microgram of $ACTH_{1-24}$, or certain other behaviourally active neuropeptides, is injected into the forebrain ventricular system of rat brain (intracerebroventricular, i.c.v., injections) and the rat is placed into an open field or into a small compartment where it is left undisturbed for an hour or longer, it will spend a majority of the time in self-grooming. The sequence of events exhibited by the animals is essentially that of animals exhibiting spontaneous grooming patterns in their home cages when they are acting to maintain a normal, clean condition (Spruijt and Gispen 1983).

The structure of ACTH-induced grooming   In an attempt to see whether or not ACTH-induced grooming differed in structure from stress- or novelty-related grooming, detailed element/duration, frequency, and transition analyses were made. The behaviour was recorded for a period of 55 min, 15 min following injection of either saline or $ACTH_{1-24}$ ($3 \mu g/3 \mu l$) and subsequent to placement in the observation cages (see Gispen *et al.* 1975). The following elements were scored: vibration, face-washing, body-washing, body-grooming, anogenital grooming, body-shake, tail-sniffing, and the combination of scratching/licking paw (see Gispen and Isaacson 1981).

Previously, it was documented that, when placed into a novel observation box, non-cannulated rats and those with cannulae placed chronically into the ventricular system (with or without a saline injection) displayed similar responses to handling, transport, and placement in a novel situation. No change in grooming behaviour could be detected between such groups of rats (Jolles *et al.* 1979a; Gispen and Isaacson 1981). Rats injected i.c.v. with appropriate neuropeptides spent more time grooming than the saline-treated rats. However, if the data are converted to proportion of time spent per grooming element as a percentage of the total time spent grooming, no sig-

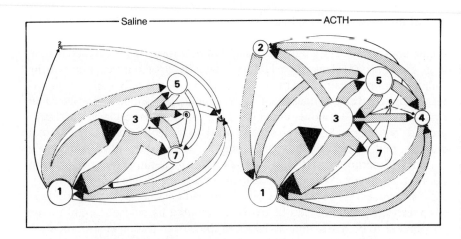

Fig. 5.1. Pathway diagram of grooming behaviour after i.c.v. saline (left) or after i.c.v. ACTH (right). Element durations and transition directions indicated by point of arrows and width of the arrows is proportional to square root of transition frequencies. Elements (circles) indicated as follows: 1, head-washing; 2, body-shakes; 3, body-grooming; 4, forepaw-vibrations; 5, scratching, paw-licking; 6, tail-sniffing; 7, anogenital grooming. (After Spruijt and Gispen (1983.))

nificant changes could be detected between the two groups of rats (Gispen and Isaacson 1981). Thus it appears that ACTH enhances the display of grooming behaviour without changing the composition of the behavioural response relative to saline-injected control rats. For both peptide- and saline-treated rats matrices of transitions between elements were composed (Fig. 5.1). The circles represent the log of the relative duration in seconds spent per behavioural element, whereas the arrows indicate transition directions; the width of the arrows is proportional to the square root of the number of transitions. Transitions occurring as less than 1 per cent of the total number of transitions are drawn as lines. The transitions occurring between 1 and 2.5 per cent are represented by open arrows. In saline-treated rats the most frequent transitions are face-washing to body-grooming and vice versa, forepaw-vibration to face-washing, body-grooming to anogenital grooming and vice versa, face-washing to scratching, body-grooming to scratching, and body-grooming to sniffing tail. Most grooming bouts tend to start with forepaw-vibrations or face-washing and end with scratching or tail-sniffing (Fig. 5.1(left)).

The structure of grooming seen under these conditions in saline-treated rats is comparable with that described for home-cage grooming behaviour by Richmond and Sachs (1980)—basically, a cephalocaudal progression of grooming acts within each bout. Also, in their experiments, scratching with the hindpaws occurred at unpredictable points in the grooming sequence and often interrupted it.

Considering the transition matrix of grooming exhibited by ACTH-treated rats (Fig. 5.1(right)), it is apparent that the major transitions within the grooming bout are similar to those seen in Fig. 5.1(left). However, as seen in Fig. 5.1(right), in ACTH-induced grooming, scratching is not a concluding element of the grooming bout. Instead, there are important new transitions between scratching and body-grooming and between scratching and vibration. Both of these elements, in turn, lead to body-shakes and face-washings and, thus, a continuation of grooming. It should be remembered that the total number of grooming bouts is very similar for saline- and ACTH-treated rats: the effect of i.c.v. ACTH is to prolong bout duration (Gispen and Isaacson 1981; Zwiers et al. 1981). It is possible that the effect of i.c.v. ACTH is to prevent scratching from being a terminal event in the usual sequence of grooming elements and, as a consequence, cause it to induce forepaw-vibrations and body-grooming.

The temporal characteristics of excessive grooming   The temporal distribution of the excessive grooming response produced by i.c.v. administration of ACTH has been recognized as an important aspect of the response (Isaacson *et al.* 1983). It is now apparent that the excessive grooming induced by neuropeptide administration produces at least two phases that are partially independent. The first phase lasts for the first 20–30 min after i.c.v. injection and is relatively independent of most pharmacological interventions. The second phase is sensitive to systemic neuroleptic and opiate antagonistic administration. In general, ACTH dose–response relationships are most easily seen in the second phase.

Neuropeptides that induce grooming   Although ACTH was the first peptide reported to induce excessive grooming, a great variety of peptides have been reported to enhance the display of excessive grooming (Table 5.1). One should bear in mind that not all publications have reported on the response in sufficient detail to allow proper comparisons. From those with sufficient details provided, it emerges that one should be cautious in generalizing the behavioural effects across peptides. To date, only ACTH/MSH and low doses of dynorphin$_{1-13}$ produce a grooming response that does not differ in structure from that seen in untreated rats when placed in a novel observation box. Thus, if central peptidergic networks or neurohumoral supply is of physiological importance in the initiation of grooming behaviour, it is assumed that the endogenous active principle is a peptide with features common to these two peptides (Spruijt and Gispen 1983).

The grooming response to i.c.v. injection of ACTH has been very useful

Table 5.1 Peptides and excessive grooming in rodents, based on Gispen and Zwiers (1985) with the addition of corticotrophin releasing factor (CRF) based on the report of Morley and Levine (1982)

Peptide	Activity*
ACTH	+
$ACTH_{1-24}$	+
$ACTH_{4-10}$	−
[D-Phe^7]$ACTH_{4-10}$	+
Org 2766	−
α-MSH	+
β-MSH	+
γ-MSH	−
Somatostatin	+ / −
TRH	±
Vasopressin	±
Oxytocin	±
Prolactin	+
β-LPH	?
CRF	+
β-endorphin	+
γ-endorphin	−
α-endorphin	±
Encephalins	−
$Dynorphin_{1-23}$	+
[dT]β-endorphin	+
[dT]$dynorphin_{1-13}$	+
Substance P	+
Eledoisin	+
Bombesin	+
Neurotensin	−
Angiotensin	−

* +, activity; ±, minor activity; −, no activity; ?, questionable.

in demonstrating the complexity with which information is encoded in peptides. $ACTH_{1-24}$ but not its composing sequences 1–10 or 11–24 induces grooming; the equimolar combination of the composing sequences will not. The fact that $ACTH_{1-24}$, α-MSH, and β-MSH were effective may be due to the common presence of the 4–10 sequence; γ-MSH, which contains the sequence Met–Gly–His–Phe–Arg did not, however, induce the response.

The administration of the 4–10 sequence *per se* is without effect. Gradual shortening at the C-terminus or at the N-terminus revealed that the message site is somewhere in the region 5–13, possibly the sequence 5–7. The inactivity of 7–10 but the activity of 5–14 and 4–7 are in support of this view. However, the [7-D-Phe]$ACTH_{4-10}$ analogue is unique among D-enantiomer substitutions in that it is active in inducing excessive grooming, although most of the excessive grooming occurs early in the observation period (Isaacson and Thomas 1986).

The role of the environment   The amount of excessive grooming induced by $ACTH_{1-24}$ does not depend on the physical nature of the observation chambers. In enriched environments as much grooming is elicited by i.c.v. $ACTH_{1-24}$ as in the small environmentally restricted test chambers most frequently used (Jolles *et al.* 1979*b*). ACTH is also effective in eliciting excessive grooming in an open-field situation in which grooming had previously been shown to have a low frequency of occurrence without the administration of the peptide (Isaacson and Green 1978). To interfere with excessive grooming, relatively stress-inducing conditions must be presented to the animals, e.g. high levels of food or water deprivation or the administration of intermittent foot shock (reviewed by Gispen and Isaacson 1986). Furthermore, if an animal is left in the environment in which foot shock was administered, all forms of grooming are suppressed for a long period of time (Hannigan and Isaacson 1981). Therefore, the presence of stress-related stimuli counteracts those conditions that lead to excessive grooming. We must emphasize, however, that, while the behaviour is predictable and comes to dominate the animals' activity, it does not occur at the expense of other behaviours. Since animals are alone in isolated, sound-attenuated chambers, the acts are not maladaptive except insofar as they represent a relatively minor expenditure of muscular energy.

In one sense it would be possible to conclude the chapter at this point by arguing that ACTH-induced excessive grooming is not a true stereotypy of behaviour. However, by considering the role of excessive grooming more generally, additional insights can be obtained regarding the role of neuropeptides and stereotyped reactions. This is due to the evidence that leads to the assumption that the neural mechanisms underlying excessive grooming are ones also responsible for a *reduction* in the brain's prior activation by environmental stressors.

The significance of excessive grooming

Originally, excessive grooming was thought to reflect an activated, aroused, or even a stressed condition. For example, Bindra and Spinner (1958) reported that exposure to novel circumstances induced grooming. Subsequently, the roles played by transporting animals from one location to another, by handling, and by other experimental procedures were systematically studied by Jolles *et al.* (1979*b*). Other stressful procedures have been found to lead to excessive grooming, including water immersion and exposure to cold (see Gispen and Isaacson 1981). From a variety of studies, however, it has become apparent that excessive grooming does not occur during stress itself, but rather after the termination of the stressful stimuli or circumstances. In fact, the continued application of stressful stimuli or stimuli associated with stress actually suppresses excessive grooming occurring as an after-effect of an earlier stress or as an after-effect to the i.c.v. administration of ACTH (Jolles *et al.* 1979*a*). The fundamental conclusion from all of the studies—one that cannot be overly stressed—is that excessive grooming reflects the activity of systems directed toward the reduction of central nervous system activation, in particular the reduction of that activity in central nervous systems that precedes or *causes* the release of ACTH. Adding support to this view are the demonstrations of the effectiveness of i.c.v. corticotrophin-releasing factor (CRF) itself, in eliciting excessive grooming (Morley and Levine 1982), and of the effectiveness of the ACTH fragments that elicit grooming when given i.c.v., thus releasing endogenous ACTH (Wiegant *et al.* 1979). Consequently, it is our opinion that excessive grooming is a behavioural correlate of neural activity directed toward decreasing further CRF and ACTH release and directed, in addition, to the restoration of conditions in the brain prevailing before the activation.

In essence, we believe that the reduction of the neurochemical and neurophysiological bases of activation is helpful to the animal in its adaptation to environmental change, an idea also proposed earlier by de Wied and Jolles (1982). If this is the case, it is important to learn the precise neural systems involved.

The neural substrates for excessive grooming

Previous studies from this and other laboratories pointed to an important role of dopaminergic systems in general and the substantia nigra in particular in ACTH-induced excessive grooming in the rat (Wiegant *et al.* 1977; Traber *et al.* 1982; Cools *et al.* 1978; Drago and Bohus 1981; Guild and Dunn 1981; Chesher and Jackson 1981; Isaacson *et al.* 1983). The modulation of peptide-induced excessive grooming by manipulation of both a dopaminergic excitation-mediating system (DA_e) and a dopaminergic inhibiting-mediating system (DA_i) (Cools *et al.* 1978) has been demonstrated. Excessive grooming seen after i.c.v. application of $ACTH_{1-24}$ was suppressed by local administration of dopaminergic agonists/antagonists in the nucleus accumbens (DA_i) or in the neostriatum (DA_e). There is evidence suggesting the involvement of the nigrostriatal dopaminergic pathway and the striatonigral GABA-ergic pathway in the expression of rigidity (Cools 1985), body posture, circling, stereotypy (Scheel-Krüger, 1982), and catalepsy (DiChiara *et al.* 1978). The striatonigral fibres are assumed to serve as a feedback system on nigrostriatal dopaminergic fibres originating in the pars compacta. In addition, they feed the three distinctive output systems of the substantia nigra (pars reticulata), projecting to the superior colliculus, certain thalamic nuclei, and the reticular formation.

We have investigated whether ACTH-induced excessive grooming, elicited locally in the substantia nigra, could be modulated by manipulation of the DA_e and DA_i receptor systems, possibly via the aforementioned GABA-ergic pathway. If haloperidol decreases dopaminergic activity in the neostriatum, which results in a decreased GABA-ergic activity in the substantia nigra, then a potentiation of grooming elicited in the substantia nigra should be noticed. Since the DA_i agonists/antagonists may also have α-noradrenergic activity, additional experiments were undertaken in order to determine if there was a specific dopamine component in the nucleus accumbens (and not a noradrenergic influence) related to excessive grooming. Specifically, we sought to determine whether the effects of the DA_i antagonist ergometrine (which also has α-noradrenergic activity) would be counteracted by an α-noradrenergic agonist or by a DA_i agonist.

The inhibitory effects of haloperidol and apomorphine on excessive grooming when applied into the neostriatum were not observed when ACTH was given into the substantia nigra, as opposed to the more common i.c.v. route (Spruijt *et al.* 1986*a*). Inhibition of the output of the substantia nigra by the neostriatum presumes the involvement of the GABA-ergic inhibitory pathway from striatum to substantia nigra. This is in agreement with the hypothesis that enhanced dopaminergic activity in the neostriatum increases the activity of the GABA-ergic striatonigral pathway (Scheel-Krüger 1982; Scheel-Krüger *et al.* 1981; Starr *et al.* 1983).

Whether or not dopaminergic agents applied to the basal ganglia reduce neuropeptide-induced excessive grooming depends on the route of administration of the neuropeptide. This may be due to complex relationships between GABA-ergic activity within the substantia nigra (pars reticulata) and the superior colliculus. The relation between GABA-ergic activity in the substantia nigra and the superior colliculus is apparent from the ability of GABA agonists to inhibit seizures when injected into the substantia nigra (Iadarola and Gale 1982), whereas GABA antagonists in the superior colliculus induce explosive running and, in higher doses, seizures and convulsions. Moreover, this explosive motor running elicited in the superior colliculus is sensitive to manipulations of the dopaminergic activities in the caudate nucleus (Cools *et al.* 1984). Since the substantia nigra is probably not as easily reached from the ventricular system as is the periaqueductal grey, intraventricular ACTH may be acting through the latter area, which may explain the different effects of dopaminergic agents on nigral and i.c.v. ACTH-induced grooming. If the forebrain dopaminergic modulation of ACTH-induced excessive grooming is exerted by the striatonigrocollicular pathway, the local application of GABA-ergic agents into the superior colliculus should alter intraventricularly (i.c.v.) elicited excessive grooming. Local administration of the GABA-ergic compounds picrotoxin and muscimol indeed suppressed or enhanced, respectively, excessive grooming (Spruijt *et al.* 1986b). In addition, localized lesions in this region demonstrated that the superior colliculus is not the primary site of action of ACTH. This structure is a prerequisite for exploration and orientation towards new stimuli, but not for ACTH-induced excessive grooming. Further experiments suggested that the periaqueductal grey, however, is essential to ACTH-induced grooming (Spruijt *et al.* 1986c). The local injection of ACTH into the periaqueductal grey induced excessive grooming and lesions in this structure markedly suppressed it (Spruijt *et al.* 1986c).

Therefore, the periaqueductal grey appears to be one site of action of ACTH as it influences excessive grooming and that dopaminergic and GABA-ergic structures participate in the regulation of the output of this structure.

We know other facts about the neural and hormonal systems related to excessive grooming. For example, these systems are independent of the feedback inhibitory actions of ACTH acting via the glucocorticoids (Jolles *et al.* 1978), but are partially dependent on naloxone-sensitive systems. Data from short-term tolerance studies in which two doses of ACTH were given 4–24 hours apart provide evidence for the involvement of multiple systems in excessive grooming and the assumed reduction of stress-induced activation. Short-term tolerance to ACTH-induced grooming involves a diminution of grooming during the second half of the hour-long observation period during the second test session. Grooming during the first part of the observation period of the session is unaffected. The last half of the test period is that time during which low doses of naloxone can abolish or reduce excessive grooming induced by i.c.v. ACTH and it is also that period of time in which i.c.v. morphine induces excessive grooming (Isaacson *et al.* 1983). Fitting this interpretation is the observation that, although naloxone pre-treatment greatly reduces ACTH-induced excessive grooming, it does not abolish the effect entirely (Jolles *et al.* 1978). The neuropeptide still produces a small increment in grooming. This would be expected because the grooming exhibited in the first half of the observation period should not be reduced and that exhibited during the second half should be greatly reduced. The net effect for the entire observation period is a less than complete reduction of the total grooming score. However, this is not the case with β-endorphin excessive grooming. Naloxone pre-treatment before i.c.v. 0.3 µg β-endorphin produces no more grooming than does i.c.v. saline (Wiegant *et al.* 1978).

In addition, we know that lesions of other brain regions diminish the excessive grooming produced by i.c.v. ACTH. These include the hippocampus and the medial portions of the nucleus accumbens. The effect of these lesions is to reduce the duration of grooming bouts. The lesions do not eliminate the responsiveness of the animals to i.c.v. ACTH; rather, they reduce the sensitivity of the animals to the neuropeptide (Elstein *et al.* 1981). Moreover, lesions in areas of the brain known to reduce or eliminate other neuropeptide effects on behaviours do *not* reduce ACTH-induced excessive grooming. These include: the septal area and various of its subregions, the medial or lateral pre-optic areas, the anterior hypothalamus, the amygdala, the parafascicular nucleus of the thalamus, the superior colliculi, and either dorsal or ventral portions of the hippocampus alone (Colbern *et al.* 1977). For hippocampal lesions to reduce ACTH sensitivity for excessive grooming, the lesion must involve *both* dorsal and ventral portions (nearly total lesions).

The dopaminergic components of excessive grooming

As noted above, on the basis of evidence from a number of divergent approaches (e.g. Versteeg 1980; Wiegant *et al.* 1977), there is reason to presume that the ascending dopamine systems reaching the basal ganglia in the forebrain have a strong relation to mechanisms involved with excessive grooming, probably involving the regulation of descending GABA-ergic pathways. Furthermore, injections of ACTH into the medial nucleus accumbens (but not the lateral) induce excessive grooming that is similar in amount and in its short-term tolerance parameters to the excessive grooming found after i.c.v. administration (Ryan and Isaacson 1983). Lesions of this area abolish excessive grooming in response to i.c.v. ACTH (Springer *et al.* 1983). Spruijt (1985) has found that the microinjection of either haloperidol or apomorphine into the caudate reduces the excessive grooming induced by i.c.v. ACTH by about 40 per cent. The introduction of ergometrine or 3, 4-dihydroxyphenylamino-2-imidazoline (DPI) into the nucleus accumbens reduces excessive grooming even more so (reductions of greater than 60 per cent). The specificity of the haloperidol or apomorphine treatments to the caudate or of the DPI or ergometrine treatments to the nucleus accumbens was tested by cross-administration of the drugs into the other structure in these studies. However, phentolamine injected into the nucleus accumbens did not affect the i.c.v. induced excessive grooming, thus reinforcing the idea that it is the dopaminergic activity in these forebrain structures that is essential to neuropeptide-induced excessive grooming. Spruijt *et al.* (1986*a*) also investigated the short-term tolerance produced by injection of the neuropeptide injected into two brain regions after a 4-hour interval. The sites studied were substantia nigra, the periaqueductal grey, and the interventricular foramen (i.c.v.). When ACTH was given i.c.v. or into the periaqueductal grey initially, a second injection 4 hours later into any of the other regions resulted in reduced excessive grooming. Initial injections into the substantia nigra unilaterally, produced a reduced responsiveness for a subsequent injection into the same site and also for a subsequent injection into the periaqueductal grey. It did not produce a reduction in responsiveness for a subsequent injection of the substantia nigra on the opposite side of the brain or for a subsequent i.c.v. injection. Therefore, while it is clear that dopaminergic systems projecting to the forebrain basal ganglia structures, the regions of origin of their dopaminergic afferents, and regions surrounding the aqueduct are involved in the expression of excessive grooming, the complex interactions among these systems remain to be fully explicated. A diagrammatic summary of some of the system's involved in excessive grooming is given in Fig. 5.2.

As noted above, both the systemic and local central nervous system administration of certain dopaminergic antagonists block the expression of excessive grooming. However, not all dopaminergic antagonists are equally effective in reducing the neuropeptide-induced excessive grooming. For

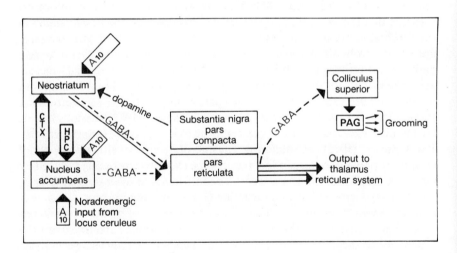

Fig. 5.2. Schematic representation of certain of the anatomical regions associated with excessive grooming in the rat. Some of the presumed transmitters of certain anatomical pathways are also indicated. Abbreviations: A10, the mesolimbic dopamine projections arising from the A10, ventral tegmental area cell group; CTX, afferents arising from neocortical areas; HPC, afferents from hippocampal formation and subiculum; GABA, γ-amino butyric acid; PAG, periaqueductal grey. (Modified from Gispen and Zwiers (1985)).

example, sulpiride, a dopaminergic antagonist with special affinity for receptors in the hippocampus, fails to reduce excessive grooming (Traber *et al*. 1982). It is an imbalance among dopaminergic systems that disrupts excessive grooming, and it is likely that disturbances of the relatively minor dopaminergic innervation of the hippocampus fail to alter the balance of the more significant systems sufficiently to disrupt excessive grooming.

We believe that a more complete understanding of the significance of excessive grooming and its neural substrates will reveal important information about how the brain attempts to restore near-normal conditions after stress. The evidence is clear that these will involve the ascending dopaminergic systems, and these systems have already been linked to mechanisms underlying aberrant mental and behavioural states.

Dopaminergic influences on behaviour

The initiating conditions, the neurochemical or environmental manipulations which precede the excessive grooming, are ones that produce a variety of changes in many neural systems. Different sorts of stressors act in different ways to create individual patterns of activation (e.g. Yuwiler 1971). At a behavioural level, conditions of stress or pharmacological interventions that produce stress-like conditions in the central nervous system change the breadth of attentional processes and the variety of motor responses an individual exhibits. Surprisingly, perhaps, such changes are not easily categorized and depend in part on the nature of the test used and characteristics of the testing situations.

One likely aspect of the effects of an acute stressor is increased activity in the forebrain dopaminergic systems, although such changes are not the only or, perhaps, even the most prominent important ones. Regardless of their relationship to stress, the effects of enhanced dopaminergic activities have not been easy to characterize. Lyon and Robbins (1975) have suggested that amphetamine, primarily acting via its dopaminergic effects, increases response rates but narrows the range of responses exhibited. (See Chapter 2, this volume, for discussion.) Others (e.g. Cools 1980) have suggested that in normal activities dopaminergic activities of the basal ganglia allow the adaptive interruption of ongoing behavioural acts by unexpected events, but in abnormal conditions either excessive perseveration or an enhanced tendency for the breakdown of existing behavioural programmes could occur.

There are many reasons why the disruption of dopaminergic activities in the brain has been difficult to characterize. In extreme cases, those of massive pharmacological dopaminergic stimulation, the problem is least difficult, for often the behaviours exhibited fit the criteria of obvious stereotypy. Similar behaviours occur in animals and in people during periods of extreme stress and may represent a natural response to such conditions.

There are, however, considerable individual differences in regard to the nature of the effects of dopaminergic stimulation. For example, a dose–response genetic analysis of the effects of apomorphine on two strains of mice indicates that they responded differently in the expression of some stereotyped behaviours but were equally sensitive in the induction of other responses. For example, one behaviour (i.e. wall-climbing) was induced by the drug in one strain but not exhibited at any dose of apomorphine in the other (Seale *et al*. 1984). These results are important because they indicate that the stereotypies induced by dopamine agonists will vary among animals of different genetic constitutions. Furthermore, additional variation can be expected in what constitutes an extreme form of stress and in regard to the time required for normal internal conditons and overt activities to be restored after the termination of the stressor. Whether differences found among individuals of the same species arise more because of variations in their genetic inheritances or because of contributions of prior environmental experiences is idle speculation. Both factors are contributory and will interact with each other to different degrees in each individual. At the human level, variations in response to stress are widely acknowledged but little has been done by way of determining differences in the environmental stimuli that initiate stress reactions or their intensity when they occur. Furthermore, we know very little about the individual differences found in the mental and behavioural correlates of the various hormonal and autonomic reactions associated with stressful responses.

Adding to our ignorance, we should note that factors related to the duration of stress-induced responses have been little studied. Clearly, differences in the duration of stress-related responses exist among people. Some of the consequences of extreme chronic or acute stressors last a lifetime, as found in those permanently impaired by the wartime experiences, the holocaust, or internment in prison camps. Some people never 'recover' from the loss of a loved friend, lover, or child, or from a 'near accident' or other trauma. While these 'lifelong' reactions may be exceptional, there can be little doubt that there is great variability among people in their ability to restore themselves after a stress experience.

We believe that the excessive grooming studied so intensively by us and by others provides the basis for understanding how rapidly an individual animal begins to recover from a stressful experience and can provide useful insights into the mechanisms that produce the recovery. By inference, we also believe that the onset of post-stress excessive grooming is contingent upon the restoration of an appropriate balance among the dopaminergic systems of the forebrain.

The prefrontal cortex and dopaminergic systems

The prefrontal cortex of the rat, as well as of many other species, receives fibres from the 'mesolimbic' dopaminergic system, the one that also innervates the nucleus accumbens and other subcortical sites (e.g. Bannon and Roth 1983). Furthermore, there are extensive projections *from* the prefrontal cortex to both the caudate and the nucleus accumbens. In general, frontal decortication enhances the stereotypy induced by apomorphine (Scatton *et al.* 1982), probably by effects in the caudate nucleus. There is direct evidence of a hippocampal modulation of dopaminergic activity in the nucleus accumbens (Springer and Isaacson 1982). While undoubtedly an oversimplification, it might appear that the neocortex is a major regulator of dopaminergic neostriatal activities, while the limbic system exerts predominant influences on dopaminergic activities in the nucleus accumbens. However, for the present purposes, it is enough that prefrontal cortical regions are subject to strong dopaminergic regulation; when this system of afferents does not function in an appropriate fashion behavioural aberrations should be anticipated.

The prefrontal cortex and 'higher functions'   The systemic administration of dopaminergic antagonists produces behavioural changes that seem to represent interruptions of 'higher-level' cognitive activities. For example, haloperidol acts to reduce transitions in motor actions of cats that are intrinsically mediated but not those guided by external stimuli (Jaspers *et al.* 1984). In rats, pimozide and spiperone inhibit the demonstration of schedule-induced drinking, but not that produced by cellular dehydration (Porter *et al.* 1984). These observations fit in with the notion that the dopaminergic systems are important for the acquisition of schedule-induced behaviours (Robbins and Koob 1980), but not behaviours tightly bound to the activities of a specific motivational system such as normal food or water consumption (Koob *et al.* 1978). Disturbances of dopaminergic functions do not disrupt the automatic or homeostatic mechanisms which might be presumed to be associated with basal ganglia function but rather produce disturbances of acquired behaviours and behaviours requiring advanced cognitive processes, ones typically associated with prefrontal cortical functions.

Disturbances of prefrontal functions   While not wishing to endorse the idea that any prefrontal neocortical region is the physical site of higher intellectual or cognitive actions, there is abundant evidence that these regions are involved in an essential fashion with neuronal systems at various levels of the nervous system that do mediate such behaviours. They are, we believe, involved with the development of a hierarchical regulation of behavioural acts (as advocated by Jackson 1884), and, when these areas are injured or diseased, there will be a loss of this hierarchical organization. The idea of the importance of the prefrontal areas in the higher levels of mental activity was also promoted by Jackson. Further, he believed that the functions of these regions continued to develop over the life span of the indiviual as well as over the course of evolution (Jackson 1887). This notion fits remarkably well with the developmental notions of the socially oriented Gestalt psychologist, Kurt Lewin (1935). He proposed an increasingly differentiated 'life space' over development, as a direct result of experience and interaction with the environment. To maintain a unified individual, this increasing differentiation necessitated the development of hierarchical processes.

What is of special interest in this context is that actual damage to the prefrontal lobes in people often produces behavioural and mental consequences similar to those found in schizophrenia (e.g. Lishman 1978; Levin 1984; Müller 1985). The inappropriate functions of the prefrontal areas can lead to a regression in the hierarchical control such that behaviour becomes based on a less well-differentiated world and actions are based more closely on acquired stimulus–response associations without regard to 'higher-order' contingencies. The loss of differentiation in the 'life space' results in a tendency to respond to many different events or stimuli in an equivalent fashion, thus leading to both maladaptive perceptions and performance, i.e. stereotypies.

In our view, these same sort of changes occur during conditions of stress. With intense or chronic conditions of stress and a loss of normal control, foresight is shortened and behaviour becomes less differential and restricted to highly learned responses. Under extreme stress, other signs of a transient elimination of frontal lobe functions can be observed. Müller (1985) has suggested that it is as if intense stress can induce a transient shutdown of prefrontal lobe activity, producing, perhaps, a catastrophic reaction. Such an occasion involves total panic, immobilization, or hyperreactivity, depending upon the individual. A complete loss of normal planning and regulatory controls occurs, and only basic, thoughtless reflex actions survive.

A comparison with the effects of traumatic brain damage   It may be of special interest, in this regard, to remember that Goldstein (1942) pointed out that patients with wartime brain injuries, regardless of their neural location, were especially prone to periods in which control and planning abilities were lost. Goldstein believed that the fear of 'losing control', and suffering a catastrophic reaction, was such a predominant motive force in head trauma patients that much of their waking actions were directed toward reducing the occurrence of unexpected or upsetting events. This accounted for the patients striving to maintain a consistent environment with almost an obsessional need to have all of their clothes and personal objects in a regular place and in a regular order. The enhanced fear of 'loss of control' was correlated with a greatly enhanced variability (lability) of both autonomic and somatic activities in his brain-damaged patients. The variability occurred both spontaneously or subsequent to mild exertion or some unanticipated stimulus.

With damage to the frontal lobes, an absence of spontaneity and an associated diminution of all activities would often alternate with states of hyperactivity and restlessness (Goldstein 1942, p. 58). Other frontal lobe patients survive in an almost catatonic state. Both forms of behaviour could have as their objective the elimination of unanticipated events. While the need to achieve a constant environment free from surprises is frequently found after frontal lobe damage, it can occur with other forms of damage, and Goldstein clearly indicated that he did not believe in any narrow view of localization of functions. For example, 'Localization of a performance means to me not an excitation in a certain place, but a dynamic process which occurs in the entire nervous system, even in the whole organism, and which has a definite configuration for each performance.' (Goldstein 1942, p. 84).

It is likely that catastrophic reactions can occur in anyone subjected to sufficient stress and to the brain-impaired individual with less provocation, but it is also likely that all forms and levels of stress tend to produce a disruption or dysfunction of brain activities that may or may not produce such clearly observable effects on behaviour. In terms of dopamine–prefrontal lobe activities, lower levels of stress may produce a dysregulation of these neural systems rather than their suppression.

Dysregulation of neural systems

When proposing a dysregulation hypothesis of depression, Siever and Davis (1985) suggested several criteria for indicating when dysregulation occurs. These include:

(1) an impairment in one or more homeostatic (feedback) control mechanisms;

(2) the basal output of the system(s) is (are) erratic;

(3) normal periodicities of function are lost;

(4) responsiveness is less selective to environmental conditions;

(5) there is a slow return to baseline conditions after a perturbing event.

These authors go on to suggest that while many, if not all, neurohormonal or neurochemical systems can become dysregulated, there is substantial evidence that the catecholaminergic systems may be most prominently changed in the affective disorders. Furthermore, they argue that, with a dysregulation approach, the inconsistencies in the literature about levels or turnover of specific transmitters in different disease states and under different conditions would be anticipated. It is not that a particular transmitter or modulator is chronically high or low, but rather that it is not under normal regulatory influences. Once the particular biologically active agent escapes the normal regulatory controls, an unstable and erratic pattern of activity results. The escape from normal homeostatic mechanisms can be due to alterations in pre- and post-synaptic receptor numbers or sensitivity, receptor affinities in receptor-mediated membrane mechanisms, changes in transmitter release, end-product inhibition, changes in the synergistic effects of transmitters coexisting in the same cells, the interactions of nerve cells with endogenous or locally active neurohormones, or to poorly understood factors such as how the amino acid adenosine may be released from the post-synaptic cell membrane to modulate pre-synaptic release (Fredholm 1981).

Stereotypy revisited

At the beginning of this chapter, we undertook to define behavioural stereotypy in a broad fashion, concentrating on the maladaptive effects of restricted attentional, motivational, or performance (motor) capabilities. Essentially, we considered stereotypy to represent a failure to react appropriately to changes in the environment. We emphasized that neuropeptide-induced excessive grooming itself, failed to meet these specifications for stereotypy. Indeed, as discussed, it probably represents the antithesis of stereotyped reactions. We pointed out that excessive grooming occurs as an animal is overcoming neural perturbations (dysfunctions) caused by environmental stressors and by the pharmacological imitation of such conditions by intracerebral administration of certain neuropeptides. Because of this we would argue that it is the product of neuronal systems that are attempting to restore normal homeostatic conditions in the brain.

Restrictions on adaptive reactions

The usual adaptiveness of mental and behavioural processes is reduced under a variety of conditions by an overall reduction in the variability of behaviour that can occur as consequences of restrictions in attentional, cognitive, or performance characteristics. At least certain of these changes are included in what we term 'stereotyped' behaviours, ones associated with abnormal dopaminergic activities in the forebrain. Furthermore, there are at least several classes of these behavioural and mental restrictions that are associated with the malfunction of mechanisms of the prefrontal areas. These range from what can be thought of as a generalized, chronic reduction in the activity of prefrontal systems (hypofunction) as may occur in psychotic disorders to a dysregulation of the same (or related) systems in depression or under conditions of chronic stress. We postulate that the behavioural limitations are associated with aberrancies in the normal regulatory mechanisms of dopaminergic and opiate-related systems, espe- .

cially in the brainstem, portions of the basal ganglia, and prefrontal cortical region, but sources of aberrancies could include all of the regions that exert regulatory influences on dopaminergic systems. It is difficult, if indeed possible, to ascertain in a particular instance or individual which of the components of the 'system' initiates the dysregulation. Probably the location of the initial malfunction will vary from disease to disease or from individual to individual with the same disease. Each of the components continually exerts regulatory influences on the others.

Homeostasis and grooming

The connection of these forms of aberrant neural regulation with the phenomenon of excessive grooming is in the fact that excessive grooming is correlated with neural activities that are directed toward the restoration of homeostatic mechanisms in the forebrain. By observing the animals we can determine when such mechanisms begin and, most likely, their duration. As noted above, from our observations of the time course of excessive grooming after an acute stressor it is clear that at least two such mechanisms are involved. Furthermore, by the study of pharmacological interventions that promote or reduce excessive grooming after an acute stress condition, insight can be gained as to the neurochemical systems that are strongly involved with the restoration of normal homeostatic processes. To date, there has been more progress made in discovering interventions that reduce excessive grooming, and the presumed restorative mechanisms underlying it, than in agents that enhance it. It is now well established that naloxone, haloperidol (high dose levels), and neurotensin (Van Wimersma Greidanus and Rinkel 1983) are effective in reducing neuropeptide-induced excessive grooming.

Grooming has been enhanced after mild stress conditions (handling, transport, and movement to a novel environment) by a modest amount of ethanol in mice genetically selected to be relatively resistant to the drug (Allan and Isaacson 1985) and by manipulation of the histaminergic system (O'Callaghan *et al.* 1982). However, in these studies it is difficult to dissociate an increase in some form of a central stress-related response (and a resultant increase in counteracting systems) from a direct enhancement of the counteracting systems *per se*. In all of the instances of neuropeptide-induced excessive grooming, the i.c.v. administration of the agents (i.e. Table 5.1), there is an induction of a central representation of an aspect of acute stress and excessive grooming occurs as counteracting neural mechanisms become engaged. Dose–response curves indicate that the greater the stress-like intervention, the longer the delay before grooming begins and the longer it persists, once started. A possible exception to this may be the excessive grooming induced by the administration of the experimental codeione R X 336-M that has a remarkable, age- and sex-related ability to induce excessive grooming after peripheral administration. This drug, closely related in structure to the opiates, may have the ability to engage restorative mechanism directly in young animals, especially males (Cowan 1981; Isaacson *et al.* 1987). Recently, a similar response has been found to occur after the systemic administration of codeine itself (Isaacson *et al.* 1988). The issue of how to distinguish a direct enhancement of homeostatic regulatory influences from an enhanced stress reaction is not easily resolved. One possibility would be the evaluation of the latency of the excessive grooming after i.c.v. or central nervous system administration. When ACTH is administered in this fashion, excessive grooming only begins 15–20 min later even though its half-life is only a few minutes. This further supports the idea that it is a rebound phenomenon of the neuropeptide's initial actions that is being measured by excessive grooming. Presumably, the activation of the rebound-counteracting mechanisms would produce an immediate (or nearly so) period of excessive grooming.

If excessive grooming does, as we think, reflect the operation of restorative neural mechanisms, behaviour should change from being restricted or 'stereotyped' during the 'stress activation period' to more flexible, adaptive behaviour during or after the grooming period. Perhaps different degrees of enchanced flexibility could be determined after each of the two restorative mechanisms presumed to exist on the basis of the time-course studies. It is difficult to measure any reduced flexibility of behaviour that occurs the after i.c.v. administration of the ACTH/MSH fragments because their half-life in the brain is so short. The activation produced by moderate-to-large doses of amphetamine is easily measured (the prolonged stereotypy) as is the prolonged excessive grooming after the activation period. However, at this time it is not possible to say that every neuropeptide that induces excessive grooming also induces a period of maladaptive behaviour, although this would be expected.

Future directions

One of the most exciting possibilities that has arisen from the studies of excessive grooming is the possibility that certain human disorders, such as psychosis or depression, arise from the failure of one or another of the restorative mechanisms reflected in the excessive grooming of the laboratory rat. However, the measurement of similar restorative processes, if they exist, in other species has eluded us, except for obviously similar responses in the mouse and the cat. It would be particularly useful to determine the behavioural correlates of restorative processes occurring after acute stress of the central pharmacological équivalents in the non-human primate. Possibly an approach that would require minimal intervention with such animals would be the systemic administration of the codeione RX 336-M or codeine to immature animals in order to determine if a consistent pattern of behaviour would be elicited and, if so, if components of this response, whatever it may be, would be found as a naturally occurring response to mild stressors after the animals were back in a 'safe' environment. In this way the degree to which behaviours correlated with the re-establishment of a normal homeostatic condition in non-human primates could be established. This might serve as a guide to what would be expected to occur as a similar correlate of a return from homeostatic disruptions in people. Such knowledge could be of value in determining the adaptive characteristics of an individual at any point in time.

References

Allan, A.M. and Isaacson, R.L. (1985). Ethanol-induced grooming in mice selectively bred for differential sensitivity to ethanol. *Behav. neural Biol.* **44**, 386–92.

Bannon, M.J. and Roth, R.H. (1983). Pharmacology of mesocortical dopamine neurones. *Pharmacol. Rev.* **35**, 53–68.

Bindra, D. and Spinner, N. (1958). Response to different degrees of novelty: the incidence of various activities. *J. Exp. Anal. Behav.* **1**, 341–50.

Chesher, G.B. and Jackson, D.M. (1981). Swim-induced grooming in mice is mediated by a dopaminergic substrate. *J. neural Transmission* **50**, 47–55.

Colbern, D., Isaacson, R.L., Bohus, B., and Gispen, W.H. (1977). Limbic-midbrain lesions and ACTH-induced excessive grooming. *Life Sci.* **21**, 393–402.

Cools A.R. (1980) Role of neostriatal dopaminergic activity in sequencing and selecting behavioural strategies: facilitation of processes involved in selecting the best strategy in a stressful situation. *Behav. Brain Res.* **1**, 361–78.

Cools, A.R. (1985). Brain and behaviour: hierarchy of feedback systems and control of its input. *Perspectives in Ethology* **6**, (eds. P. Klopfer and P. Bateman), pp. 109–68. New York, Plenum.

Cools, A.R., Wiegent, V.M., and Gispen, W.H. (1978). Distinct dopaminergic systems in ACTH induced grooming. *Eur. J. Pharmacol.* **50**, 265–8.

Cools, A.R., Coolen, J.M.M., Smit, J.C.A., and Ellenbrock, B.A. (1984). The striato-nigral-collicular pathway and explosive running behavior: functional interaction between neostriatal dopamine and collicular GABA. *Eur. J. Pharmacol.* **100**, 71–7.

Cowan, A. (1981). RX 336-M, a new chemical tool in the analysis of the quasimorphine withdrawal syndrome. *Fed. Proc.* **40**, 1497–501.

Delgado-Escueta, A.V. and Walsh, G.O. (1983). The selection process for surgery of intractable complex partial seizures: surface EEG and depth electrography. In *Epilepsy* (eds. A.A. Ward, J.K. Penry, and D.P. Purpura), pp. 295–326. Raven Press, New York.

de Wied, D. and Jolles, J. (1982). Neuropeptides derived from proopiocortin: behavioural, physiological, and neurochemical effects. *Physiol. Rev.* **62**, 967–1059.

Di Chiara, G., Morelli, M., Porceddu, M.L., and Gessa, G.L. (1978). Evidence that nigral GABA mediates behavioural responses elicited by striatal dopamine receptor stimulation. *Life Sci.* **23**, 2045–50.

Douglas, R.J. (1967). The hippocampus and behavior. *Psychol. Bull.* **67**, 416–42.

Drago, F. and Bohus, B. (1981). Hyperprolactinemia-induced excessive grooming in the rat: time-course and element analysis. *Behav. neural Biol.* **33**, 117–22.

Elstein, K., Hannigan, J.H., Jr, and Isaacson, R.L. (1981). Repeated intracerebroventricular injections of ACTH(1–24) in rats with hippocampal lesions. *Behav. neural Biol.* **32**, 248–54.

Fredholm, B.B. (1981). Trans-synaptic modulation of transmitter release with special reference to adenosine. In *Chemical transmission* (ed. L. Stjarne, P. Hedqvist, H. Lagercrantz, and A. Wennmalm). pp. 211–22. Academic Press, New York.

Gaffan, D., Gaffan, E.A., and Harrison, S. (1984*a*). Effects of fornix transection on spontaneous and trained non-matching by monkeys. *Quart. J. exp. Psychol.* **36B**, 285–303.

Gaffan, D., Shields, C., and Harrison, S. (1984*b*). Delayed matching by fornix-transected monkeys: the sample, the push, and the bait. *Quart. J. exp. Psychol.* **36B**, 305–17.

Gispen, W.H. and Isaacson, R.L. (1981). ACTH-induced excessive grooming in the rat. *Pharmacol. Ther.* **12**, 209–46.

Gispen, W.H. and Isaacson, R.L. (1986). Excessive grooming in response to ACTH. *Encycloped. Pharmacol. Ther.* 273–312.

Gispen, W.H. and Zwiers, H. (1985). Behavioural and neurochemical effects of ACTH. In *Handbook of neurochemistry* (ed. A. Lajtha), pp. 375–412. Plenum, New York.

Gispen, W.H., Wigant, V.M., Greven, H.M., and de Wied, D. (1975). The induction of excessive grooming in the rat by intraventricular application of peptides derived from ACTH: structure–activity studies. *Life Sci.* **17**, 645–52.

Goldstein, K. (1942). *After effects of brain injury in war. Their evaluation and treatment.* Grune and Stratton, New York.

Guild, A.L. and Dunn, A.J. (1981). Dopamine involvement in ACTH-induced grooming behavior. *Pharmacol. Biochem. Behav.* **17**, 13–36.

Hannigan, J.H., Jr and Isaacson, R.L. (1981). Conditioned excessive grooming in the rat after footshock: effect of naloxone and situational cues. *Behav. neural Biol.* **33**, 280–92.

Iadarola, M.J. and Gale, K. (1982). Substantia nigra: site of anticonvulsant activity mediated by γ-aminobutyric acid. *Science* **218**, 1237–40.

Isaacson, R.L. and Green, E.J. (1978). The effect of ACTH(1–24) on locomotion, exploration, rearing, and grooming. *Behav. Biol.* **24**, 118–22.

Isaacson, R.L. and Thomas, J. (1986). The character of (D-Phe-7)- and $ACTH_{4-10}$-induced excessive grooming. *Exp. Neurol.* **93**, 657–61.

Isaacson, R.L., Hardy, C-A., and Hannigan, J.H., Jr. (1987). Age and sex-related induction of excessive grooming by RX 336-M in the rat. *Behav. Neurol Biol.* **47**, 250–61.

Isaacson, R.L., Hannigan, J.H., Jr, and Gispen, W.H. (1983). The time course of excessive grooming after neuropeptide administration. *Brain Res. Bull.* **11**, 289–93.

Isaacson, R. L., Danks, A. M., Brakkee, J., Schefman, K., and Gispen, W. H. (1988). Excessive grooming induced by the administration of codeine and morphine. *Behav. Neurol Biol.* **50**, 37–45.

Jackson, J. H. (1884). Evolution and dissolution of the nervous system. In *Selected writings of John Hughlings Jackson, Vol. II* (ed. J. Taylor), pp. 45–53. Hodder & Stoughton, Ltd, London. (This edition published in 1932.)

Jackson, J. H. (1887). Remarks on evolution and dissolution of the nervous system. In *Selected writings of John Hughlings Jackson, Vol. II* (ed. J. Taylor), pp. 92–118. Hodder & Stoughton, Ltd, London. (This edition published in 1932.)

Jaspers, R., Schwarz, M., Sontag, K. H., and Cools, A. R. (1984). Caudate nucleus and programming behaviour in cats: role of dopamine in switching motor patterns. *Behav. Brain Res.* **14**, 17–28.

Jolles J., Wiegant, V. M., and Gispen, W. H. (1978). Reduced behavioral effects with ACTH(1–24) after a second administration. *Neurosci. Lett.* **9**, 261–6.

Jolles, J., Rompa-Barendregt, J., and Gispen, W. H. (1979a). Novelty and grooming behavior in the rat. *Behav. neural Biol.* **25**, 563–72.

Jolles, J., Rompa-Barendregt, J., and Gispen, W. H. (1979b). ACTH-induced excessive grooming in the rat: the influence of environmental and motivational factors. *Hormones Behav.* **12**, 60–72.

Koob, G. F., Riley, S. J., Smith, S. C., and Robbins, T. W. (1978). Effects of 6-hydroxydopamine lesions of the nucleus accumbens septi and olfactory tubercle on feeding, locomotor activity, and amphetamine anorexia in the rat. *J. comp. physiol. Psychol.* **92**, 917–27.

Levin, S. (1984). Frontal lobe dysfunction in schizophrenia-II. Impairments of psychological and brain functions. *J. psychiat. Res.* **18**, 57–72.

Lewin, K. (1935). *A dynamic theory of personality.* McGraw-Hill, New York.

Lishman, W. A. (1978). *Organic psychiatry.* Blackwell, Oxford.

Lyon, M. and Robbins, T. W. (1975). The action of central nervous system drugs: a general theory concerning amphetamine effects. In *Current developments in psychopharmacology, Vol. 2* (ed. W. Essman and L. Valzelli), pp. 81–163. Spectrum, New York.

Morley, J. E. and Levine, A. S. (1982). Corticotrophin releasing factor, grooming, and ingestive behavior. *Life Sci.* **31**, 1459–64.

Müller, H. F. (1985). Prefrontal cortex dysfunction as a common factor in psychosis. *Acta psychiat. scand.* **71**, 431–40.

O'Callaghan, M., Horowitz, G. P., and Isaacson, R. L. (1982). An investigation of the involvement of histaminergic systems in novelty-induced grooming in the mouse. *Behav. neural Biol.* **35**, 368–74.

Porter, H. H., Goldsmith, P. A., McDonough, J. J., Heath, G. F., and Johnson, D. N. (1984). Differential effects of dopamine blockers on the acquisition of schedule-induced drinking and deprivation-induced drinking. *Physiol. Psychol.* **12**, 302–6.

Richmond, G. and Sachs, B. D. (1980). Grooming in Norway rats: the development and adult expression of a complex motor pattern behavior. *Behaviour* **75**, 82–95.

Robbins, T. W. and Koob, G. F. (1980). Selective disruption of displacement behaviour by lesions of the mesolimbic dopamine system. *Nature* **285** 409–11.

Ryan, J. P. and Isaacson, R. L. (1983). Intra-accumbens injections of ACTH induce excessive grooming in rats. *Physiol. Psychol.* **11**, 54–8.

Scatton, B., Worms, P., Lloyd, K. G., and Bartholini, G. (1982). Cortical modulation of striatal function. *Brain Res.* **232**, 331–43.

Scheel-Krüger, J. (1982). GABA in the striato-nigral and striato-pallidal systems as moderator and mediator of striatal functions. *Neurosci. Lett.* **Suppl. 10**, S433.

Scheel-Krüger, J., Magelund, G. and Olianas, M. C. (1981). Role of GABA in the striatal output system: globus pallidus, nucleus entopeduncularis, substantia nigra, and nucleus subthalamicus. *Advances biochem. Psychopharmacol.* **30**, 165.

Seale, T. W., McLanahan, K., Johnson, P., Carney, J. M., and Rennert, O. (1984). Systematic comparison of apomorphine-induced changes in two mouse strains with inherited differences in brain dopamine receptors. *Pharmacol. Biochem. Behav.* **21**, 237–44.

Siever, L. J. and Davis, K. L. (1985). Overview: toward a dysregulation hypothesis of depression. *Am. J. Psychiat.* **142**, 1017–31.

Springer, J. E. and Isaacson, R. L. (1982). Catecholamine alterations in basal ganglia after hippocampal lesions. *Brain Res.* **252**, 185–8.

Springer, J. E., Isaacson, R. L., Ryan, J. P., and Hannigan, J. H., Jr. (1983). Dopamine depletion in nucleus acumbens reduces ACTH(1–24)-induced excessive grooming. *Life Sci.* **33**, 207–11.

Spruijt, B. M. (1985). ACTH and behavior: mechanisms and function. PhD thesis, State University of Utrecht, Utrecht, The Netherlands.

Spruijt, B. M. and Gispen, W. H. (1983). ACTH and grooming behaviour in the rat. In *Hormones and vertebrates* (ed. J. Balthazar, E. Prove, and R. Gilles), pp. 118–36. Springer-Verlag, Berlin.

Spruijt, B. M., Cools, A. R., and Gispen, W. H. (1986a). Dopaminergic modulation of ACTH-induced excessive grooming. *Eur. J. Pharmacol.* **120**, 249–56.

Spruijt, B., Cools, A. R., and Gispen, W. H. (1986b). The colliculus superior modulates ACTH-induced excessive grooming. *Life Sci.* **39**, 461–70.

Spruijt, B. M., Cools, A. R., and Gispen, W. H. (1986c). The periaqueductal gray: a prerequisite for ACTH-induced excessive grooming. *Behav. Brain Res.* **20**, 19–25.

Starr, M. S., Summerhayes, M., and Kilpatrick, I. C. (1983). Interactions between dopamine and γ-aminobutyrate in the substantia nigra: implications for the striatonigral output hypothesis. *Neuroscience* **8**, 547.

Traber, J., Klein, H. R., and Gispen, W. H. (1982). Actions of antidepressant and neuroleptic drugs on ACTH- and novelty-induced behavior in the rat. *Eur. J. Pharmacol.* **80**, 407–14.

Van Wimersma Greidanus, Tj. B. and Rinkel, G. J. E. (1983). Neurotensin suppresses ACTH-induced grooming. *Eur. J. Pharmacol.* **88**, 117–20.

Versteeg, D. H. G. (1980). Interaction of peptides related to ACTH, MSH, and β-LPH with neurotransmitters in the brain. *Pharmacol. Ther.* **11**, 535–57.

Wiegant, V. M., Cools, A. R., and Gispen, W. H. (1977). ACTH-induced excessive grooming involves brain dopamine. *Eur. J. Pharmacol.* **41**, 343–5.

Wiegant, V. M., Jolles, J., Colbern, D., Zimmerman, E., and Gispen, W. H. (1979).

Intracerebroventricular ACTH activates the pituitary–adrenal system: dissociation from a behavioral response. *Life Sci.* **25**, 1791–6.

Wiegant, V.M., Jolles, J., and Gispen, W.H. (1978). β-Endorphin grooming in the rat: single dose tolerance. In *Characteristics and Functions of opioids. Developments in neuroscience, vol. 4* (eds. J.M. van Ree and L. Terenius) pp. 447–50. Elsevier, Amsterdam.

Yuwiler, A. (1971). Stress. In *Handbook of neurochemistry, Vol. 6* (ed. A. Lajtha) pp. 103–71. Plenum Press, New York.

Zwiers, H., Aloyo, V.J., and Gispen, W.H. (1981). Behavioral and neurochemical effects of the new opioid peptide dynorphin(1–13): Comparison with other neuropeptides. *Life Sci.* **31**, 2545–51.

6

Stereotyped and other motor responses to 5-hydroxytryptamine receptor activation

GERALD CURZON

Introduction

Pharmacological stimulation of postsynaptic 5-hydroxytryptamine (5-HT) receptors in rodents leads to complex behavioural syndromes. Their components may include hindlimb abduction, 'wet-dog' or body-shakes (paroxysmal shaking of the head and trunk, side-to-side head-weaving, reciprocal forepaw-treading ('piano playing'), tremor, Straub tail, and increased reactivity to stimuli (reviewed in Jacobs 1976; Gerson and Baldessarini 1980; Green and Heal 1985). Head-weaving and forepaw-treading are stereotyped inasmuch as they are apparently meaningless and repetitive fragments of normal behaviour.

The 5-HT syndrome can be induced by numerous drug treatments, e.g. by giving the amino acid L-tryptophan, (the dietary precursor of 5-HT) after pre-treatment with a monoamine oxidase inhibitor (MAOI; Hess and Doepfner 1961; Grahame-Smith 1971a) or by injecting 5-hydroxytryptophan (5-HTP), a tryptophan metabolite and the immediate precursor of 5-HT. The effect of the latter treatment is potentiated by drugs which either inhibit the neuronal re-uptake of 5-HT or prevent its destruction (Ortmann *et al.* 1980; Ortmann 1984). The syndrome is also elicited by giving a 5-HT re-uptake inhibitor after pre-treatment with the MAOI tranylcypromine (Ashkenazi *et al.* 1983) or by the MAOI phenelzine alone. This drug causes classical dopamine (DA)-dependent behaviour followed some hours later by the 5-HT syndrome (Dourish *et al.* 1982). The syndrome is also induced by 5-HT releasers such as *p*-chloroamphetamine and fenfluramine (Trulson and Jacobs 1976), phenylethylamines (Hwang and Van Woert 1979, 1980a, b; Dourish 1982), and α-methyltryptamine (Marsden 1980), as well as by drugs which stimulate postsynaptic 5-HT receptors directly, e.g. 5-methoxy-N,N-dimethyltryptamine (5-MeODMT; Grahame-Smith

1971*b*), LSD (Trulson *et al.* 1976*b*), and 8-hydroxy-2-(di-n-propylamino) tetralin (8-OH-DPAT; Tricklebank *et al.* 1984; Dourish *et al.* 1985). The agonist quipazine also causes the syndrome (Green *et al.* 1976) although this may partly reflect presynaptic actions of the drug (Fuller *et al.* 1981).

Many drugs used to elicit the 5-HT syndrome also have other central effects which may have direct behavioural consequences or may enhance or inhibit components of the 5-HT syndrome. For example, the 5-HT releasers *p*-chloroamphetamine and fenfluramine and the DA releaser amphetamine when given at high dosage lose their specificity of action and release both transmitters so that complex behavioural patterns occur which include classical DA-dependent components, components of the 5-HT syndrome, and backward walking (Taylor *et al.* 1974; Sloviter *et al.* 1978*a*; Lees *et al.* 1979; Curzon *et al.* 1979; Fernando *et al.* 1980). Furthermore, some drugs only elicit part of the 5-HT syndrome. Thus, phencyclidine causes head-weaving (plus backward walking and circling) but not forepaw-treading and hindlimb-abduction (Nabeshima *et al.* 1984), and N,N-dimethyltryptamine causes hindlimb-abduction, Straub tail (and backward walking), but not forepaw-treading and head-weaving (Jenner *et al.* 1980). The drug 8-OH-DPAT causes forepaw-treading and head-weaving but not tremor, Straub tail, or hindlimb-abduction and elicits two behavioural components which are not part of the syndrome as described by early workers, i.e. flat body posture and episodic tonic extension of a single hindlimb (Tricklebank *et al.* 1984; Dourish *et al.* 1985).

The 5-HT syndrome provides a convenient way of studying postsynaptic responses to drugs affecting serotonergic systems by means of their behavioural effects. However, as it does not occur spontaneously, it obviously does not result from the normal release of 5-HT. Similarly, although the syndrome can occur on giving 5-HTP (when 5-HT synthesis no longer depends on the normal rate-limiting hydroxylation of tryptophan), it is not induced by tryptophan (the normal dietary 5-HT precursor) which only moderately increases brain 5-HT (Carlsson and Lindqvist 1978).

Certain individual components of the 5-HT syndrome, as broadly defined in the first paragraph of this chapter, and related behavioural effects have been proposed as specific indices of responses at 5-HT receptors. The rapid lateral head-twitches or shakes which are similar to pinna reflexes and are shown by mice given 5-HTP (Corne *et al.* 1963) have the advantage of ease of scoring and much evidence indicates that they result from a central effect of 5-HT (Matthews and Smith 1980; Nakamura and Fukushima 1978). They are much more rapid than head-weaving and appear not to be simply a concomitant of whole-body tremor as this is reported to have a strikingly different relationship with 5-HTP dosage (Martin *et al.* 1985). The 'wet-dog' shakes shown by rats are not clearly differentiated from head twitches and have also been proposed as an index of 5-HT receptor stimulation

(Bedard and Pycock 1977). Work by others strengthens this claim (Drust *et al.* 1979; Yap and Taylor 1983). However, 'wet-dog' shakes can be mediated by numerous mechanisms that do not primarily involve 5-HT (Kleinrok and Turski 1980; Turski *et al.* 1984; Drust and Connor 1983). Whether this behaviour, when elicited by dipping rats into cold water (Wei *et al.* 1973), depends on 5-HT is unclear.

Another motor behaviour of related interest occurs in guinea-pigs given 5-HTP (Klawans *et al.* 1973), L-tryptophan + MAOI, or 5-HT agonists (Chadwick *et al.* 1978). These animals show synchronous fore- and hindlimb myoclonic jerks. 5-HTP causes somewhat similar behaviour in human infants (Coleman 1971) and exacerbates various myoclonic disorders (Growdon *et al.* 1976) but alleviates post-anoxic intention myoclonus, a condition associated with defective central 5-HT metabolism (Chadwick *et al.* 1975; Growdon *et al.* 1976). (See Stoessl, Chapter 10, this volume, for discussion.)

Treating rats with 1-(3-chlorophenyl) piperazine (mCPP) or 1-[3-(trifluoromethyl)phenyl]piperazine (TFMPP), drugs thought previously to act mainly as 5-HT_{1B} receptor agonists, causes not motor behaviour but hypolocomotion (Lucki and Frazer 1982*a*). These substances have now been shown to cause hypolocomotion (Kennett and Curzon 1988*a*), hypophagia (Kennett and Curzon 1988*b*), and anxiety-like behaviour (Kennett *et al.* 1989) mainly by action at 5-HT_{1C} receptors. This agrees with recent binding data (Hoyer 1988*a*).

Evaluating the 5-HT syndrome

The behavioural complexity of the 5-HT syndrome has long been recognized (Hess and Doepfner 1961; Grahame-Smith 1971*a*). Furthermore, some of the earlier descriptions may have incorporated behavioural effects of the MAOI drugs given which were not specifically related to 5-HT changes. They also sometimes included the gross toxicological effects which eventually resulted from these treatments. Much valuable work has been done (especially before the present decade, e.g. Green and Grahame-Smith 1976*a*, 1978) in which the syndrome was assessed simply in terms of increased locomotion measured with commercial activity meters. However, these were often hardly influenced by many components of the 5-HT syndrome and largely reflected the hyperactivity caused by many drug treatments which provoke the syndrome. The hyperactivity is at least partly mediated by associated activation of dopaminergic systems (Crow and Deakin 1977; Jenner *et al.* 1980; Marsden 1980; Deakin and Dashwood 1981). It often exhibits a very different time course from that of the other behavioural components and can even be potentiated by 5-HT receptor antagonists

(Dourish 1982). Uncertainties in the interpretation of this kind of data are compounded by pharmacological evidence that 5-HT inhibits DA-dependent locomotion (Warbritton *et al.* 1978; Jones *et al.* 1981) and by the proposal (albeit contested) that it can also cause locomotor hyperactivity by action at certain 5-HT receptors (see below). In view of these complexities it is not surprising that the 5-HT syndrome as elicited by different means is associated with very different intensities of locomotion.

An 'all-or-none' procedure (Method I) for assessing the 5-HT syndrome (Trulson and Jacobs 1976; Sloviter *et al.* 1980) represents an advance on methods based on the use of activity meters as it depends specifically on behaviour resulting from activation of 5-HT receptors. Trulson and Jacobs considered the syndrome to be present if the rat showed at least four of the following six signs: tremor, rigidity, reciprocal forepaw-treading, Straub tail, hindlimb-abduction, and lateral head-weaving. Sloviter *et al.* (1978*a, b*) defined the syndrome as present if rats simultaneously exhibited forepaw-treading, head-weaving (or head tremor), and hindlimb-abduction. However, as has been pointed out for amphetamine-induced behaviour (Thomas and Handley 1978; Fray *et al.* 1980), methods based on summating groups of behavioural components obscure or ignore changes of specific components and involve the assumption that all components reflect different degrees of activation of a common mechanism. Similar criticisms are applicable to 5-HT-dependent behaviour. For example, although the behavioural syndrome after *p*-chloroamphetamine treatment has been assessed by summating different components (Trulson and Jacobs 1976), these have different time courses (Deakin and Green 1978) and dose dependencies (Fernando and Curzon 1981). Other limitations of methods based on combining scores for a defined group of components of the 5-HT syndrome derive from the fact that some drugs only induce certain components (see Introduction to this chapter). Some of the above problems are also relevant to the procedure (Method II) used by Fernando and Curzon (1981) in which four individual behavioural components (forepaw-treading, hindlimb-abduction, body shakes, Straub tail) were scored separately but summated.

A procedure (Method III) based on Andrews *et al.* (1982) in which individual components are separately assessed in each of a number of observation periods is as follows. Each intermittent behavioural component (head-weaving, forepaw-treading) was assessed on a 0–4 scale; 0 absent; 1 present once; 2 present several times; 3 present frequently; 4 present continuously. Continuous behavioural components (hindlimb-abduction, Straub tail, tremor) were assessed on a 0–4 intensity scale. 0 absent; 1 perceptible; 2 weak; 3 medium; 4 maximal.

Although between-observer concordance is high for method III, it involves an element of subjectivity. An alternative procedure which is less vulnerable to this criticism involves the recording of total times spent in the

performance of each behavioural component using hand-held counters and
stopwatches (Dourish *et al.* 1985) or computer-supported analysis of
videotape recordings of behaviour (Dourish *et al.* 1986).

Table 6.1 strikingly illustrates that different components of the 5-HT
syndrome are mediated by different mechanisms and that methods I, II, and
III can lead to different conclusions. According to method I, the DA agonist
apomorphine significantly inhibited the syndrome elicited by 5-MeODMT.
However, method II indicated that it was without effect, while independent
assessment of each component by Method III revealed that apomorphine
significantly inhibited hindlimb-abduction and Straub tail but significantly
enhanced forepaw treading.

Mechanisms mediating the 5-HT syndrome and related behaviour

The requirement for 5-HT

Investigations of presynaptic aspects of treatments which cause the 5-HT
syndrome underline its essentially pharmacological rather than physiological
importance. For example, it is not reported to appear following raphe
stimulation which presumably leads to 5-HT release from vesicles by an
exocytotic mechanism similar to that occurring on spontaneous neuronal
firing. The syndrome is, however, elicited by the 5-HT releaser *p*-
chloroamphetamine even after vesicular storage is disrupted by reserpine
(Kuhn *et al.* 1985). Furthermore, tryptophan + MAOI produce the
syndrome by a grossly non-physiological mechanism highly dependent on
tryptamine (Marsden and Curzon 1978; 1979; Atterwill and Green 1980)
which increases manyfold under these conditions (Durden and Philip 1980).
The mechanism by which the syndrome occurs may involve a synergistic
interaction between tryptamine and 5-HT (Dourish and Greenshaw 1983).
Both amines may also contribute to the myoclonus induced in guinea-pigs by
tryptophan + the MAOI pargyline (Luscombe *et al.* 1983).

The above synergism may explain why behaviour induced by tryptophan
+ the MAOI tranylcypromine is prevented not only by pre-treatment with
the 5-HT synthesis inhibitor *p*-chlorophenylalanine (Grahame-Smith 1971*a*)
but also by a dose of the aromatic amino acid decarboxylase inhibitor
Ro4–4062 sufficient to markedly reduce brain levels of tryptamine but not
5-HT (Marsden and Curzon 1979). The involvement of presynaptic 5-HT in
the syndrome is also indicated by the ability of *p*-chlorophenylalanine
to prevent its production by the 5-HT releasers *p*-chloroamphetamine,
fenfluramine, and *p*-methoxyphenylethylamine (Trulson and Jacobs 1976;
Segal and Weinstock 1983). Work by Dickinson and Curzon (1983) in which
individual behavioural components were scored was in general agreement

Table 6.1 Effect of apomorphine on behaviour induced by 5-MeODMT: assessment by three methods (data from Dickinson et al. 1983)

	Method I	Method II	Method III					
	No. of rats with 5-HT syndrome: no. of rats observed	Summated scores	Individual behavioural scores					
			Hindlimb-abduction	Forepaw-treading	Head-weaving	Straub tail	Tremor
5-MeODMT	8:8	7.8 ± 0.4	10.5 ± 0.6	6.1 ± 0.7	2.7 ± 0.6	1.9 ± 0.3	1.9 ± 0.3
5-MeODMT + apomorphine	2:5†	8.4 ± 0.4	7.0 ± 0.9‡	8.8 ± 0.8*	1.0 ± 0.9	0.3 ± 0.2‡	2.2 ± 0.7
Apomorphine	0:7	1.0 ± 0.6	1.2 ± 0.7	0.1 ± 0.1	0	0	0

Rats were given 5-MeODMT (8 mg/kg intraperitoneally) and/or apomorphine (1.25 mg/kg intraperitoneally) and their behaviour assessed by methods I, II, and III as described in the text. Scores are means ± SEM. Differences from values for rats given 5-MeODMT alone: †$p < 0.05$, Fisher's exact probability test. *$p < 0.05$, **$p < 0.01$, Mann–Whitney U test, 2-tailed.

with the above findings although *p*-chloroamphetamine and amphetamine still caused hindlimb-abduction after 5-HT was depleted by 80 per cent.

A number of studies have concerned the 5-HT neurones which mediate the 5-HT syndrome and related responses. Transection of the neuraxis before administration of MAOI and tryptophan indicates that the syndrome as a whole, (apart from 'wet dog' shakes which were not noted) and hindlimb-abduction, may require neuronal systems in the pons, medulla oblongata, and spinal cord, and that spinal mechanisms alone are responsible for tremor and Straub tail (Jacobs and Klemfuss 1975).

Dickinson *et al.* (1984) investigated the effects of lesions produced by injecting the 5-HT neurotoxin, 5, 7-dihydroxytryptamine (5, 7-DHT), into the spinal cord, striatum, nucleus accumbens, and substantia nigra on 5-HT-dependent responses elicited by amphetamine at high dosage or by 5-MeODMT. Injections into the two latter regions did not alter the behavioural responses substantially. Also, intraspinal 5, 7-DHT treatment did not significantly alter the effects of amphetamine although a reduction of the score for Straub tail occurred which just failed to reach significance. Straub tail elicited by the 5-HT agonist 5-MeODMT was, however, significantly increased by intraspinal 5, 7-DHT. These findings imply that Straub tail is mediated by spinal 5-HT, the 5, 7-DHT pre-treatment enhancing post-synaptic receptor sensitivity (Trulson *et al.* 1976*a*) so that induction of Straub tail behaviour by the agonist is promoted.

Dickinson *et al.* (1984) also found that 5, 7-DHT pre-treatment increased tremor but not other components of behaviour elicited by 5-MeODMT. These findings are consistent with the transection experiments of Jacobs and Klemfuss (1975) and with the report by Deakin and Green (1978) that Straub tail induced by tranylcypromine + 5-MeODMT, is enhanced by treatment with 5, 7-DHT in the spinal cord. They do not confirm the increased hindlimb-abduction which was also described by the latter authors. This difference may be because Dickinson *et al.* injected 5, 7-DHT at T13 whereas Deakin and Green injected it more rostrally at C1–C2 which probably led to depletion of 5-HT in some supraspinal regions. The mediation of tremor, Straub tail, and hindlimb-abduction by 5-HT in the spinal cord or adjacent areas is also indicated by their appearance following intrathecal injection of 5-HT (Larson and Kondzielski 1982).

When Dickinson *et al.* (1984) injected 5, 7-DHT into the striatum, so that 5-HT was depleted in this region but not in the nucleus accumbens, two 5-HT-dependent effects of amphetamine—'wet dog' shakes and backward walking—were inhibited. The inhibition of 'wet dog' shakes points to striatal 5-HT terminals being needed for this behaviour and is consistent with the finding of Bedard and Pycock (1977) that 'wet dog' shakes, induced by 5-HTP, were abolished by section at the level of the posterior, but not the anterior commissure.

The inhibition of backward walking by striatal 5, 7-DHT is consistent with its induction when 5-HT was injected into the striatum of the cat (Cools 1973). In rats, backward walking was elicited by intrastriatal injections of DA or p-hydroxyamphetamine (Fog and Pakkenberg 1971) in doses likely not only to have dopaminergic effects but also to release 5-HT (Sloviter et al. 1978b; Hwang and Van Woert 1980a). The lack of effect of lesions induced by intrastriatal 5, 7-DHT on head-weaving (Dickinson et al. 1984) even though it is abolished by striatalectomy (Jacobs and Klemfuss 1975) is explicable by the finding that this behaviour is prevented by destruction of striatal DA terminals by 6-hydroxydopamine (6-OHDA; Andrews et al. 1982).

The above experiments as a whole suggest that 5-HT-induced behaviour can be divided into three groups requiring (1) striatal 5-HT ('wet dog' shakes and backward walking); (2) spinal 5-HT (Straub tail and tremor); and (3) 5-HT in other but unknown regions (head-weaving, forepaw-treading, hindlimb-abduction).

The role of 5-HT receptors

The previous section concerned the brain loci at which 5-HT elicits different components of the 5-HT syndrome. The inhibition of the syndrome by numerous 5-HT antagonists indicates a requirement for 5-HT receptors (Sloviter et al. 1978a, b; Marsden 1980; Green et al. 1981; Dourish 1982). It is, however, intriguing that, while methysergide blocks the 5-HT syndrome induced by the 5-HT releaser p-methoxyphenylethylamine in the mouse (Hwang and Van Woert 1979), methysergide and other 5-HT antagonists are somewhat surprisingly reported to enhance the behavioural effects of the releaser in the rat (Segal and Weinstock 1983).

Evidence points to at least three types of postsynaptic 5-HT receptor in the brain. Early studies distinguished between $5-HT_1$ and $5-HT_2$ receptors by their high affinities for $[^3H]$-5-HT and $[^3H]$-spiperone respectively (Peroutka and Snyder 1979). Subsequently, the $5-HT_1$ type was divided into $5-HT_{1A}$ and $5-HT_{1B}$ from which $[^3H]$-5-HT was respectively more and less readily displaced by spiperone (Pedigo et al. 1981; Schnellmann et al. 1984). More recent evidence has suggested that the 5-HT sites may be heterogeneous (Asarch et al. 1985; Blurton and Wood 1986) and central $5-HT_{1C}$, $5-HT_{1D}$ and $5-HT_3$ sites have now been identified (Fozard 1987; Hoyer et al. 1988; Hoyer 1988; Kilpatrick et al. 1987). As drugs are identified or developed which bind selectively to the various sites they can be used to distinguish between the mechanisms mediating different components of the syndrome.

Even before drugs which were selective for the different receptors were available, Green et al. (1981) found that 5-HT antagonists had different effects on different components of the syndrome and suggested that the receptors mediating forepaw-treading and head-weaving were not of the same type as those mediating hindlimb-abduction and reactivity. More recently, Lucki et al. (1984) reported that low doses of methysergide and metergoline inhibited numerous components of the 5-HT syndrome elicited by 5-MeODMT with the striking exception of head-weaving. They also used selective 5-HT$_2$ receptor antagonists to distinguish between the 5-HT syndrome defined essentially as by Trulson and Jacobs (1976) and head-twitches. The syndrome was blocked by antagonists which bind comparably at both 5-HT$_1$ and 5-HT$_2$ receptors (i.e. metergoline and methysergide) but not by antagonists which bind much more effectively at 5-HT$_2$ receptors (i.e. ketanserin and pipamperone). It thus appears to depend on 5-HT$_1$ receptors which agrees with the finding that drug treatments which decreased their number also decreased the ability of 5-MeODMT to produce the syndrome (Lucki and Frazer 1982). Head-twitches (elicited by 5-HTP) were blocked by all the 5-HT agonists tested and thus appear to depend on 5-HT$_2$ receptors.

As Lucki et al. point out, head-twitch has tended to be equated with the 5-HT syndrome even though it was not included in standard descriptions (Grahame-Smith 1971a, b; Trulson and Jacobs 1976). The demonstration that different 5-HT-dependent behavioural models may be mediated by different receptors should help to avoid the repetition of past confusions. For example, evidence that 5-HTP-induced head twitches (Peroutka et al. 1981) or tryptamine-induced clonic seizures (Leysen et al. 1978) depend on 5-HT$_2$ receptors has been taken to indicate that these receptors mediate in the 5-HT syndrome.

Although Green et al. (1983) found that the 5-HT syndrome was inhibited by the selective 5-HT$_2$ antagonist pirenperone, this could be due to other effects of the drug (Tricklebank et al. 1984). The latter authors point out that the induction of many components of the syndrome by the agonist 8-OH-DPAT strongly indicates mediation by 5-HT$_{1A}$ receptors as its affinity for these sites is orders of magnitude greater than that for 5-HT$_{1B}$ or 5-HT$_2$ sites (Middlemiss and Fozard 1983). Mediation by 5-HT$_{1B}$ and 5-HT$_{1C}$ receptors appears unlikely since the 5-HT$_{1C}$ selective agonist m-chlorophenylpiperazine (mCPP) and the 5-HT$_{1B}$ selective agonist RU 24969 have little 5-HT syndrome-inducing activity (Sills et al. 1985; Tricklebank et al. 1986). Tricklebank et al. (1984) also showed that haloperidol and other drugs interfering with catecholaminergic transmission reduced 8-OH-DPAT-dependent locomotion, head-weaving, and forepaw-treading. This is consistent with catecholamines also being required for these behavioural components. It is therefore of interest that reserpine pre-treatment did not prevent induction of forepaw-treading or flat body postures by 8-OH-DPAT. Their blockade by the 5-HT$_1$ antagonist (−) pindolol and the 5-HT$_{1A}$ antagonist spiperone point to 5-HT$_{1A}$ receptors being involved. This possibility is strengthened by the inability of α_1-adrenoreceptor, DA-receptor, or 5-HT$_2$-receptor antagonists to prevent forepaw-treading or flat body posture

(Tricklebank *et al.* 1984). Essentially similar results were obtained when the 5-HT syndrome was induced by 5 MeODMT (Tricklcbank *et al.* 1985). These two studies however reveal an apparent paradox which demands further investigation, i.e. how can these two 5-HT agonists elicit behaviour which is blocked by haloperidol in normal rats but not in reserpine-treated animals?

In common with the 5-HT syndrome, the myoclonic jerks of brainstem origin shown by guinea-pigs given 5-HTP (Chadwick *et al.* 1978) may depend on the stimulation of $5\text{-}HT_1$ receptors. This is indicated by the finding by Luscombe *et al.* (1984) that agonists such as 5-MeODMT and dimethyltryptamine which are relatively selective for these receptors (Sills *et al.* 1984) are also highly potent inducers of myoclonus while piperazine-containing agonists, which Sills *et al.* find to be selective for $5\text{-}HT_{1B}$ receptors, are much less potent. However this topic needs further investigation in the light of present knowledge on the effects of agonists and antagonists at 5-HT receptor subtypes.

The question of how drug-provoked 5-HT- and DA-dependent changes interact to elicit locomotor activity has been briefly mentioned in the discussion of methods of evaluating the 5-HT syndrome. Recent work on the behavioural effects of the drug RU 24969 is of some relevance. RU 24969 is a $5\text{-}HT_1$ agonist with some selectivity for the $5\text{-}HT_{1B}$ subtype (Sills *et al.* 1984; Tricklebank *et al.* 1986). Rats given RU 24969 show little 5-HT syndrome-like activity unless they are pre-treated with reserpine when forepaw-treading and flat body posture are enhanced (Tricklebank *et al.* 1986). However, RU 24969 causes profound locomotor stimulation. Green *et al.* (1984) suggest that this occurs through action at $5\text{-}HT_1$ receptors but Tricklebank *et al.* (1986) were unable to prevent the behaviour using drugs having $5\text{-}HT_1$- and $5\text{-}HT_2$-receptor blocking activity. Indeed, in agreement with Green *et al.* they noted that metergoline (a drug with high affinity for both types of receptor) tended to enhance the locomotor activity induced by RU 24969. In general, the locomotor activity induced by serotonergic drugs, such as RU 24969 (Green *et al.* 1984; Tricklebank *et al.* 1986), 8-OH-DPAT (Tricklebank *et al.* 1984), and 5-MeODMT (Tricklebank *et al.* 1985), is readily shown to be inhibited by drugs which are antagonists at catecholamine receptors. It has not been convincingly shown to depend on 5-HT.

Requirement for DA

The involvement of DA in the 5-HT syndrome has been the subject of controversy in the earlier literature (Jacobs *et al.* 1975; Heal *et al.* 1976; Sloviter *et al.* 1978*a*; Curzon *et al.* 1979; Fernando *et al.* 1980). Much of this disagreement derives from the inadequacies of the behavioural scoring methods used and from the misinterpretation of the effects of non-specific drugs. More recently Andrews *et al.* (1982) reinvestigated the role of DA in 5-HT-dependent behaviour by determining the effects of injecting the DA neurotoxin 6-hydroxydopamine (6-OHDA) into the substantia nigra, ventral tegmentum, striatum, and nucleus accumbens on 5-HT-dependent responses elicited by amphetamine at high dosage.

Results of the above study are shown in Table 6.2. None of the classical 5-HT behavioural components induced by amphetamine were altered in intensity when DA in the accumbens was specifically depleted but each of the other lesions caused a characteristic spectrum of changes. Head-weaving was significantly decreased by these three lesions, all of which decreased striatal DA. This agrees with Jacobs and Klemfuss (1975) who found that head-weaving was decreased after striatalectomy. Reciprocal forepaw-treading was significantly decreased only by the nigral and tegmental lesions. These decreased DA in both the striatum and accumbens. The results are consistent with DA being needed for the above two repetitive behaviours. Whether DA specifically contained in the above terminal regions is required for reciprocal forepaw-treading is unclear; the ability of pargyline + L-tryptophan to induce it after striatalectomy (Jacobs and Klemfuss 1975) argues otherwise. The results of Andrews *et al.* (1982) agree with the report that head-weaving and forepaw-treading due to the 5-HT agonist 8-OH-DPAT are inhibited by haloperidol and other drugs which interfere with catecholaminergic transmission (Tricklebank *et al.* 1984). They are also consistent with the enhancement by apomorphine of forepaw-treading due to 5-MeODMT (Dickinson and Curzon 1983). However, apomorphine inhibited the associated head-weaving. Nevertheless, the above findings as a whole suggest that 5-HT-dependent stereotyped behaviour (head-weaving and reciprocal forepaw-treading) is also dependent on DA. This is of some interest in view of the role of DA in classical stereotyped behaviour and the finding by Andrews *et al.* (1982) that 5-HT-induced behaviour without obvious stereotyped character (body-shakes and hindlimb-abduction) appeared to require neither striatal nor accumbens DA. Indeed they tended to increase when DA levels were reduced, suggesting that, on the contrary, they were inhibited by DA.

The increase of body-shakes noted by Andrews *et al.* (1982) in nigrally lesioned rats agrees with Bedard and Pycock (1977) who showed that body-shakes provoked by 5-HTP were decreased by DA agonists or by amphetamine (given at 4 mg/kg—a much lower dose than that needed to elicit the 5-HT syndrome). The myoclonus induced in the guinea-pig by 5-HTP (Volkman *et al.* 1978; Weiner *et al.* 1979) is similarly inhibited by DA. Hindlimb-abduction, the other 5-HT-dependent behaviour induced by amphetamine, appears to be inhibited by striatal DA as it was significantly increased by striatal lesions but not by lesions of the accumbens (Andrews *et al.* 1982). However, interpretation of the effects of the other

Table 6.2 Effects of 6-OHDA lesions on 5-HT-dependent responses to D-amphetamine (25 mg/kg intraperitoneally) (data from Andrews et al. 1982)

Lesion site	Decrease of DA (per cent)		Behaviour				
	Nucleus accumbens	Striatum	Head-weaving	Forepaw-treading	Body-shakes	Hindlimb-abduction	Backward walking
Substantia nigra	35	70	↓	↓	↑	NS	↓
Ventral tegmentum	56	55	↓	↓	NS	↑	↓
Striatum	NS	61	↓	↑	NS	↑	↓
Nucleus accumbens	50	NS	NS	NS	NS	NS	N

The arrows indicate statistically significant increases and decreases. NS, not significant.

6-OHDA lesions on hindlimb-abduction is less clear as it was increased by ventral tegmental but not by nigral lesions even though both considerably decreased striatal DA. This apparent anomaly may reflect 'response incompability' (Robbins and Iversen 1973) as hindlimb-abduction and the increased locomotion in the nigrally lesioned rats would tend to be mutually exclusive.

Evidence that non-stereotyped components of 5-HT-dependent behaviour were inhibited by increased activity at DA-receptors was also obtained by Dickinson, Jackson, and Curzon (1983). Thus, apomorphine inhibited the induction of both hindlimb-abduction and Straub tail by 5-MeODMT. Similarly, Deakin and Dashwood (1981) showed that the hindlimb-abduction elicited by p-chloroamphetamine was enhanced by the catecholamine depletor α-methyl-p-tyrosine. However, unlike 6-OHDA, it did not impair forepaw-treading or head-weaving. This difference could be because 6-OHDA has an 'all-or-none' effect on DA neurons while α-methyl-p-tyrosine causes a general, but not necessarily complete inhibition of catecholamine synthesis throughout the brain.

The role of DA in backward walking is indicated by its occurence together with more commonly seen components of the 5-HT syndrome when high doses are given of drugs which can lead to stimulation of both 5-HT- and DA-receptors e.g. amphetamine, fenfluramine, or p-chloroamphetamine (Lees et al. 1979; Curzon et al. 1979; Fernando et al. 1980), β-phenylethylamine (Dourish 1982), LSD (Bonetti and Bondiolotti 1980), N,N-dimethyltryptamine (Jenner et al. 1980), 5-HTP (Shimomura et al. 1981), and 2, 5-dimethoxy-4-methylamphetamine (Yamamato and Ueki 1981). The blockade of backward walking by DA-antagonists is also consistent with a requirement for DA (Lees et al. 1979; Fernando et al. 1980; Shimomura et al. 1981) although the relative effects of a series of DA antagonists were also explicable in terms of blockade of 5-HT-receptors (Fernando et al. 1980). However, involvement of both transmitters is indicated by the induction of backward walking when 5-HT- and DA-releasers are given together at doses which are separately ineffective (Curzon et al. 1979). Furthermore, Andrews et al. (1982) showed that backward locomotion after injection of amphetamine was strikingly inhibited in rats with 6-OHDA lesions which significantly decreased striatal DA. It was unaffected when DA depletion was restricted to the nucleus accumbens (Table 6.2). These results could be due to striatal DA being specifically required for backward walking. Alternatively, 'response incompatibility' could be involved as striatal and ventral tegmental lesions which prevented backward walking also increased an incompatible behaviour, hindlimb-abduction.

As DA appears to be needed for some 5-HT-dependent behavioural components and appears to inhibit others, it is hardly surprising that there has been disagreement on its role in 5-HT behaviour when assessed globally. Thus, some groups (Trulson and Jacobs 1976; Sloviter *et al.* 1978*b*; Fernando *et al.* 1980) found no evidence for DA involvement while others (Silbergeld and Hruska 1979; Marsden 1980) found that neuroleptics blocked 5-HT-dependent behaviours.

5-HT and DA requirements of different components of 5-HT behaviour in the rat

The investigations described above permit tentative distinctions to be made between the components of the 5-HT syndrome according to their requirement for 5-HT in different brain regions and for different 5-HT receptors and their different relationships with DA (Table 6.3). This scheme is consistent with much of the data in the literature although, as indicated above, some apparently contradictory findings have also been reported. These may well reflect problems of drug specificity or the possibility that DA at different sites has different effects on 5-HT-dependent behaviour or even that the behaviour can be mediated by more than one receptor mechanism (Goodwin and Green 1985).

Table 6.3 reveals the strikingly different dependencies of various components of 5-HT-elicited behaviour. It also indicates some of the more obvious gaps in our knowledge and should, if confirmed by future findings, be of use in the study of how drug, environmental, and other influences affect aminergic outputs.

The role of noradrenalin (NA)

The 5-HT syndrome elicited by the MAOI tranylcypromine + tryptophan is blocked by the adrenergic β-antagonist (–) propranolol (Green and Grahame-Smith 1976*b*) and other non-specific (i.e. β_1 + β_2) adrenergic blockers which penetrate readily to the brain (Costain and Green 1978). However, as these drugs in their (–) forms are also antagonists at 5-HT$_{1A}$ and 5-HT$_{1B}$ receptors (Middlemiss *et al.* 1977; Nahorski and Wilcocks 1983) and only the (–) but not the (+) form of one of them (pindolol) blocked the 5-HT-dependent behaviour elicited by 8-OH-DPAT and 5-MeODMT (Tricklebank *et al.* 1984, 1985) it is likely that actions at 5-HT- rather than NA-receptors are responsible for their effects on the 5-HT syndrome. More direct evidence is also against NA neuronal activity being obligatory for the syndrome as 6-OHDA lesions of central NA pathways decreased neither the intensity nor the duration of head-weaving, forepaw-treading, hindlimb-abduction, and Straub tail elicited by the 5-HT agonist quipazine (Nimgaonkar *et al.* 1983).

Although NA does not seem to be obligatory for the 5-HT syndrome, Ortmann *et al.* (1981) showed that the syndrome induced by 5-HTP was potentiated by β-agonists when injected either peripherally or centrally and

Table 6.3 Characteristics of components of 5-HT-dependent behaviour in rodents

| Behaviour | 5-HT requirements | | Effects of DA on response[3] | Inhibition by low dose of metergoline[4] | Induction by 5-HT agonist after reserpine[5] |
	Region[1]	Receptors[2]			
Head weaving		5-HT_{1A}	+	No	No
Forepaw treading		5-HT_{1A}	+	Yes	Yes
Hindlimb abduction			–	Yes	
Flat body posture		5-HT_{1A}		Yes	Yes
Straub tail	Spinal	5-HT_1	–	Yes	
Tremor	Spinal	5-HT_1		Yes	
Head twitches		5-HT_2			
Body shakes	Striatum		–		
Backward walking	Striatum		+		

The following are principal references. See text for fuller evidence for and against the above classification. [1] Dickinson et al. (1984). [2] Lucki et al. (1984); Tricklebank et al. (1984, 1985). [3] Andrews et al. (1983); Dickinson and Curzon (1983). [4] Lucki et al. (1984). [5] Tricklebank et al. (1984, 1985).

Cowen *et al.* (1982) showed that the syndrome induced by quipazine was potentiated by the β-agonist clenbuterol. As this drug did not elicit the 5-HT syndrome when given alone and as the potentiation was blocked by the central β_1 antagonist metoprolol but not by the peripheral β_1-antagonist atenolol or the β_2-antagonist butoxamine, it probably acts by facilitating central β_1-dependent noradrenergic transmission and not by a direct effect on 5-HT receptors.

A similar mechanism is probably responsible for the potentiating effect of the above drugs on 5-HT-dependent head twitches in mice (Ortmann *et al.* 1981; Cowen *et al.* 1982). While agonist action at central β_1-receptors facilitates head twitch, α_2-adrenoreceptor agonists inhibited the twitches induced by central 5-HT injection and α_2-antagonists potentiated them (Handley and Brown 1982). As for the role of NA in backward walking, drug experiments on the amphetamine-(Sloviter *et al.* 1978a; Curzon *et al.* 1980) and 5-HTP-(Shimomura *et al.* 1981) induced behaviour are not clearly interpretable.

Behavioural responses to 5-HT receptor activation as experimental tools

The behavioural effects of 5-HT receptor stimulation as discussed in this chapter provide a valuable means of detecting and investigating 5-HT-dependent changes of brain function *in vivo*. The following brief account is intended primarily as a signpost to the substantial literature describing these applications.

For example, Grahame-Smith, Green and their colleagues have used the above behavioural approach to study the effect of ECT on depressive illness. When rats were given an electroconvulsive shock each day for approximately 10 days, they showed increased behavioural and electrophysiological responses to drug treatments which increased 5-HT-dependent behaviour (Green and Heal 1985; Vetulani *et al.* 1981; DeMontigny 1984; Wielosz 1985). Various other changes also occurred but the important point in the present context is that the results suggest that the antidepressant action of ECT may depend on enhancement of 5-HT-dependent responses.

In somewhat related work, behavioural deficits following immobilization stress have been used as a rat model of depression and enhancement of components of the 5-HT syndrome on repeated immobilization has been used as an index of adaptive changes which normally oppose the development of depression (Kennett *et al.* 1985a). Both normalization of behaviour and enhancement of response to 5-MeODMT on repeated immobilization were opposed by corticosterone (Dickinson *et al.* 1985; Kennett *et al.* 1985b) and by female sex (Kennett *et al.* 1986). These findings strengthen the

analogy to depressive illness as this is associated with elevated glucocorticoids and has a higher incidence in women than in men.

The two examples described above are mutually consistent as they suggest
that enhanced behavioural responses to agonist action at 5-HT receptors are
indices of both the antidepressant action of ECT and of the effectiveness of
normal mechanisms which oppose stress-induced depression. The 5-HT
syndrome has also been used to study antidepressant drug action. Here,
results are less clear-cut. Although the syndrome when elicited by tranylcypromine + tryptophan is enhanced by acute treatment with 5-HT re-uptake
inhibitors, their antidepressant effects require chronic administration and in
these circumstances some workers report that the syndrome is attenuated
(Hwang et al. 1980) and others that it is unimpaired (Lucki and Frazer 1982).
Furthermore, Ogren et al. (1985) find that chronic antidepressant treatment
can increase or decrease the head twitch response to 5-MeODMT according
to dosage and time schedules. It should be noted that these three studies
differ with respect to species, experimental design, and behaviour observed.

5-HT-dependent behaviour has also been used in the investigation of
hallucinogenic drugs. Sloviter et al. (1980) found that their potencies in man
were largely paralleled by their ability to induce the 5-HT syndrome in the
rat as indicated by an 'all-or none' method and it has been suggested that
the backward walking which results from concurrent release of 5-HT and
DA may directly reflect hallucinogenic activity. Thus, high doses of
amphetamine cause backward walking in the rat and schizophrenia-like
symptoms including both aural and visual hallucinations in man (Woodrow
et al. 1978). Furthermore, Cools (1973) noted that injecting amphetamine
into the anteroventral part of the cat caudate had similar effects to 5-HT
which caused backward walking and activities resembling hunting of non-
existent prey. Numerous other drugs which cause backward walking also
cause hallucinations (reviewed Curzon et al. 1980). The proposal that backward walking in laboratory animals is a response to hallucination (Davis
et al. 1978) thus appears attractive.

The 5-HT syndrome has been applied to the study of anticonvulsant drug
action. Thus, chronic treatment with phenytoin caused apparent subsensitivity of 5-HT receptors insofar as the response to 5-MeODMT was
decreased (Lalonde and Botez 1985). This finding has some consistency with
the opposite effects of both electroconvulsive shock and convulsant drug
treatments as these increase the response to 5-MeODMT (Green and
Grahame-Smith 1978). It is also of interest in view of pharmacological
evidence of an inverse relationship between serotoninergic activity and
seizure susceptibility (Wada et al. 1972).

A few investigators have used 5-HT-dependent behaviour to investigate
central abnormalities in metabolic and neurological disorders. For example,
Trulson and MacKenzie (1981) report that the 5-HT syndrome is attenuated

in rats with streptozotocin-induced diabetes. This, however, is probably largely a result of impaired transport to the brain of the drugs used to induce the syndrome. Another group (Goudsmit *et al.* 1981) find that infection with scrapie markedly enhances the 5-HT syndrome-like behaviour shown by hamsters given either 5-HTP or quipazine.

A number of reports reveal that 5-HT-dependent behaviour can be influenced by endocrine changes, e.g. the impairment of the 5-HT syndrome when induced by 5-MeODMT after chronic corticosterone treatment (Dickinson *et al.* 1985). There are also various indications that thyroid activity enhances responses to 5-HT (Atterwill 1981; Brochet *et al.* 1985). These results imply that the 5-HT syndrome may be of considerable value as a means of studying central consequences of normal and pathological endocrine changes.

Finally, very recent work provides putative behavioural tests of activation of 5-HT$_1$ receptor subtypes. Thus, the hyperphagic effect of 8-OH-DPAT (Dourish *et al.* 1985), the hypophagic effect of RU 24969 (Kennett *et al.* 1987) and the hypolocomotor effect of mCPP (Kennett and Curzon 1988*a*) provide indices of the activation of presynaptic 5-HT$_{1A}$, postsynaptic 5-HT$_{1B}$ and postsynaptic 5-HT$_{1C}$ receptors respectively. These three receptor selective behavioural probes may be expected to have many applications, when one considers how valuable measurements even of the global 5-HT syndrome have been.

Acknowledgements

A. R. Green and G. A. Kennett are thanked for helpful discussions.

References

Andrews, C. D., Fernando, J. C. R., and Curzon, G. (1982). Differential involvement of dopamine-containing tracts in 5-hydroxytryptamine-dependent behaviours caused by amphetamine in large doses. *Neuropharmacology* **21**, 63–8.

Asarch, K. B., Ransom, R. W., and Shih, J. C. (1985). 5-HT-1a and 5-HT-1b selectivity of two phenylpiperazine derivatives: evidence for 5-HT-1b heterogeneity. *Life Sci.* **36**, 1265–73.

Ashkenazi, R., Finberg, J. P. M., and Youdim, M. B. H. (1983). Behavioural hyperactivity in rats treated with selective monoamine oxidase inhibitors and LM5008, a selective 5-hydroxytryptamine uptake blocker. *Br. J. Pharmacol.* **79**, 765–70.

Atterwill, C. K. (1981). Effect of acute and chronic tri-iodothyronine (T$_3$) administration to rats on central 5-HT- and dopamine-mediated behavioural responses and related brain biochemistry. *Neuropharmacology* **20**, 131–44.

Atterwill, C.K. and Green, A.R. (1980). Responses of developing rats to L-tryptophan plus an MAOI. I. monitoring changes in behaviour, brain 5HT and tryptophan. *Neuropharmacology* **19**, 325–35.

Bedard, P. and Pycock, C.J. (1977). 'Wet-dog' shake behaviour in the rat: a possible quantitative model of central 5-hydroxytryptamine activity. *Neuropharmacology* **16**, 663–70.

Blurton, P.A. and Wood, M.D. (1986). Identification of multiple binding sites for ³H-5-hydroxytryptamine in the rat CNS. *J. Neurochem.* **46**, 1392–8.

Bonetti, E.P. and Bondiolotti, G. (1980). Backward locomotion in rats, a specific stereotyped behaviour. *Experientia* **36**, 705.

Brochet, D., Martin, P., Soubrie, P., and Simon, P. (1985). Effects of triiodothyronine on the 5-hydroxytryptophan-induced head twitch and its potentiation by antidepressants in mice. *Eur.J.Pharmacol.* **112**, 411–14.

Carlsson, A. and Lindqvist, M. (1978). Dependence of 5-HT and catecholamine synthesis on concentrations of precursor amino acids in rat brain. *Naunyn-Schmiedeberg's Arch.Pharmacol.* **303**, 157–64.

Chadwick, D., Harris, R., Jenner, P., Reynolds, E.H., and Marsden, C.D. (1975). Manipulation of brain serotonin in the treatment of myoclonus. *Lancet* **ii**, 434–5.

Chadwick, D., Hallett, M., Jenner, P., and Marsden, C.D. (1978). 5-Hydroxytryptophan-induced myoclonus in guinea-pig. *J.neurol.Sci.* **35**, 157–65.

Coleman, M. (1971). Infantile spasms associated with 5-hydroxytryptophan administration in patients with Down's syndrome. *Neurology* **21**, 911–19.

Cools, A.R. (1973). Serotonin: a behaviourally active compound in the caudate nucleus of cats. *Isr. J.med.Sci.* **9**, 5–16.

Corne, S.J., Pickering, R.W., and Warner, B.T. (1963). A method for assessing the effects of drugs on the central actions of 5-hydroxytryptamine. *Br.J.Pharmacol.* **20**, 106–20.

Costain, D.W. and Green, A.R. (1978). β-adrenoreceptor antagonists inhibit the behavioural responses of rats to increased brain 5-hydroxytryptamine. *Br.J.Pharmacol.* **64**, 193–200.

Cowen, P.J., Grahame-Smith, D.G., Green, A.R., and Heal, D.J. (1982). β-adrenoreceptor agonists enhance 5-hydroxytryptamine-mediated behavioural responses. *Br.J.Pharmacol.* **76**, 265–70.

Crow, T.J. and Deakin, J.W.F. (1977). Role of tryptaminergic mechanisms in the elements of the behavioural syndrome evoked by tryptophan and a monoamine oxidase inhibitor. *Br.J.Pharmacol.* **59**, 461.

Curzon, G., Fernando, J.C.R., and Lees, A.J. (1979). Backward walking and circling: behavioural responses induced by drug treatments which cause simultaneous release of catecholamines and 5-hydroxytryptamine. *Br.J.Pharmacol.* **66**, 573–9.

Curzon, G., Fernando, J.C.R., and Lees, A.J. (1980). Behaviour provoked by simultaneous release of dopamine and serotonin: possible relevance to psychotic behavior. In *Enzymes and neurotransmitters in mental disease* (ed. E. Usdin, T.L. Sourkes, and M.B.H. Youdim), pp. 411–30. John Wiley & Sons, New York.

Davis, W.M., Bedford, W.A., Buelke, J.L., Guinn, M.M., Hatoum, H.T., Waters, I.W., Wilson, M.C., and Braude, M.C. (1978). Acute toxicity and gross behavioural effects of amphetamine, four methoxyamphetamines and mescaline in rodents, dogs and monkeys. *Toxicol.appl. Pharmacol.* **45**, 49–62.

Deakin, J.W.F. and Dashwood, M.R. (1981). The differential neurochemical bases of the behaviours elicited by serotonergic agents and by a combination of a monoamine oxidase inhibitor and L-dopa. *Neuropharmacology* **20**, 123–30.

Deakin, J.F.W. and Green, A.R. (1978). The effects of putative 5-hydroxytryptamine antagonists on the behaviour produced by administration of tranylcypromine and L-DOPA to rats. *Br.J.Pharmacol.* **64**, 201–9.

DeMontigny, C. (1984). Electroconvulsive shock treatments enhance responsiveness of forebrain neurons to serotonin. *J.Pharmacol.exp. Ther.* **228**, 230–4.

Dickinson, S.L. and Curzon, G. (1983). Roles of dopamine and 5-hydroxytryptamine in stereotyped and non-stereotyped behaviour. *Neuropharmacology* **22**, 805–12.

Dickinson, S.L., Jackson, A., and Curzon, G. (1983). Effect of apomorphine on behaviour induced by 5-methoxy-N,N-dimethyltryptamine; three different scoring methods give three different conclusions. *Psychopharmacology* **80**, 196–7.

Dickinson, S.L., Andrews, C.D., and Curzon, G. (1984). The effects of lesions produced by 5,7-dihydroxytryptamine on 5-hydroxytryptamine-mediated behaviour induced by amphetamine in large doses in the rat. *Neuropharmacology* **23**, 423–9.

Dickinson, S., Kennett, G.A., and Curzon, G. (1985). Reduced 5-hydroxytryptamine dependent behaviour in rats following chronic corticosterone treatment. *Brain Res.* **345**, 10–18.

Dourish, C.T. (1982). A pharmacological analysis of the hyperactivity syndrome induced by β-phenylethylamine in the mouse. *Br.J.Pharmacol.* **77**, 129–39.

Dourish, C.T., Boulton, A.A., and Dyck, L.E. (1982). Biphasic behavioural stimulation induced by a monoamine oxidase-inhibiting antidepressant. *Prog.Neuropsychopharmacol.* **6**, 382–8.

Dourish, C.T. and Greenshaw, A.J. (1983). Effects of intraventricular tryptamine and 5-hydroxytryptamine on spontaneous motor activity in the rat. *Res.Commun.Psychol.Psychiat.Behav.* **8**, 1–9.

Dourish, C.T., Hutson, P.H. and Curzon, G. (1985). Low doses of the putative serotonin agonist 8-hydroxy-2-(di-n-propylamino) tetralin (8-OH-DPAT) elicit feeding in the rat. *Psychopharmacology* **86**, 197–204.

Dourish, C.T. Hutson, P.H. and Curzon G. (1986). Parachlorophenylalanine prevents feeding induced by the serotonin agonist 8-hydroxy-2-(di-n-propylamino) tetralin (8-OH-DPAT). *Psychopharmacology* **89**, 467–471.

Drust, E.G. and Connor, J.D. (1983). Pharmacological analysis of shaking behaviour induced by enkephalins, thyrotropin-releasing hormone or serotonin in rats: evidence for different mechanisms. *J.Pharmacol.exp.Ther.* **224**, 148–54.

Drust, E.G., Sloviter, R.S., and Connor, J.D. (1979). Effect of morphine on 'wet-dog' shakes caused by cerebroventricular injection of serotonin. *Pharmacology* **18**, 299–305.

Durden, D. A. and Philips, S. R. (1980). Kinetic measurements of the turnover rates of phenylethylamine and tryptamine *in vivo* in the rat brain. *J.Neurochem.* **34**, 1725–32.

Fernando, J. C. R. and Curzon, G. (1981). Behavioural responses to drugs releasing 5-hydroxytryptamine and catecholamines: effects of treatments altering precursor concentrations in brain. *Neuropharmacology* **20**, 115–22.

Fernando, J. C. R., Lees, A. J., and Curzon, G. (1980). Differential antagonism by neuroleptics of backward-walking and other behaviours caused by amphetamine at high dosage. *Neuropharmacology* **19**, 549–53.

Fog, R. and Pakkenberg, H. (1971). Behavioural effects of dopamine and *p*-hydroxyamphetamine injected into corpus striatum of rats. *Exp.Neurol.* **31**, 75–86.

Fozard, J. R. (1987). 5-HT: the enigma variations. *TIPS* **8**, 501–6.

Fray, P. J., Sahakian, B. J., Robbins, T. W., Koob, G. F., and Iversen, S. D. (1980). An observational method for quantifying the behavioural effects of dopamine agonists: contrasting effects of *d*-amphetamine and apomorphine. *Psychopharmacology* **69**, 253–9.

Fuller, R. W., Snoddy, H. D., Mason, N. R., Hemrick-Luecke, S. K., and Clemens, J. A. (1981). Substituted piperazines as central serotonin agonists: comparative specificity of the postsynaptic actions of quipazine and *m*-trifluoromethyl-phenylpiperazine. *J.Pharmacol. exp. Ther.* **218**, 636–41.

Gerson, S. C. and Baldessarini, R. J. (1980). Motor effects of serotonin in the central nervous system. *Life Sci.* **27**, 1435–51.

Goodwin, G. M. and Green, A. R. (1985). A behavioural and biochemical study in mice and rats of putative selective agonists and antagonists for 5-HT_1 and 5-HT_2 receptors. *Br.J.Pharmacol.* **84**, 743–53.

Goudsmit, J., Rohwer, R. G., Silbergeld, E. K., and Gajdusek, D. C. (1981). Hypersensitivity to central receptor activation in scrapie-infected hamsters and the effect of serotonergic drugs on scrapie symptoms. *Brain Res.* **220**, 372–7.

Grahame-Smith, D. G. (1971*a*). Studies *in vivo* on the relationship between brain tryptophan, brain 5-HT synthesis and hyperactivity in rats treated with a monoamine oxidase inhibitor and L-tryptophan. *J.Neurochem.* **18**, 1053–66.

Grahame-Smith, D. G. (1971*b*). Inhibitory effect of chlorpromazine on the syndrome of hyperactivity produced by L-tryptophan or 5-methoxy -N, N-dimethyltryptamine in rats treated with a monoamine oxidase inhibitor. *Br.J.Pharmacol.* **3**, 856–64.

Green, A. R. and Grahame-Smith, D. G. (1976*a*). Effects of drugs on the processes regulating the functional activity of brain 5-hydroxytryptamine. *Nature* **260**, 487–491.

Green, A. R. and Grahame-Smith, D. G. (1976*b*). (–) Propranolol inhibits the behavioural response of rats to increased 5-hydroxytryptamine in the central nervous system. *Nature* **262**, 594–6.

Green, A. R. and Grahame-Smith, D. G. (1978). Processes regulating the functional activity of brain 5-hydroxytryptamine: results of animal experimentation and their relevance to the understanding and treatment of depression. *Pharmakopsychiatrie* **11**, 3–16.

Green, A.R. and Heal, D.J. (1985). The effects of drugs on serotonin-mediated behavioural models. In *Neuropharmacology of serotonin* (ed. A.R. Green), pp. 326–65, Oxford University Press, Oxford.

Green, A.R., Youdim, M.B.H., and Grahame-Smith, D.G. (1976). Quipazine: its effects on rat brain 5-hydroxytryptamine metabolism, monoamine oxidase activity and behaviour. *Neuropharmacology* **15**, 173–9.

Green, A.R., Hall, J.E., and Rees, A.R. (1981). A behavioural and biochemical study in rats of 5-hydroxytryptamine receptor agonists and antagonists, with observations on structure–activity requirements for the agonists. *Br.J.Pharmacol.* **73**, 703–19.

Green, A.R., O'Shaugnessy, K., Hammond, M., Schacter, M., and Grahame-Smith, D.G. (1983). Inhibition of 5-hydroxytryptamine-mediated behaviour by the putative 5-HT$_2$ antagonist pirenperone. *Neuropharmacology* **22**, 573–8.

Green, A.R., Guy, A.P., and Gardner, C.R. (1984). The behavioural effects of RU 24969, a suggested 5HT$_1$ receptor agonist in rodents and the effect on the behaviour of treatment with antidepressants. *Neuropharmacology* **23**, 655–661.

Growdon, J.H., Young, R.R., and Shahani, B.T. (1976). L-5-hydroxytryptophan in treatment of several different syndromes in which myoclonus is prominent. *Neurology* **26**, 1135–40.

Handley, S.L. and Brown, J. (1982). Effects on the 5-hydroxytryptamine induced head-twitch of drugs with selective actions on alpha$_1$- and alpha$_2$-adrenoreceptors. *Neuropharmacology* **21**, 507–10.

Heal, D.G., Green, A.R., Boullin, D.J., and Grahame-Smith, D.G. (1976). Single and repeated administration of neuroleptic drugs to rats: effects on striatal dopamine-sensitive adenylcyclase and locomotor activity produced by tranylcypromine and L-tryptophan or L-dopa. *Psychopharmacology* **49**, 287–300.

Hoyer, D. (1988*a*). Functional correlates of serotonin 5-HT$_1$ recognition sites. *J.Receptor Res.* **8**, 59–81.

Hoyer, D. (1988*b*). Molecular pharmacology and biology of 5-HT$_{1C}$ receptors. *TIPS* **9**, 89–94.

Hoyer, D., Waeser, C., Pazos, A., Probst, A., and Palacios, J.M. (1988). Identification of a 5-HT$_1$ recognition site in human brain membranes different from 5-HT$_{1A}$, 5-HT$_{1B}$ and 5-HT$_{1C}$ sites. Neurosci Lett. **85**, 357–62.

Hess, S.M. and Doepfner, W. (1961). Behavioural effects and brain amine content in rats. *Arch.int.Pharmacodyn.* **134**, 89–99.

Hwang, E.C. and Van Woert, M.H. (1979). Behavioural and biochemical effects of para-methoxyphenylethylamine. *Res.Commun.Chem.Pathol.Pharmacol.* **23**, 419–30.

Hwang, E.C. and Van Woert, M.H. (1980*a*). Comparative effects of substituted phenylethylamines on brain serotonergic mechanisms. *J.Pharmacol.exp.Ther.* **213**, 254–60.

Hwang, E.C. and Van Woert, M.H. (1980*b*). Comparative effects of various serotonin releasing agents in mice. *Biochem.Pharmacol.* **29**, 3163–7.

Hwang, E.C., Magnussen, I. and Van Woert, M.H. (1980). Effect of chronic fluoxetine administration on serotonin metabolism. *Res.Commun.Chem.Pathol.Pharmacol.* **29**, 79–98.

Jacobs, B. L. (1976). Minireview. An animal behaviour model for studying central serotonergic synapses. *Life Sci.* **19**, 777–86.

Jacobs, B. L. and Klemfuss, H. (1975). Brain stem and spinal cord mediation of a serotonergic behavioural syndrome. *Brain Res.* **100**, 450–7.

Jacobs, B. L., Wise, W. D. and Taylor, K. M. (1975). Is there a catecholamine serotonin interaction in the control of motor activity? *Neuropharmacology* **14**, 501–6.

Jenner, P., Marsden, C. D., and Thanki, C. M. (1980). Behavioural changes induced by N,N-dimethyltryptamine in rodents. *Br.J.Pharmacol.* **69**, 69–80.

Jones, D. L., Mogenson, G. J., and Wu, M. (1981). Injections of dopaminergic, cholinergic, serotonergic and GABA-ergic drugs into the nucleus accumbens: effects on locomotor activity in the rat. *Neuropharmacology* **20**, 29–38.

Kennett, G. A., Chaouloff, F., Marcou, M., and Curzon, G. (1986). Female rats are more vulnerable than males in an animal model of depression: the possible role of serotonin. *Brain Res.* **382**, 416–21.

Kennett, G. A. and Curzon, G. (1988a). Evidence that mCPP may have behavioural effects mediated by central 5-HT$_{1C}$ receptors. *Br.J.Pharmacol.* **94**, 137–47.

Kennett, G. A. and Curzon, G. (1988b). Evidence that hypophagia induced by mCPP and TFMPP requires 5-HT$_{1C}$ receptors: hypophagia induced by RU 24969 only requires 5-HT$_{1B}$ receptors. *Psychopharmacology*, **96**, 93–100.

Kennett, G. A., Dickinson, S. L. and Curzon, G. (1985a). Enhancement of some 5-HT-dependent behavioural responses following repeated immobilization in rats. *Brain Res.* **330**, 253–63.

Kennett, G., Dickinson, S., and Curzon, G. (1985b). Central serotonergic responses and behavioural adaptation to repeated immobilisation: the effect of the corticosterone synthesis inhibitor metyrapone. *Eur.J.Pharmacol.* **119**, 143–52.

Kennett, G. A., Dourish, C. T., and Curzon, G. (1987). 5-HT$_{1B}$ agonists induce anorexia at a postsynaptic site. *Eur.J.Pharmacol.* **141**, 429–35.

Kennett, G. A., Whitton, P., Shah, K., and Curzon, G. (1989). Anxiogenic-like effects of mCPP and TFMPP in animal models are opposed by 5-H$_{1C}$ receptor antagonists. *Eur. J. Pharmacol.* **164**, 445–54.

Kilpatrick, G. J., Jones, B. J., and Tyers, M. B. (1987). Identification and distribution of 5-HT$_3$ receptors in rat brain using radioligand binding. *Nature* **330**, 746–8.

Klawans, H. L., Goetz, C., and Weiner, W. J. (1973). 5-Hydroxytryptophan-induced myoclonus in guinea pigs and the possible role of serotonin in infantile myoclonus. *Neurology* **23**, 1234–40.

Kleinrok, Z. and Turski, L. (1980). Kainic acid-induced wet dog shakes in rats. *Naunyn-Schmiedeberg's Arch. Pharmacol.* **314**, 37–46.

Kuhn, D. M., Wolf, W. A., and Youdim, M. B. H. (1985). 5-Hydroxytryptamine release *in vivo* from a cytoplasmic pool: studies on the 5-HT behavioural syndrome in reserpinized rats. *Br.J.Pharmacol.* **84**, 121–9.

Lalonde, R. and Botez, I. M. (1985). Chronic phenytoin and the stereotyped motor response induced by 5-methoxy-N,N-dimethyltryptamine in rats. *Brain Res.* **326**, 388–91.

Larson, A. A. and Kondzielski, M. H. (1982). Serotonin induced gnawing in mice:

comparison with tail pinch-induced gnawing. *Pharmacol.Biochem.Behav.* **16**, 407–9.

Lees, A. J., Fernando, J. C. R., and Curzon, G. (1979). Serotonergic involvement in behavioural responses to amphetamine at high dosage. *Neuropharmacology* **18**, 153–8.

Leysen, J. E. (1985). Characterization of serotonin receptor binding sites. In *Neuropharmacology of serotonin* (ed. A. R. Green), pp. 79–109. Oxford University Press, Oxford.

Leysen, J. E., Niemegeers, C. J. E., Tollenaere, J. P., and Laduron, P. M. (1978). Serotonergic component of neuroleptic receptors. *Nature* **272**, 168–71.

Lucki, I. and Frazer, A. (1982*a*). Behavioural effects of indole and piperazine type serotonin receptor agonists. *Soc.Neurosci.Abst.* **8**, 101.

Lucki, I. and Frazer, A. (1982*b*). Prevention of the serotonin syndrome in rats by repeated administration of monoamine oxidase inhibitors but not tricyclic antidepressants. *Psychopharmacology* **77**, 205–11.

Lucki, I., Nobler, M. S., and Frazer, A. (1984). Differential actions of serotonin antagonists on two behavioural models of serotonin receptor activation in the rat. *J.Pharmacol. exp. Ther.* **228**, 133–9.

Luscombe, G., Jenner, P., and Marsden, C. D. (1983). Alterations in brain 5HT and tryptamine content during indoleamine-induced myoclonus in guinea pigs. *Biochem.Pharmacol.* **32**, 1857–64.

Luscombe, G., Jenner, P., and Marsden, C. D. (1984). Correlation of [^{3}H]5-hydroxytryptamine (5-HT) binding to brain stem preparations and the production and prevention of myoclonus in guinea pig by 5-HT agonists and antagonists. *Eur.J.Pharmacol.* **104**, 235–44.

Marsden, C. A. (1980). Involvement of 5-hydroxytryptamine and dopamine neurones in the behavioural effects of α-methyltryptamine. *Neuropharmacology* **19**, 691–8.

Marsden, C. A. and Curzon, G. (1978). The contribution of tryptamine to the behavioural effects of L-tryptophan in tranylcypromine-treated rats. *Psychopharmacology* **57**, 71–6.

Marsden, C. A. and Curzon, G. (1979). The role of tryptamine in the behavioural effects of tranylcypromine + L-tryptophan. *Neuropharmacology* **18**, 159–64.

Martin, P., Frances, H., and Simon, P. (1985). Dissociation of head twitches and tremors during the study of interactions with 5-hydroxytryptophan in mice. *J.pharmacol.methods* **13**, 193–200.

Matthews, W. D. and Smith, C. D. (1980). Pharmacological profile of a model for central serotonin activation. *Life Sci.* **26**, 1397–403.

Middlemiss, D. N. and Fozard, J. R. (1983). 8-hydroxy-2-(di-n-propylamino) tetralin discriminates between subtypes of the 5-HT$_1$ recognition site. *Eur.J.Pharmacol.* **90**, 151–3.

Middlemiss, D. N., Blakeborough, L., and Leather, S. R. (1977). Direct evidence for an interaction of β-adrenergic blockers with the 5-HT receptor. *Nature* **267**, 289–90.

Nabeshima, T., Yamaguchi, K., Hiramatsu, M., Amano, M., Furukawa, H. and

Kameyama, T. (1984). Serotonergic involvement in phenycylidine-induced behaviours. *Pharmacol.Biochem.Behav.* **21**, 401-8.

Nahorski, S.R. and Wilcocks, A.L. (1983). Interactions of β-adrenoceptor antagonists with 5-hydroxytryptamine receptor subtypes in the rat cerebral cortex. *Br.J.Pharmacol.* **78**, 107P.

Nakamura, M. and Fukushima, H. (1978). Effect of 5, 6-dihydroxytryptamine on the head twitches induced by 5-HTP, 5-HT, mescaline and fludiazepam in mice. *J.Pharm.Pharmacol.* **30**, 56-8.

Nimgaonkar, V.L., Green, A.R., Cowen, P.J., Heal, D.J., Grahame-Smith, D.G., and Deakin, J.W.F. (1983). Studies on the mechanisms by which clenbuterol a β-adrenoreceptor agonist enhances 5-HT-mediated behaviour and increases metabolism of 5-HT in the brain of the rat. *Neuropharmacology* **22**, 739-49.

Ogren, S.O., Fuxe, K., and Agnati, L. (1985). The importance of brain serotonin receptor mechanisms for the action of antidepressant drugs. *Pharmacopsychiatry* **18**, 209-13.

Ortmann, R. (1984). The 5-HT syndrome in rats as tool for the screening of psychoactive drugs. *Drug Develop. Res.* **4**, 593-606.

Ortmann, R., Waldmeier, P.C., Radeke, E., Felner, A., and Delini-Stula, A. (1980). The effects of 5HT uptake- and MAO-inhibitors on L-5-HTP-induced excitation in rats. *Naunyn-Schmiedeberg's Arch. Pharmacol.* **311**, 185-92.

Ortmann, R., Martin, S., Radeke, E. and Delini-Stula, A. (1981). Interaction of β-adrenoreceptor agonists with the serotonergic system in rat brain. A behavioural study using the L-5-HTP syndrome. *Naunyn-Schmiedeberg's Arch.Pharmacol.* **316**, 225-30.

Pedigo, N.W., Yamamura, H.I., and Nelson, D.L. (1981). Discrimination of multiple [^{3}H] 5-hydroxytryptamine binding sites by the neuroleptic spiperone in rat brain. *J.Neurochem.* **36**, 220-6.

Peroutka, S.J. and Snyder, S.H. (1979). Multiple serotonin receptors: differential binding of [^{3}H] 5-hydroxytryptamine, [^{3}H] lysergic acid diethylamide and [^{3}H] spiroperidol. *Mol.Pharmacol.* **16**, 687-99.

Peroutka, S.J., Lebovitz, R.M., and Snyder, S.H. (1981). Two distinct central serotonin receptors with different physiological functions. *Science* **212**, 827-9.

Robbins, T. and Iversen, S.D. (1973). A dissociation of the effects of D-amphetamine on locomotor activity and exploration in rats. *Psychopharmacology* **28**, 155-64.

Schnellmann, R.G., Waters, S.J., and Nelson, D.L. (1984). [^{3}H] 5-hydroxytryptamine binding sites: species and tissue variation. *J.Neurochem.* **42**, 65-70.

Segal, M. and Weinstock, M. (1983). Differential effects of 5-hydroxytryptamine antagonists on behaviours resulting from activation of different pathways arising from the raphe nuclei. *Psychopharmacology* **79**, 72-8.

Shimomura, K., Mori, J. and Honda, F. (1981). Backward walking induced by L-5-hydroxytryptophan in mice. *Jap.J.Pharmacol.* **31**, 39-46.

Silbergeld, E.K. and Hruska, R.E. (1979). Lisuride and LSD: Dopaminergic and serotonergic interactions in the "serotonin syndrome". *Psychopharmacology* **65**, 233-7.

Sills, M.A., Wolfe, B.B., and Frazer, A. (1984). Determination of selective and non-selective compounds for the 5-HT$_{1A}$ and 5-HT$_{1B}$ receptor subtypes in rat frontal cortex. *J.Pharmacol.exp.Ther.* **231**, 480–7.

Sills, M.A., Lucki, I. and Frazer, A. (1985). Development of selective tolerance to the serotonin behavioural syndrome and suppression of locomotor activity after repeated administration of either 5-MeODMT or mCPP. *Life Sci.* **36**, 2463–9.

Sloviter, R.S., Drust, E.G., and Connor, J.D. (1978*a*). Evidence that serotonin mediates some behavioural effects of amphetamine. *J.Pharmacol.exp.Ther.* **206**, 348–52.

Sloviter, R.S., Drust, E.G., and Connor, J.D. (1978*b*). Specificity of a rat behavioural model for serotonin receptor activation. *J.Pharmacol. exp.Ther.* **206**, 339–52.

Sloviter, R.S., Drust, E.G., Damiano, B.P., and Connor, J.D. (1980). A common mechanism for lysergic acid, indolealkylamine and phenethylamine hallucinogens: serotonergic mediation of behavioural effects in rats. *J.Pharmacol.exp.Ther.* **214**, 231–8.

Taylor, M., Goudie, A.J., Mortimore, S., and Wheeler, T.J. (1974). Comparison between behaviours elicited by high doses of amphetamine and fenfluramine: implications for the concept of stereotypy. *Psychopharmacologia* **40**, 249–58.

Thomas, K.V. and Handley, S.L. (1978). On the mechanism of amphetamine-induced behavioural changes. I. An observational analysis of dexamphetamine. *Arzneimittel-Forsch.* **28**, 827–33.

Tricklebank, M.D., Forler, C., and Fozard, J.R. (1984). The involvement of subtypes of the 5-HT$_1$ receptor and of catecholaminergic systems in the behavioural response to 8-hydroxy-2-(di-n-propylamino) tetralin in the rat. *Eur.J.Pharmacol.* **106**, 271–82.

Tricklebank, M.D., Forler, C., Middlemiss, D.N., and Fozard, J.R. (1985). Subtypes of the 5-HT receptor mediating the behavioural responses to 5-methoxy-N,N-dimethyltryptamine in the rat. *Eur.J.Pharmacol.* **117**, 15–24.

Tricklebank, M.D., Middlemiss, D.N., and Neill, J. (1986). Pharmacological analysis of the behavioural and thermoregulatory effects of the putative 5-HT$_1$ receptor agonist, RU 24969 in the rat. *Neuropharmacology.* **25**, 877–86.

Trulson, M.E. and Jacobs, B.L. (1976). Behavioural evidence for the rapid release of CNS serotonin by PCA and fenfluramine. *Eur.J.Pharmacol.* **36**, 149–54.

Trulson, M.E. and MacKenzie, R.G. (1981). Subsensitivity to 5-hydroxytryptamine agonists occurs in streptozocin-diabetic rats with no change in [^{3}H] 5-HT receptor binding. *J.Pharm.Pharmacol.* **33**, 472–4.

Trulson, M.E., Eubanks, E.E., and Jacobs, B.L. (1976*a*). Behavioural evidence for supersensitivity following destruction of central serotonergic nerve terminals by 5, 7-dihydroxytryptamine. *J.Pharmacol.exp.Ther.* **198**, 23–32.

Trulson, M.E., Ross, C.A., and Jacobs, B.L. (1976*b*). Behavioural evidence for the stimulation of CNS serotonin receptors by high doses of LSD. *Psychopharmacol.Commun.* **2**, 149–64.

Turski, W.A., Czuczwar, S.J., Turski, L., Sieklucka-Dziuba, M., and Kleinrok, Z. (1984). Studies on the mechanism of wet dog shakes produced by carbachol in rats. *Pharmacology* **28**, 112–20.

Vetulani, J., Lebrecht, U., and Pilc A. (1981). Enhancement of responsiveness of the central serotonergic system and serotonin-2 receptor density in rat frontal cortex by electroconvulsive treatment. *Eur.J.Pharmacol.* **76**, 81–5.

Volkman, P.H., Lorens, S.A., Kindel, G.H., and Ginos, J.Z. (1978). L-5-Hydroxytryptophan-induced myoclonus in guinea pigs. A model for the study of central serotonin-dopamine interactions. *Neuropharmacology* **17**, 947–955.

Wada, J.A., Balzamo, E., Meldrum, B.S., and Naquet, R. (1972). Behavioural and electrographic effects of L-5-hydroxytryptophan and D,L-parachlorophenylalanine on epileptic Senegalese baboons (Papio papio). *Electroencephalogr.clin.Neurophysiol.* **33**, 520–6.

Warbritton, J.D., Stewart, R.M., and Baldessarini, R.J. (1978). Decreased locomotor activity and attenuation of amphetamine hyperactivity with intraventricular infusion of serotonin in the rat. *Brain Res.* **143**, 373–82.

Wei, E., Loh, H.H., and Way, E.L. (1973). Neuroanatomical correlates of wet shake behaviour in the rat. *Life Sci.* **12**, (2), 489–96.

Weiner, W.J., Carvey, P.M., Nausieda, P.A., and Klawans, H.L. (1979). Dopaminergic antagonism of L-5-hydroxytryptophan-induced myoclonic jumping behaviour. *Neurology* **29**, 1622–5.

Wielosz, M. (1985). Increased sensitivity to serotonergic agonists after repeated electroconvulsive shock in rats. *Pharmacol.Biochem.Behav.* **22**, 683–7.

Woodrow, K.M., Reifman, A., and Wyatt, R.J. (1978). Amphetamine psychosis—a model for paranoid schizophrenia. In *Neuropharmacology and behaviour* (ed B. Haber and M.H. Aprison), pp. 1–22. Plenum Press, New York.

Yamamoto, T. and Ueki, S. (1981) The role of central serotonergic mechanisms on head-twitch and backward locomotion induced by hallucinogenic drugs. *Pharmacol.Biochem.Behav.* **14**, 89–95.

Yap, C.Y. and Taylor, D.A. (1983). Involvement of $5-HT_2$ receptors in the wet-dog shake behaviour induced by 5-hydroxytryptophan in the rat. *Neuropharmacology* **22**, 801–4.

7

Disintegration into stereotypy induced by drugs or brain damage: a microdescriptive behavioural analysis

PHILIP TEITELBAUM, SERGIO M. PELLIS, and
TERRY L. DeVIETTI

Introduction

Implicit in the phenomenon of stereotyped behaviour is a puzzle: the term
stereotype applies to a behavioural act that is repeated again and again, but
unlike a motivated act, it makes no sense because it does not seem to achieve
an adaptive outcome.* Drug-induced stereotypy, such as that produced
by high doses of central stimulants, has that character. The wide variety
of seemingly unrelated independent stereotypies generated by central
stimulants is also puzzling. In rodents, for instance, drugs such as
apomorphine and amphetamine have been reported to elicit climbing,
jumping, rearing, prancing, running, walking, circling, revolving, pivoting,
gnawing, licking, nose-poking, sniffing, verticalization, side-to-side head
and paw movements, backward locomotion, and underwater swimming
without surfacing (e.g. Alander *et al*. 1983; Cole 1977; Costall and Naylor
1973; Decsi *et al*. 1979; Fray *et al*. 1980; Janssen *et al*. 1960; Jerussi and Glick
1976; Kokkinidis and Anisman 1979; Schiørring 1971; Schoenfeld *et al*.
1975; Segal *et al*. 1980; Szechtman *et al*. 1982; Teitelbaum 1986; Thomas and
Handley 1978; Voigtlander *et al*. 1975). What do they have in common?

We believe that stereotypy is a disintegrated form of behaviour. In order
to understand it, a microdescriptive behavioural analysis is required which is
different from the way one usually describes behaviour. Such an analysis can
reveal neurological movement factors common to many otherwise seemingly
unrelated stereotyped acts.

---

* We distinguish between adaptive behaviour which may be stereotyped in form, versus
stereotypy, which in addition to being repetitive, appears to be purposeless, and even
maladaptive. Many instinctive behaviours can be stereotyped in form, but are nevertheless,
adaptive.

A normal animal's behaviour is typically adaptive—the outcome of each act is beneficial for the animal's survival. Since, by our definition, a stereotype is not adaptive, we must disconnect our description of the act from its outcome, to be able to handle the disconnected character of the behaviour. In the usual analysis of behaviour, there is a perception of 'adaptive wholeness' that governs the way we describe, measure, and think about it. We merely label each 'act' in terms of its potential or actual outcome, e.g. feeding, drinking, mating, etc. We generally see no need to isolate and measure the movement of the body parts involved, because we take for granted that they are fully integrated with each other and with the appropriate aspects of the environment in achieving the outcome. But where stereotypy exists an adaptive outcome is absent, so we must apply an analysis of movement, not outcome. This is the essence of microdescriptive behavioural analysis.

Stimulant-induced stereotypy

As cited above, stimulant drugs induce many forms of locomotion as well as movements involving only part of the body. The latter, including biting, licking, head-bobbing and -weaving, paw-movements, sniffing, and nose-poking are often considered as a stereotype, whereas locomotion is not (Segal and Schuckit 1983). We believe this is a mistake, caused by the perceptual illusion of 'adaptive wholeness'. When an animal moves from one place to another, as in an open field, for instance, it moves as a whole, and therefore its behaviour looks as though it is goal-directed—the animal seems to be exploring the environment purposively, either looking for reinforcing stimuli (e.g. food, water, warmth, shelter, or a mate) or going somewhere. But when the animal performs repeated movements of only part of its body, without moving as a whole from one place to another, the behaviour may often be labelled as a stereotype (for a general reference, see Segal and Schuckit 1983). Repeated movement of a part of the body without an adaptive outcome violates the illusion of adaptive wholeness, leading it to be called stereotypy, whereas locomotion, seeming whole, appears adaptively purposive. Chewing and licking, if they were accompanied by swallowing, would be thought adaptive if the substance were beneficial (food or water). Then the drug would be said to induce hyperphagia or hyperdipsia. But if no swallowing accompanies the act, then the behaviour is interpreted as abnormal—in this case, as a stereotype. Our work, as well as that of others (Schiørring 1979), indicates that drug-induced locomotion in an open field can also be a stereotype, so we will begin our analysis by looking for factors of movement common to the many seemingly unrelated locomotor 'acts' generated by the dopaminergic agonists, apomorphine and amphetamine.

An 'open' field usually has walls to prevent the animal from leaving it. Walls complicate the movements a rat will display, particularly under the influence of stimulant drugs (Schiørring 1979; Szechtman et al. 1985). To simplify the behaviour as much as possible at first, a wall-less open field was used—a large transparent sheet of glass placed several feet above the floor. The height prevented the animal from walking off the surface, the smoothness of the glass decreased the likelihood that surface irregularity would trigger biting (which interrupts and distorts locomotion), and the transparency allowed views of the movement of the body parts simultaneously from the side and below (Szechtman, et al. 1980, 1985). Instead of counting the number of 'acts' per unit time after drug injection (e.g. crossings from side to side, rearings) as is commonly done automatically by light-beam interruption indicators (Dourish and Cooper 1984; Sanberg et al. 1983), the behaviour was videotaped or filmed and the size and direction of head and body movements per 15 second interval were measured continuously throughout the course of the drug's action (Szechtman et al. 1985). The Eshkol–Wachmann movement notation system (EWMN) was used to write down and think about the movements and positions of each part of the animal's body (Eshkol and Wachmann 1958). EWMN provides movement symbols and concepts in a format suited to the analysis of body movement (e.g. Golani 1976; Golani et al. 1979; Pellis 1981, 1985; Szechtman et al. 1985).

Within 2 to 3 minutes or so after the subcutaneous neck injection of 1.25 mg/kg apomorphine hydrochloride, all spontaneous rearing and grooming movements disappear—the animal puts its snout to the ground and moves along the surface. Then, as shown in Fig. 7.1 (see rat B3 for the clearest example), forward steps appear, reaching a peak frequency within the first 5 minutes after drug injection. After that they typically decline, to a point where they may disappear entirely. With a greater latency after drug injection, lateral turning movements appear, superimposed on the waxing and then waning forward movement. As shown in Fig. 7.2, as movements along these dimensions sum algebraically, forward locomotion, circling, revolving in tight circles (forward walking still present), and pivoting (without forward walking; see below) are generated successively during the course of action of the drug. Finally, when both hindlegs are rooted to the ground, only movements of the forequarters are possible, yielding side-to-side head and forequarter movements (Szechtman et al. 1985). Throughout the period when the snout is in light contact with the floor, no spontaneous upward movement of the head is seen. At that time, however, in an enclosure with walls, the animal scans and rears upward while maintaining snout

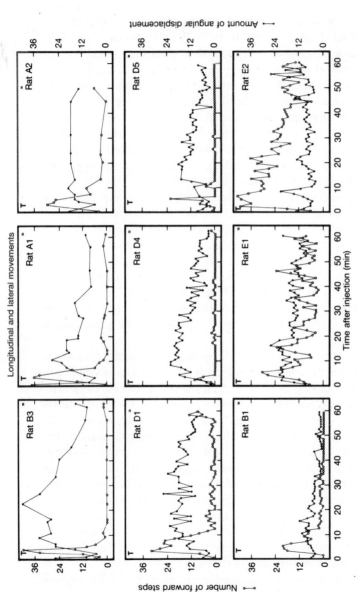

Fig. 7.1. Time course of lateral angular displacement of the head and of forward progression in individual rats injected with 1.25 mg/kg of apomorphine. Forward progression was measured in terms of forward steps. Lateral angular displacement was measured in units of 45° (1 = 45°). For rats B3, A1, and A2, selected portions of their behaviour were filmed (16 mm movie). These filmed sequences were notated using the Eshkol–Wachman Movement Notation; each graph point corresponds to 15 seconds of activity. For the remaining rats, data were obtained from continuous videorecords of the rats' behaviour; these graphs provide a complete summary of the animals' activity. For each component every data point represents the value in the minute interval at the indicated time—the score was divided by 4 to correspond to the 15 second intervals employed for the rats in the top row. In this and in all subsequent graphs, the position of the sign 'T' indicates the time at which uninterrupted snout contact was established, and the position of the sign ' = ', the time at which snout contact was released. If snout contact was released after 65 minutes, the release sign (=) was positioned at the extreme right of the

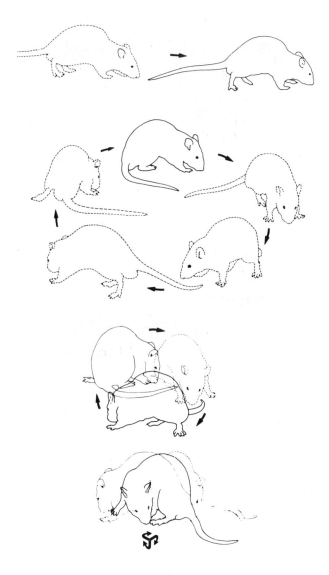

Fig. 7.2. A schematic illustration of four successive composite stereotypies generated in the course of action of apomorphine. From top to bottom: forward walking, circling, revolving, and pivoting. It should be noted that during 'circling' the animals typically locomote along circular paths without completing 360° before changing direction. (From Szechtman *et al.* 1985.)

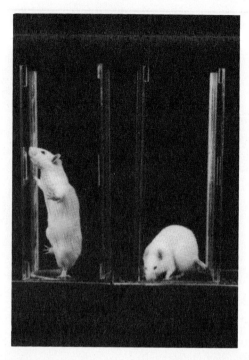

Fig. 7.3. After injection (intraperitoneal) of apomorphine (10 mg/kg) the rat on the left climbs the smooth walls of the container, whereas the rat on the right continuously gnaws the wire mesh on the floor. (From Szechtman *et al.* 1982.)

contact with the wall (see Fig. 7.3 (on left)) (Szechtman *et al.* 1982). If, however, the floor is a wire grid, directed mouthing movements are triggered and the pattern of locomotion seen clearly on the sheet of glass will be interrupted and obscured by chewing and licking.

A large dose of amphetamine reveals another aspect of dopamine's action on movement. About 20 minutes after injection of 20 mg/kg of *d*-amphetamine sulphate, rats start backing up very rapidly, sometimes right off the table (Curzon *et al.* 1979). In water, however, such animals swim forward underwater horizontally or dive to the bottom of the tank, never swimming to the surface as an undrugged animal does (Fig. 7.4). If not plucked from the water in less than a minute, such a rat will drown (Alander, Servidio, Schallert, and Teitelbaum 1983; described briefly in Teitelbaum 1986; Petree and DeVietti 1989). How are underwater swimming and 'backing up' related? In the course of the drug's action, when the animal is placed in an open field, away from walls, several very different 'acts' appear. As shown in Fig. 7.5, within a minute or so after injection, exaggerated

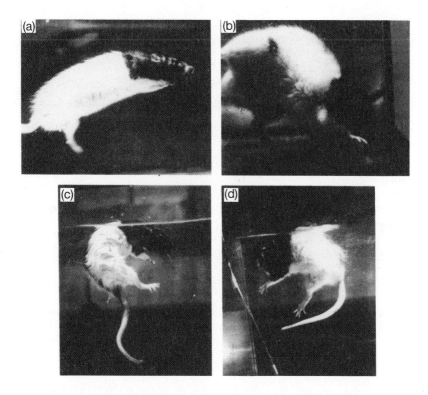

Fig. 7.4. Twenty minutes or so after the injection of a large dose of amphetamine, a rat swims underwater or dives to the bottom. It never swims to the surface as a normal rat does; if not plucked from the water within a minute or so, it will drown. (From Teitelbaum 1986.)

upward 'rearing' was seen. At 2 minutes, a form of 'prancing' was observed, with the animal walking forward on its hindlegs, its forelegs in the air. By 3.5 minutes, vigorous forward 'running' appeared. By 10 minutes, lateral 'head-scanning' was seen, and by 24 minutes, 'nosing' and 'sniffing' the ground were evident. But our analysis shows that each stereotyped 'act' was formed as a composite aggregate of three subcomponent dimensions of movement, which are acted upon by the drug: vertical, longitudinal, and lateral. These appear with a different latency after drug injection, and wax and wane separately. One effect of the drug's action is on the orientation of the head—from vertically up to vertically down. Thus 'rearing' is maximal upward vertical movement of the head involving recruitment of the body, without any forward or lateral movement. 'Running' is forward locomotion interacting with the maintenance of a horizontal position of the head,

Amphetamine

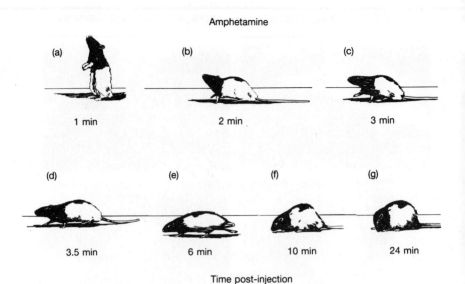

Time post-injection

Fig. 7.5. The continuous monitoring, from the time of injection, of the effects of amphetamine (20 mg/kg) on the locomotor behaviour of a rat in an open field. See text for explanation. (From Teitelbaum 1986.)

without lateral turning, etc. When placed in water at 20 min. or so after injection, such animals swam horizontally underwater or dove down—they could not direct their swimming upward at that time, though they could do so in the early minutes of the drug's action (Alander *et al.* 1983; Petree and DeVietti 1989). What about backing up? On the ground, as the head is progressively ventroflexed downward during the action of amphetamine, a point is reached where the snout, now in contact with the ground, flexes ventrally toward the abdomen. Forward walking has ceased completely by this time, and the rat is standing in a hunched posture. Our impression is that when the snout flexes toward the body, it contacts the feet, eliciting a quick two-step backwards. These backward steps are quickly repeated, yielding 'backing up'. But this should be analysed further, by movement notation, using high-speed film.

The above examples show that, after a high dose of a central stimulant drug, a stereotyped 'act' is not an integrated unit where the whole animal is achieving an adaptive outcome, but rather a composite aggregate of subsystems which mediate movement along independent spatial dimensions. The composite form of the 'act' is determined by the algebraic summation of the directions and amplitudes of movement that have differentially been induced by the drug. So compelling is our tendency to label behaviour in terms of adaptive 'acts', that we mistakenly see each as separate, unitary, and not connected with the other 'acts' induced by the drug.

Dopaminergic movement subsystems and their gradient of integration as evident in recovery from catalepsy

Dopamine integrates movement cephalocaudally from head to tail (Golani *et al.* 1979). It acts on separate subcomponents of exploration, which we call movement subsystems (Schallert *et al.* 1978c; Teitelbaum *et al.* 1980). Both aspects of its action are evident in the effects of damage or chemical blockade of the dopaminergic system and in its subsequent spontaneous or drug-induced recovery. By studying these, one can more meaningfully interpret how stereotyped acts are produced by central stimulant drugs.

Full catalepsy: defence of body stability isolated from exploration

If we give a rat a high dose (5 mg/kg) of haloperidol (a dopamine receptor blocker), we produce dopamine-deficiency catalepsy,* a 'zero condition' (Magnus 1926) for exploratory movement (Teitelbaum 1982a). Postural support remains functionally intact, but all forms of movement related to orientation to the outside world are suppressed, including head-scanning, head-orienting, directed mouthing (biting and licking at external objects), and forward locomotion. (Sniffing also seems absent, but we have not analysed it, and will not discuss it here.) The aggregate of allied reflexes that maintain stable static equilibrium (standing, clinging), defend it (crouching, bracing), or prepare for it (contact-placing (Wolgin 1985), righting in air, contact-righting) make up the postural support subsystem (Teitelbaum *et al.* 1980, 1982). This remains intact under haloperidol and is therefore non-dopaminergic. (It may be serotonergic: methysergide, a serotonin blocker, abolishes static standing in akinetic lateral hypothalamic-damaged animals (Chesire and Teitelbaum 1982) as well as in normal animals (S. Pellis, V. Pellis and Teitelbaum, in preparation.)) Each of the subcomponent postural support reflexes can be further fractionated (Chen *et al.* 1986; Pellis *et al.* 1985, 1986, 1987a), but, for our purposes here, the postural support subsystem can serve as a reference zero point from which to view the subcomponents of exploratory movement. Postural support is a whole-body response—all of the segments of the body and limbs are integrated into the

* We use the term catalepsy to denote the immobility that goes along with dopamine deficiency, as described here. Morphine induces a state that has also been called catalepsy or catatonia (e.g. Costall and Naylor 1974; Kuschinsky and Hornykiewicz 1972). We use the term morphine-induced immobility to differentiate that state from dopamine-deficiency-induced catalepsy. We have shown that they are quite different—indeed they are complementary rather than alike (DeRyck and Teitelbaum 1983, 1984; DeRyck *et al.* 1980; Pellis *et al.* 1986).

defence of its stability. The cataleptic animal tolerates awkward postures for long periods without moving, as long as they provide stable support. Disturb that support, however, and the cataleptic animal comes to life until stable support is once again achieved. Dopamine-deficiency-induced full catalepsy, therefore, represents the isolated action of the postural support subsystem, which is non-dopaminergic, while all the subcomponents of exploratory movement, being dopaminergic, are suppressed.

Partial catalepsy with head-scanning: cephalocaudal recruitment of the body into scanning without locomotion

An appropriate amount of bilateral lateral hypothalamic (L H) damage disrupts the ascending dopaminergic systems, also producing catalepsy.[*] It allows very slow recovery, revealing more clearly the reactivation and reintegration of separate subcomponents of exploration. With very large electrolytic lesions (probably involving serotonergic systems as well, see above), postural support is affected briefly, recovering quickly. Also early in recovery, exploratory tactile scanning movements of the head appear, the snout sweeping in light contact along the ground. These head sweeps compete with postural support for control over the body (Teitelbaum 1982*b*). Tactile head-scanning recruits the segments of the body away from static support rostrocaudally into exploratory movement. Such head-scanning recovers at different rates along three dimensions, first laterally (to the left and right; Fig. 7.6(a), (b), and, more slowly, longitudinally in the midline (Fig. 7.7(a)–(c)). Only much later does vertical head movement appear, first scanning along vertical surfaces and, eventually, in the air independent of surfaces (Golani *et al.* 1979). At first, the forelegs and hindlegs remain rooted to the ground in postural support, resisting the scanning actions of the head, resulting in exaggerated lateral bending (Fig. 7.6(b)) and forward midline stretching (Fig. 7.7(c)) of the head and neck. Later, the forelegs cooperate in scanning, leaving only the hindlegs rooted. The exaggerated bending and stretching now shifts to the pelvis (Fig. 7.6(c)). Thus, in dopamine deficiency, due to the conflict between the recovering control system (scanning) and the previously dominant mode of control (postural support), a form of behavioural disintegration exists. The cephalocaudal progression of active conflict between the two mutually antagonistic control

---

[*] We know that the treatments we are using, e.g. lateral hypothalamic damage, high-dose haloperidol, 6-OHDA without desmethylimipramine, all involve additional systems besides dopamine. We believe the weight of the evidence implicates dopamine in the symptoms we are describing (e.g. Marshall *et al.* 1974; Oltmans and Harvey 1972; Sanberg 1980; Ungerstedt 1971; Zigmond and Stricker 1973), so for convenience we say dopamine deficiency when, to be precise, we should say catecholamine or even monoamine deficiency. We do not mean to exclude other transmitters from consideration—indeed, we believe their role in these phenomena should be more carefully analysed.

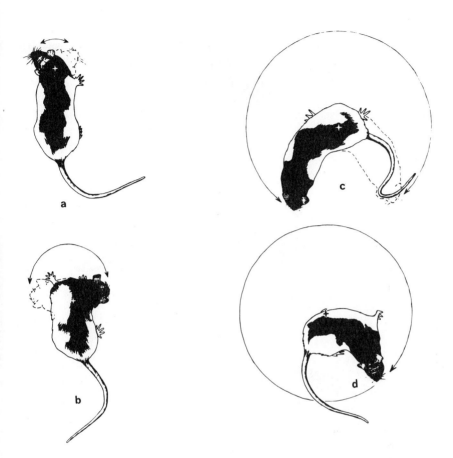

Fig. 7.6. Top view of an L H-damaged rat performing increasingly larger-amplitude horizontal lateral movements during four successive phases of recovery. Dashed line and solid line drawings indicate the extreme positions that the rat assumes during each phase. The arrows indicate the amplitude of the movements. The plus sign indicates the root of the movement, beyond which there is practically no recruitment of limb and body segments for movement. During increasingly larger lateral movements (b, c, d), the limb and body segments are recruited in a cephalocaudal order. (From Golani *et al.* 1979.)

systems is indicated by the place along the body where exaggerated bending or stretching appears.

Partial catalepsy with pivoting: head-scanning recruits only one hindleg at a time, in postural adjustment steps

Once the forelegs co-operate in head-scanning, the two types of scans (midline and lateral) can be added to each other. When a ventral head tuck (a

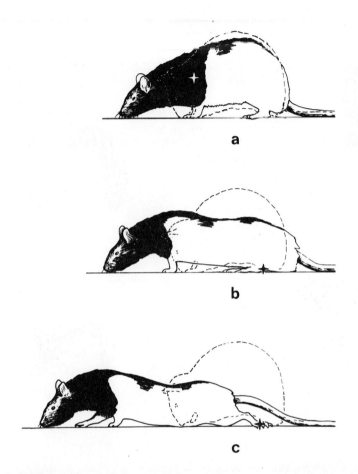

Fig. 7.7. Side view of an L H-damaged rat performing increasingly larger-amplitude longitudinal snout movements during three successive phases of recovery. Dashed line and solid line drawings indicate the extreme positions that the rat assumes during each phase. The plus sign indicates the root of movement. (From Golani *et al.* 1979.)

longitudinal midline tactile scan flexing towards the abdomen) precedes or follows a lateral scan, the animal's weight is shifted backward considerably. To maintain stable equilibrium, the hindleg on the side toward which the head has turned is then recruited, in backward postural adjustment steps, causing the animal to pivot in tight circles (see Fig. 7.6(d)). In such backward pivoting, the hindleg contralateral to the turn remains rooted to the ground, in postural support. Later in recovery, when a midline-forward tactile-guided head stretch is added to a lateral scanning movement, opening it wider, the body weight is shifted forward while . pivoting. Now the contralateral hindleg steps forward to prevent the body from falling, while the ipsilateral hindleg serves as the pivot point. Thus, although the animal seems quite mobile while pivoting, we believe that it is not actually walking, but is merely maintaining postural stability while scanning laterally from a fixed point.

Partial catalepsy with head-orienting: recruitment of head and forelimbs into orienting while the hindquarters remain immobile in postural support

With anterolateral hypothalamic damage, a partial form of catalepsy can be produced, which may seem paradoxical (Teitelbaum 1982b; Teitelbaum *et al*. 1980, 1983) but is actually quite instructive. As in haloperidol-induced full catalepsy, postural support remains intact, with head-scanning and locomotion fully suppressed. Like a haloperidol-treated animal, such an animal remains unmoving, even in bizarre postures (as long as they provide

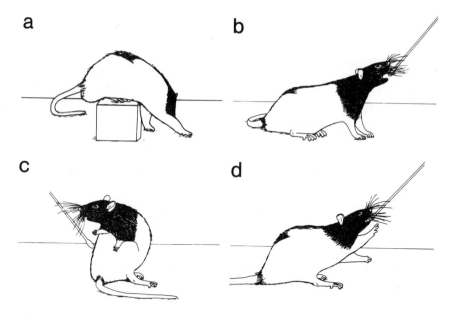

Fig. 7.8. With large anterolateral hypothalamic lesions, 'paradoxical' catalepsy is produced. (a) As long as it is in a position that provides stable equilibrium and support, the rat remains unmoving without head-scanning or locomotion, even in awkward postures. (b–d) Such a rat comes to life if a stimulus to which it can orient is moved toward it. Note the functional disconnection between hind- and frontquarters. The hindlegs remain facing forward in postural support, or even bracing backward against the displacement produced by the head, mouth, and forelegs which strain forward (b and d) or laterally (c) toward the stimulus. (From Teitelbaum 1982b.)

stable support). However, unlike an animal made cataleptic by haloperidol, or by lateral hypothalamic damage at the level of the ventromedial nucleus (Marshall *et al.* 1971; Marshall and Teitelbaum 1974), in a rat with more anterior lateral hypothalamic damage, head-orienting is not suppressed. If a moving visual or tactile stimulus is presented, its head comes to life and orients to the stimulus. The forelegs co-operate by grasping, and the mouth bites at the stimulus, but the hindlegs remain rooted in postural support, refusing to co-operate by stepping (see Fig. 7.8). Treating such an animal with haloperidol abolishes the head-orienting and directed-mouthing, and the forelegs no longer reach for and grasp objects, now serving only in support (De La Cruz, S. Pellis, and Teitelbaum, unpublished results). This illustrates that head-orienting represents a distinct subcomponent of exploratory locomotion. Closely allied and co-operating with it are directed mouthing and the directed manipulative use of the forepaws. All of these are dependent on dopamine function.

In an animal with lateral hypothalamic damage at the level of the ventromedial nucleus, as in the fully cataleptic animal produced by haloperidol, or by 6-OHDA applied intraventricularly or locally to the ascending dopaminergic systems (Marshall and Gotthelf 1979; Marshall and Teitelbaum 1974), head-orienting is abolished. This has been called sensory neglect (Marshall *et al.* 1971) and is perhaps related to the neglect produced in humans by parietal damage (Denny-Brown and Chambers 1958; Heilman 1972; Heilman *et al.* 1970) and/or in rats by tectal lesions (Redgrave *et al.* 1980). Recovery of head-orienting is gradual and rostrocaudal, illustrating that, as dopaminergic function returns, it does so along the same gradient, from head to tail, for both movement subsystems, head-scanning and head-orienting. They are independent, however, because before any appreciable recovery of orienting occurs, recovery of head-scanning may have proceeded quite far along the body gradient.

Hierarchy of thresholds of activation in dopaminergic movement subsystems

There appears to be a hierarchy in the thresholds of activation of the various dopaminergic movement subsystems. This can be seen in the slow course of spontaneous recovery from lateral hypothalamic damage, presumably based, at least in part, on progressive denervation supersensitivity of the residual intact components of the damaged dopaminergic system (e.g. Creese *et al.* 1977; Neve *et al.* 1982; Neve and Marshall 1984). The earlier the onset of recovery, the lower the presumed threshold of activation. Thus, head-scanning recovers before orienting, which in turn appears before directed mouthing. Head-scanning may be an initial component of turning and forward locomotion—in lateral hypothalamus (LH) damaged animals, it seems separate because it is superimposed on and competes with postural support, which resists the recruitment of the segments of the body into turning or walking forward. Whether they are independent subsystems or not, they are allied in their function: head-scanning recruits the segments of the body first laterally into turning, then forward into forward locomotion, and finally vertically into upward tactile scans and rearing. If the thresholds of activation of the separate dopaminergic movement subsystems are indeed organized in this manner, one would expect that apomorphine, a post-synaptic dopaminergic receptor agonist, should activate the subsystems sequentially in an order that parallels their appearance in spontaneous recovery after dopaminergic (LH) damage (Szechtman et al. 1985). This is so in animals made akinetic by local 6-OHDA destruction of ascending catecholamine systems. In such animals, whose dopaminergic caudate receptors become supersensitive due to denervation (Neve et al. 1982), very low doses of apomorphine (0.05–0.2 mg/kg) induce a series of lateral head-scanning movements prior to forward locomotion (Marshall and Gotthelf 1979), much like the 'warm-up' sequence described earlier in spontaneously recovering LH-damaged rats (Golani et al. 1979) and in normal infant rats and other infant mammals (Eilam and Golani 1988; Golani et al. 1981). But in intact animals, using the high doses of apomorphine or amphetamine necessary to produce in them the activation of locomotion and mouthing, we see quite the opposite sequence: vertical movement (rearing) appears first, forward locomotion next, and finally lateral movement (turning).

The key fact here is that, as far as forward steps are concerned, forward locomotion first waxes and then progressively wanes, until the high-dose apomorphine-treated animal no longer walks forward. Szechtman et al. (1980, 1985) have suggested that, at high doses of apomorphine, most of what is seen represents a regression to akinesia rather than an activation sequence. In other words, the apomorphine, after initially briefly stimulating the postsynaptic system (for the first 2 or 3 minutes), then appears to be reversing its action on forward locomotion—it is functionally shutting it down. A seemingly analogous reversal of the nature of the post-synaptic caudate action of high-dose amphetamine has been demonstrated electrophysiologically by Alloway and Rebec (1984) and Rebec and Segal (1980). It also accords with the findings of Ricaurte et al. (1984), which indicate that, at high doses, amphetamine damages the system. The shut-down of function is apparent behaviourally only when the effects on move-ment, not on acts, are studied. Such microdescriptive behavioural analysis reveals that the drug acts biphasically on continuous neurological variables, which affect separate movement subsystems differentially.

As we have pointed out, from evidence on animals recovering spon-taneously from damage to the dopaminergic system, dopamine recruits movement cephalocaudally. In a damaged system there is hyporecruitment, with small-amplitude movements available only to the most rostral (head and neck) segments of the body. Later in recovery, conflict between control systems is apparent in the exaggerated bending and stretching of head and neck against the forelegs, or of forequarters against hindlegs. Conversely, when the intact dopaminergic system is being hyperstimulated, one would expect, at least for a brief period, cephalocaudal hyperrecruitment of the limb and body segments. We believe we have observed this: at a certain phase of the action of a large dose of amphetamine sulphate (10–20 mg/kg), rats seem to turn *en bloc*; recruiting their front legs into the turn before the head and neck have moved very much at all (Alander *et al.* 1983). This should be measured more systematically. Cephalocaudal recruitment of movement has also been noted during the course of action of a therapeutic dose of L-dopa in patients with parkinsonism (observations from the film 'Awakenings' (Yorkshire (UK) TV; 1977), based on Sacks' work on post-encephalitic patients exhibiting parkinsonism; see Sacks 1976).

Disintegrated forms of exploratory locomotion

Once a dopamine-deficient animal has recovered forward locomotion, and therefore no longer seems even partially cataleptic, it is difficult to view its behaviour as stereotyped. It moves as a whole from place to place in the open field, scanning along the ground, and may stop to nibble at palatable food it encounters. It therefore looks as though it is exploring for food. But is it reasonable to expect, in a brain-damaged or drugged animal, that integration recovers abruptly, just because the animal can walk? Is the locomotion of such an animal actually fully integrated? If not, our problem becomes one of developing techniques to identify, isolate, and analyse the nature of the disintegrations (i.e. the functional uncoupling of the parts of the body) that produce the various forms of stereotyped locomotor behaviour. So far, we have found three useful methods for doing so. These include: (1) partial enclosures that yield 'behavioural traps' in functionally disintegrated but not in normal animals; (2) the selective disinhibition of fractional forms of walking; and (3) the use of prior experience to reverse, in varying degree, the behavioural trapping produced by some drugs.

The 'behavioural trap' as a method for revealing functional disintegration in exploratory locomotion

If a recovering L H-damaged rat happens to walk into a corner, it is trapped there, sometimes for long periods. A normal animal would simply rear up, turn, and walk out of the alley. In contrast, the lateral hypothalamic rat performs in place a repetitive series of stereotyped head-scanning movements and stepping patterns (Levitt and Teitelbaum 1975; Golani *et al.* 1979). Even when the animal is facing toward the open end of a blind alley, it seems just as likely to turn back into the dead end as to proceed out of the partial enclosure. At this stage of its recovery, it appears to lack goal-directedness, responding reflexively to each configuration of surfaces it encounters. Its snout is reacting to surfaces, while its legs engage in support or locomotion. In the open field these actions of the animal's body parts do not usually oppose each other, and we readily assume it is acting as a whole. But when the animal walks into a corner, the 'whole' seems to behave queerly. Its seemingly goal-directed holistic behaviour makes 'mistakes' that trap the animal in the partial enclosure. It does not string together sequences of movements that lead it out of the alley. We realize then that such an animal is merely a collection of parts that are acting independently and may work at cross-purposes. Therefore, dopamine deficiency produces a disintegration of goal-directed behaviour into stereotype.

Stereotyped locomotion revealed in atropine-treated intact animals by behavioural traps

Partial enclosures destroy the illusion of 'adaptive wholeness' behaviourally, not physically. The normal animal is always able to leave the situation, but the brain-damaged or drugged animal's reactions to the surfaces interrupt its forward locomotion, and the repetitive actions of only part of the body make clear the hitherto unsuspected existence of stereotypy. For instance, atropine has been shown to induce hyperactivity (Bures 1967; Herz 1967; Vanderwolf 1975) and to disrupt learned performance (Buresova *et al.* 1964; Meyers *et al.* 1964), but it has not been associated with stereotypy, as have the central stimulant drugs. We believe this is because such animals generally more freely from place to place. But when they walk into a corner or a blind alleyway, they are trapped there, quite differently from the way in which an L H-damaged recovering animal is trapped. At a certain stage in its recovery, the L H-damaged animal does not scan upward along the walls forming the dead end. Its forward locomotion is arrested by bilateral and frontal snout and whisker contact with the walls. Its head scans only laterally, and stretches forward or flexes ventrally, leading it eventually to tumble out of the alleyway, heels over head, following the head as it squeezes back under the body, ending up facing outward toward the open end of the alleyway (for an illustration of such a manoeuvre see Fig. 6 in Golani *et al.* 1979). Thus, it appears that the L H-damaged animal at that stage in recovery is trapped because it does not back up or scan upward. In contrast, the atropine-treated intact animal repeatedly scans upward along the walls of the dead end. But its hindquarters appear to switch from forward locomotion into static standing when the snout initially makes bilateral and frontal contact with the walls of the dead end. The hindlegs then do not co-operate by turning and

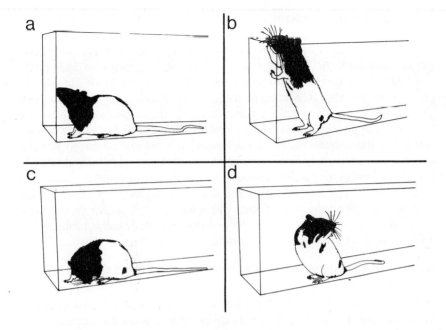

Fig. 7.9. After injection with atropine (50 mg/kg) a naive rat is trapped in a blind alley. (a) The rat repetitively scans up and down the front vertical wall of the Plexiglas alley. (b) With repeated scans, these movements increase in amplitude, sometimes as far upward as the top edge of the wall. (c) The rat also scans the floor, and (d) laterally along the side wall. Throughout all this, the hindlegs remain facing forward in postural support, being functionally disconnected from the scanning actions of the forequarters. (From Schallert *et al.* 1980.)

stepping as the head scans laterally (see Fig. 7.9) along the upper side walls of the alleyway, and the animal is behaviourally trapped. The functional disconnection between hind- and frontquarters produced by obstacles in atropine-treated intact rats is highlighted on a small platform whose top surface is a few inches off the ground. A normal animal descends within seconds, whereas the atropine-treated intact rat is trapped, sometimes for hours (DeVietti *et al.* 1985; Schallert *et al.* 1980). As its head scans downward toward the ground along the vertical surfaces of the platform, its hindlegs grip the edge and refuse to budge, or even back actively away from the edge, resisting the body instability produced by the animal's shift of weight downwards toward the floor. This defeats the exploratory forward movement and the animal is trapped. Thus, the trapping in partial enclosures in atropine-treated animals appears to be due primarily to a functional disintegration of the co-operation between body and head that is necessary for adaptive exploration in the face of obstacles.

The selective disinhibition of fractional forms of forward locomotion in otherwise akinetic animals: head-led versus hindleg-driven locomotion

Our evidence on brain-damaged rats suggests that two forms of control over forward locomotion need to be differentiated:

(1) head-led locomotion, where the head initiates tactile scanning along the ground and gradually recruits the body and legs into forward locomotion;

(2) body-initiated locomotion, where the hindlegs drive the body forward, and the front legs join in later, merely co-operating, and with the head being passively carried along or exerting only a limited 'steering' type of control.

In normal animals, these two types of control seem so balanced and well-integrated that it is difficult to dissociate them. In brain-damaged or drug-induced stereotyped behaviours, however, forward locomotion can become dissociated this way, and thus it is necessary to describe and understand how fractional forms of walking can interact with the other elements of exploratory locomotion.

If bilateral lesions are made, localized in the region of the nucleus reticularis tegmenti pontis (NRTP), a rat will display excessive forward locomotion to the point where it gallops at very high speed (Brudzinski and Mogenson 1984; Cheng *et al.* 1981; Chesire *et al.* 1983). Therefore, forward locomotion is normally controlled by an inhibitory system of which the NRTP is a necessary part. If a normal rat is made akinetic by a large (5 mg/kg) systemic dose of haloperidol, and then GABA is injected bilaterally into the NRTP (which mimics the effect of lesions there), the animal is no longer akinetic, but instead gallops rapidly forward (Cheng *et al.* 1981; Chesire *et al.* 1983). Thus dopamine-deficiency-induced akinesia appears to be indirect: its action depends on the intactness of a system that inhibits locomotion, which includes the NRTP. In dopamine deficiency, therefore, the intact NRTP system appears to inhibit forward locomotion to an excessive degree, producing akinesia (Chesire *et al.* 1983).

If so, then in dopamine-deficiency-induced akinesia, which is a model for human parkinsonian akinesia, two avenues of therapy lie open (Schallert *et al.* 1979):

(1) replacement therapy with L-dopa, the precursor of dopamine which passes the blood–brain barrier, thus counteracting the deficiency;

(2) treatment by drugs which block the inhibitory systems released by dopamine deficiency.

Anticholinergic disinhibition of locomotion in dopamine-deficient akinetic animals: head-led locomotion

Anticholinergic drugs were the earliest form of treatment of parkinsonism (Klawans 1973; Yahr *et al.* 1969) and are still used as an adjunct to L-dopa therapy. They are currently believed to ameliorate rigidity and tremor, but not akinesia (Barbeau 1972). However, in 6-OHDA-treated (dopamine-deficient) rats, made otherwise completely akinetic and cataleptic, a large dose of atropine (25 mg/kg) releases locomotion (Schallert *et al.* 1978*a*, *b*). It is abnormal in character and excessive in amount. The details of such locomotion are interesting (Schallert *et al.* 1978*a*, *b*; Pellis *et al.* 1987*b*), but, for our purposes here, it is important merely to note that atropine-released locomotion appears to be snout-led not hindleg-driven. From a standing immobile position, as the drug takes effect, the snout moves laterally or forward, in contact with the ground. In such a movement, the neck seems to stretch when the body does not co-operate in the movement. These movements are repeated, gradually increasing in amplitude, as in the 'warm-up' described above for recovering LH animals. The legs are gradually recruited and the animal walks forward. If it walks into a corner, the animal's locomotion is arrested by light bilateral and frontal snout or whisker contact, and, because it does not back, rear up along walls, or turn around, it is trapped indefinitely in the partial enclosure (the two walls of a corner, or the blind end of an alleyway). Such trapping immediately reveals that the locomotion is a simpler form, lacking some of the normal components. The arrest of forward locomotion merely by light whisker contact, and the way the snout initiates the movement with the legs lagging in their co-operation, suggests to us that such locomotion is initiated and 'led' by the snout rather than 'driven' by the hindlegs. In other forms of disintegrated locomotion, a rat may drive itself forward powerfully against the corner formed by the light walls, without being inhibited by contact with them, as is illustrated below.

Methysergide-released hindleg-driven locomotion

Cholinergic blockade by atropine does not release locomotion in animals made akinetic by electrolytic LH damage, although it does so when the destruction is produced more selectively by 6-OHDA. We interpret this to mean that the electrolytic damage transects descending striatal pathways, spared by 6-OHDA, that are necessary for anticholinergic release of locomotion. In LH-damaged animals, however, a different disintegrated form of locomotion can be released by methysergide, a serotonin receptor blocker (Chesire and Teitelbaum 1982). Early after such lesions, even before the LH-damaged animal has recovered postural support, and is otherwise completely akinetic, a large dose (45 mg/kg) of methysergide will release pure forward locomotion. Without support, such animals crawl, the hindlegs driving the body forward. The front legs lag in their co-operation, being bent far backward before stepping, as the body moves forward. The head does not scan laterally actively, being merely carried along on the body by the movement of the hindlegs. Such an animal may crawl right off the edge of the table. When the head encounters the same light plastic walls that completely inhibit the forward progression of an animal released by atropine, the methysergide-released animal continues to drive forward, pushing the walls of the corner ahead of it as it moves along the table. We conclude, therefore, that a form of hindleg-driven locomotion can be isolated, which, at a particular stage of recovery from LH damage, is not subject to guidance or inhibition by sensation coming from the head. Thus, an animal's reactions to obstacles, as illustrated by behavioural traps in partial enclosures, can shed light on many kinds of disconnections and disintegrations of neural control of exploratory locomotion.

Prior experience can reverse drug-induced behavioural trapping

An obstacle is psychological as well as physical. This is why prior experience can prevent the effect of some drugs that would otherwise induce behavioural trapping in partial enclosures. Limited experience can yield partial protection, revealing new and more subtle forms of functional disconnection and disintegration.

As mentioned above, a naive intact animal injected with a high dose of atropine (50–60 mg/kg) will be trapped in a corner or on an elevated platform. If it has had prior experience in the alleyway, it is no longer trapped there, while still being trapped on the unfamiliar platform, and vice versa (DeVietti *et al.* 1985). With only a little experience in the alleyway, it does not escape by rearing up and turning around, which is the fully normal reaction that it shows after sufficient prior experience. Instead it retreats backward out of the alley, still crouched low. Its posture in the open field is instructive. An atropine-treated animal in an unfamiliar open field stays close to the walls with its body, and explores only with snout contact along the floor or wall (see Fig. 7.10(a), (c)). Its head and body seem to be functionally disconnected, the body crouching low (with minimal leg extensor support) and refusing to co-operate with the thigmotactic scanning of the snout, so that there is exaggerated stretching and bending of the head and neck or of the torso. Conversely, with prior experience in the open field, it stands with full support (legs extended), snout in the air, and readily leaves the walls to cross the open area in a fast walk or a run (see Fig. 7.10(b), (d)). All these reactions to familiar or unfamiliar situations are shown by undrugged rats, but to a lesser degree (DeVietti *et al.* 1985). A strange open

Atropine sulphate (60 mg/kg)

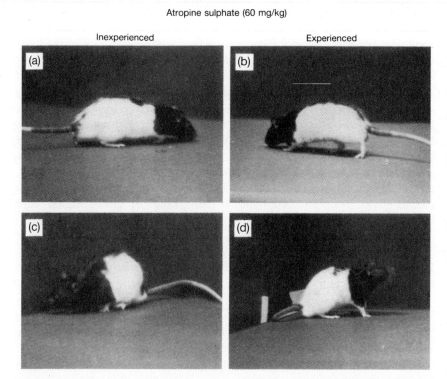

Fig. 7.10. Comparison of reactions in atropinized rats inexperienced or experienced in the open field. Movements toward a wall following placement in the centre of the open field (a and b). Immobility near a wall (c and d). Note the high posture, little or no body contact with the floor, and much less snout contact with the ground and walls in the experienced rat. In contrast, the inexperienced rat moves slowly, with inadequate co-operation by the hindlegs, and with much body and snout contact with the ground and the walls. (From DeVietti *et al.* 1985.)

field appears to be a psychological obstacle to a rat. The same subcomponent body reactions whose disintegrated actions behaviourally trap the naive atropine-treated animal in the partial enclosure are the ones that seem to act at cross-purposes in the unfamiliar open field. However, what is maladaptive in one context may be adaptive in another. It is adaptive for a rodent to freeze in fear, and to hug the surfaces of walls or of large objects that can inhibit the killing swoop of its aerial predators (e.g. Glickman and Morrison 1969; Lay 1974; Payne 1971). The problem is that other mechanisms, for alternative reactions that might offer a more appropriate way of dealing with the situation, appear to be excluded. Thus, in the face of an unfamiliar situation, atropine appears excessively to potentiate 'freezing in fear', with all the functional disconnections and disintegrations that go along with it. Conversely, with prior experience, atropine appears exaggeratedly to heighten inbuilt postures and movements appropriate when little danger appears to be present.

Something of this sort must be going on as well when amphetamine is acting. An animal that would drown (see above) because it only swims underwater in an unfamiliar tank is able to surface and stay alive if it has had prior experience there (Petree and DeVietti 1989). Perhaps this is related to the sudden drowning death described in wild rats in unfamiliar swimming situations (Richter 1957).

General discussion

We have shown that a microdescriptive behavioural analysis, which focuses on the movement of individual body parts rather than on acts, can make sense of several puzzling aspects of central stimulant-induced stereotyped behaviour. We believe that the currently maintained distinction between stereotype and locomotion is not valid, and that it is generated by what we have called the perceptual illusion of 'adaptive wholeness' which pervades the description of normal, motivated behaviour. In our view, all stereotypy is a disintegrated form of behaviour akin to that produced by brain damage. Where such disintegration exists, behavioural description in terms of adaptive outcome is inappropriate. The many seemingly unrelated 'acts' produced by amphetamine or apomorphine are not integrated acts at all, but are composite aggregate forms generated by the drugs' action independently on a few continuous neurological movement variables. Our microdescriptive behavioural analysis indicates that, in high doses, these drugs appear only briefly to stimulate the dopaminergic system before reversing their action to functionally shut it down. Recent electrophysiological evidence agrees with this (Alloway and Rebec 1984; Rebec and Segal 1980; Ricaurte et al. 1984).

Postural support, being non-dopaminergic, remains isolated but intact in dopamine deficiency. Recovery of dopaminergic function indicates that separate subsystems of exploratory movement, having different thresholds of activation, recover independently at different rates, superimposing their activity on postural support. These subsystems include head-scanning, head-orienting, directed mouthing, and manipulative use of the forepaws. Dopamine acts independently on three dimensions of head movement (lateral, longitudinal, and vertical), recruiting limb and body segments rostrocaudally. Through such recruitment, head-scanning becomes turning, forward locomotion, upward scanning, and rearing. During recovery from damage, conflict (disintegration) exists between postural support and head-scanning, yielding an exaggerated bending and stretching 'warm-up' sequence in the activation of locomotion from cataleptic standing. With more anterolateral damage to the ascending dopaminergic systems, a different form of partial catalepsy can be produced, in which conflict exists between forequarter orienting versus hindquarter immobile standing. Even though, in recovery, catalepsy disappears and locomotion seems to be relatively free in an open field, the animal's reactions to physical and psychological obstacles reveal that its neural control mechanisms are not yet fully integrated. Behavioural traps in partial enclosures reveal different disintegrated forms of locomotion, present in dopamine deficiency, in blockade of cholinergic function, and in high-dose treatment with dopaminergic agonists.

These findings in animals may have relevance for clinical neurology. It is well known that patients suffering from Parkinson's disease experience great difficulty in walking when faced with obstacles that appear innocuous to a normal person. For instance, when they approach a doorway, their locomotion may deteriorate sharply. Similarly, they may become immobilized at the curb when they must step off to cross a heavily trafficked street (P. Teitelbaum, personal observation). These observations suggest that subtle forms of disintegration of control in the face of obstacles, analogous to those shown here in animals, may exist in humans with Parkinson's disease or other disorders of locomotion. It may be fruitful to explore the use of physical and psychological obstacles as diagnostic aids in the detection of disintegration of neural control of locomotion in people.

Curzon and co-workers (Andrews *et al.* 1982; Curzon *et al.* 1979; Dickinson and Curzon 1983) have shown that both dopaminergic and serotonergic systems are necessary for the backward locomotion produced in rats by a high dose of amphetamine. (See also Chapter 6, this volume.) We have pointed out that the 'act' of backing up is quite complex, involving a dopaminergic movement component that acts on head verticality. This may interact with other, serotonergic components of movement. Their interaction at an appropriate time after injection may yield 'backing up'. It would pay to re-examine, with microdescriptive behaviour analysis, the amphetamine-induced behaviour of animals after selective serotonergic (Dickinson *et al.* 1984; Lees *et al.* 1979) or dopaminergic (Andrews *et al.* 1982) damage to see whether different independent movement factors can be revealed in such animals.

A general characteristic of the abnormal animals we have studied (e.g. amphetamine- or apomorphine-treated, atropinized, LH-damaged electro-lytically or by 6-OHDA, and NRTP-damaged) is that they all show excessive snout thigmotaxis in their exploratory locomotion. Is exaggerated snout thigmotaxis a general sign of some degree of disintegration of control of locomotion in rodents? Szechtman (1983) has shown that altering the tactile input by bandaging one side of the snout in apomorphine-treated animals systematically causes them to circle in the direction of the uncovered side. What would happen to locomotion in these various types of animals if the snout were denervated?

Finally, in their theory of the stimulatory action of amphetamine on operant behaviour, Lyon and Robbins (Lyon and Robbins 1975; Robbins 1981; Robbins and Sahakian 1981) point out that amphetamine speeds up the rate of behaviour. (See also Chapter 2, this volume.) They presume, therefore, that at higher doses, those behaviours which can be performed at higher rates will eventually crowd out slower responses, leading to a predominance of behaviours such as licking and biting. We believe their theory is correct in some respects—amphetamine does accelerate the rate of operant action. However, our evidence suggests that, at high doses, the picture may be complicated by the biphasic action of amphetamine or apomorphine—these drugs appear to stimulate at first, but later, they seem to reverse their action and depress the system, as documented above. Functional disintegration then may predominate. Some aspects of the functional disintegration of operant control of behaviour under a high dose of amphetamine have been described (Teitelbaum and Derks 1958). The challenge remains of how to diagnose the presence and interaction of the two opposing states—that of stimulated operant (integrated) behaviour versus overstimulated or damaged (disintegrated) behaviours induced by dopaminergic agonists or analogous drug actions.

Acknowledgements

We thank Dr Ilan Golani and other members of the Zoology Department of Tel Aviv University where this paper was written, with support by funds from NIH Grant NS-11671 and a John Simon Guggenheim Fellowship (to PT). Terry DeVietti was an NIH Postdoctoral Research Fellow at the University of Illinois during the time that the work on atropine stereotypy described here was done. We thank Dr Henry Szechtman of McMaster University, and Dr David L. Wolgin of Florida-Atlantic University for constructive criticisms.

References

Alander, D. H., Servidio, S., Schallert, T., and Teitelbaum, P. (1983). Possible vestibular involvement in behaviour induced by d-amphetamine sulfate. *Fed. Proc.*, **42**, 1159.

Alloway, K.D. and Rebec, G.V. (1984). Apomorphine-induced inhibition of neostriatal activity is enhanced by lesions induced by 6-hydroxydopamine but not by long-term administration of amphetamine. *Neuropharmacology* **23**, 1033–40.

Andrews, C.D., Fernando, J.C.R., and Curzon, G. (1982). Differential involvement of dopamine-containing tracts in 5-hydroxytryptamine-dependent behaviours caused by amphetamine in large doses. *Neuropharmacology* **21**, 63–8.

Barbeau, A. (1972). Contributions of levodopa therapy to the neuropharmacology of akinesia. In *Parkinson's disease* (ed. J. Siegfried), pp. 151–74. Hans Huber Publishers, Basel.

Brudzinski, S.M. and Mogenson, G.J. (1984). The role of the nucleus reticularis tegmenti pontis in locomotion. A lesion study in the rat. *Brain Res. Bull.* **12**, 513–20.

Bures, J. (1967). The effect of physostigmine and atropine on some behavioural and electrophysiological functions in rats. In *Neuro-psycho-pharmacology* (ed. H. Brill, p. 383.) Mouton and Co, Amsterdam.

Buresova, D., Bures, J., Bohdanecky, Z., and Weiss, T. (1964). Effect of atropine on learning, extinction, and retrieval in rats. *Psychopharmacologia* **5**, 255–63.

Chen, Y.-C., Pellis, S.M., Sirkin, D.W., Potegal, M., and Teitelbaum, P. (1986). Bandage-backfall: Labyrinthine and non-labyrinthine components. *Physiol. Behav.* **37**, 805–14.

Cheng, J.-T., Schallert, T., DeRyck, M., and Teitelbaum, P. (1981). Galloping induced by pontine tegmentum damage in rats: A form of 'Parkinsonian festination' not blocked by haloperidol. *Proc. Nat. Acad. Sci. USA* **78**, 3279–83.

Chesire, R.M. and Teitelbaum, P. (1982). Methysergide releases locomotion without support in lateral hypothalamic akinesia. *Physiol. Behav.* **28**, 335–47.

Chesire, R.M., Cheng, J.-T., and Teitelbaum, P. (1983). The inhibition of movement by morphine or haloperidol depends on an intact nucleus reticularis tegmenti pontis. *Physiol. Behav.* **30**, 809–18.

Cole, S.O. (1977). Interaction of arena size with different measures of amphetamine effects. *Pharmacol. Biochem. Behav.* **7**, 181–4.

Costall, B. and Naylor, R.J. (1973). The role of telencephalic dopaminergic systems in the mediation of apomorphine-stereotyped behaviour. *Eur. J. Pharmacol.* **24**, 8–24.

Costall, B. and Naylor, R. (1974). A role for the amygdala in the development of the cataleptic and stereotypic actions of the narcotic agonists and antagonists in the rat. *Psychopharmacologia* **25**, 203–13.

Creese, I., Burt, D.R., and Snyder, S.H. (1977). Dopamine receptor binding enhancement accompanies lesion-induced behavioural supersensitivity. *Science* **197**, 596–8.

Curzon, G., Fernando, J.C.R. and Lees, A.J. (1979). Backward walking and circling: Behavioural responses induced by drug treatments which cause simultaneous release of catecholamines and 5-hydroxytryptamine. *Br. J. Pharmacol.* **66**, 573–9.

Decsi, L., Gacs, E., Zambo, K., and Nagy, J. (1979). Simple device to measure stereotyped rearing of the rat in an objective and quantitative way. *Neuropharmacology* **18**, 723-5.

Denny-Brown, D. and Chambers, R.A. (1958). The parietal lobe and behaviour. *Res. Pub. Ass. Res. Nerv. Ment. Dis.* **36**, 35-117.

DeRyck, M. and Teitelbaum, P. (1983). Morphine versus haloperidol catalepsy in the rat: an electromyographic analysis of postural support mechanisms. *Exp. Neurol.* **79**, 54-76.

DeRyck, M. and Teitelbaum, P. (1984). Morphine catalepsy as an adaptive reflex state in rats. *Behav. Neurosci.* **98**, 243-61.

DeRyck, M., Schallert, T., and Teitelbaum, P. (1980). Morphine versus haloperidol catalepsy in the rat: A behavioural analysis of postural support mechanisms. *Brain Res.* **201**, 143-72.

DeVietti, T.L., Pellis, S.M., Pellis, V.C., and Teitelbaum, P. (1985). Previous experience disrupts atropine-induced stereotyped 'trapping' in rats. *Behav. Neurosci.* **99**, 1128-41.

Dickinson, S.L. and Curzon, G. (1983). Roles of dopamine and 5-hydroxytryptamine in stereotyped and non-stereotyped behaviours. *Neuropharmacology* **22**, 805-12.

Dickinson, S.L., Andrews, C.D. and Curzon, G. (1984). The effects of lesions produced by 5, 7-dihydroxytryptamine on 5-hydroxytryptamine-mediated behaviour induced by amphetamine in large doses in the rat. *Neuropharmacology* **23**, 423-30.

Dourish, C.T. and Cooper, S.J. (1984). Potentiation of total horizontal activity and ambulation in rats treated with combinations of β-phenylethylamine and naloxone. *Neuropharmacology* **23**, 1059-65.

Eilam, D. and Golani, I. (1988). The ontogeny of exploratory behaviour in the house rat (*Rattus rattus*): the mobility gradient. *Developmental Psychobiology* **21**, 679-710.

Eshkol, N. and Wachmann, A. (1958). *Movement notation*. Weidenfeld and Nicolson, London.

Fray, P.J., Sahakian, B.J., Robbins, T.W., Koob, G.F., and Iversen, S.D. (1980). An observational method for quantifying the behavioural effects of dopamine agonists: Contrasting effects of *d*-amphetamine and apomorphine. *Psychopharmacology* **69**, 253-9.

Glickman, S.E. and Morrison, B.J. (1969). Some behavioural and neural correlates of predation susceptibility in mice. *Commun. Behav. Biol.* **4**, 261-7.

Golani, I. (1976). Homeostatic motor processes in mammalian interactions: a choreography of display. In *Perspectives in ethology*, Vol. 2 (ed. P.T.G. Bateson and P.H. Klopfer), pp. 69-134. Plenum Press, New York.

Golani, I., Wolgin, D.L., and Teitelbaum, P. (1979). A proposed natural geometry of recovery from akinesia in the lateral hypothalamic rat. *Brain Res.* **164**, 237-67.

Golani, I., Bronchti, G., Moualem, D., and Teitelbaum, P. (1981). "Warm-up" along dimensions of movement in the ontogeny of exploration in rats and other infant mammals. *Proc. Nat. Acad. Sci.*, USA **78**, 7226-9.

Heilman, N. (1972). Frontal lobe neglect in man. *Neurology* **22**, 660–4.

Heilman, K. M., Pandya, D. N., and Geschwind, N. (1970). Trimodal inattention following parietal lobe ablations. *Trans. Am. Neurol. Ass.* **95**, 259–61.

Herz, A. (1967). Some actions of cholinergic and anticholinergic drugs on reactive behaviour. In *Neuro-psycho-pharmacology* (ed. H. Brill), pp. 384–5. Mouton and Co, Amsterdam.

Janssen, P. A. J., Niemegeers, C. J. C., and Jageneau, A. H. M. (1960). Apomorphine antagonism in rats. *Arzneimittel-Forsch.* **10**, 1003–5.

Jerussi, T. P. and Glick, S. D. (1976). Drug-induced rotation in rats without lesions: behavioural and neurochemical indices of a normal asymmetry in nigro-striatal function. *Psychopharmacology* **64**, 45–54.

Klawans, H. L. (1973). *The pharmacology of extrapyramidal movement disorders*, p. 8. S. Karger, New York.

Kokkinidis, L. and Anisman, H. (1979). Circling behaviour following systemic *d*-amphetamine administration: Potential noradrenergic and dopaminergic involvement. *Psychopharmacology* **64**, 45–54.

Kuschinsky, K. and Hornykiewicz, O. (1972). Morphine catalepsy in the rat: Relation to striatal dopamine metabolism. *Eur. J. Pharmacol.* **19**, 119–22.

Lay, D. M. (1974). Differential predation on gerbils (*Meriones*) by the little owl, *Athene brahma*. *J. Mammal.* **55**, 608–14.

Lees, A. J., Fernando, J. C. R., and Curzon, G. (1979). Serotonergic involvement in behavioural responses to amphetamine at high doses. *Neuropharmacology* **18**, 153–8.

Levitt, D. R. and Teitelbaum, P. (1975). Somnolence, akinesia and sensory activation of motivated behaviour in the lateral hypothalamic syndrome. *Proc. Nat. Acad. Sci. USA* **72**, 2819–23.

Lyon, M. and Robbins, T. (1975). The action of CNS stimulant drugs: A general theory concerning amphetamine effects. In *Current developments in psychopharmacology*, Vol. 2 (ed. W. B. Fessman and L. Valzelli), pp. 80–163. Spectrum Publications, New York.

Magnus, R. (1926). Some results of studies in the physiology of posture. *Lancet* **211**, 531–6, 585–8.

Marshall, J. F. and Gotthelf, T. (1979). Sensory inattention in rats with 6-hydroxydopamine-induced degeneration of ascending dopaminergic neurons: apomorphine induced reversal of deficits. *Exp. Neurol.* **65**, 398–411.

Marshall, J. F. and Teitelbaum, P. (1974). Further analysis of sensory inattention following lateral hypothalamic damage in rats. *J. Comp. Physiol. Psychol.* **86**, 375–95.

Marshall, J. F., Turner, B H., and Teitelbaum, P. (1971). Sensory neglect produced by lateral hypothalamic damage. *Science* **174**, 523–5.

Marshall, J. F., Richardson, J. S., and Teitelbaum, P. (1974). Nigrostriatal bundle damage and the lateral hypothalamic syndrome. *J. Comp. Physiol. Psychol.* **87**, 808–30.

Meyers, B., Roberts, K. H., Riciputi, R. H., and Domino, E. F. (1964). Some effects of muscarinic cholinergic blocking drugs on behaviour and the electrocorticogram. *Psychopharmacologia* **5**, 289–300.

Neve, K. A. and Marshall, J. F. (1984). The effects of denervation and chronic haloperidol treatment on neostriatal dopamine receptors density are not additive in the rat. *Neurosci. Lett.* **46**, 77–83.

Neve, K. A., Kozlowski, M. R., and Marshall, J. F. (1982). Plasticity of neostriatal dopamine receptors after nigrostriatal injury: relationship to recovery of sensorimotor functions and behavioural supersensitivity. *Brain Res.* **244**, 33–44.

Oltmans, G. A. and Harvey, J. A. (1972). L H syndrome and brain catecholamine levels after lesions of the nigrostriatal bundle. *Physiol. Behav.* **8**, 69–78.

Payne, R. S. (1971). Acoustic location of prey by barn owls. *J. Exp. Biol.* **54**, 535–73.

Pellis, S. M. (1981). A description of social play by the Australian magpie *Gymnorhina tibicen* based on Eshkol-Wachman notation. *Bird Behav.* **3**, 61–79.

Pellis, S. M. (1985). What is fixed in a fixed action pattern? A problem of methodology. *Bird Behav.* **6**, 10–15.

Pellis, S. M., Chen, Y. -c., and Teitelbaum, P. (1985). Fractionation of the cataleptic bracing response in rats. *Physiol. Behav.* **34**, 815–23.

Pellis, S. M., De La Cruz, F., Pellis, V. C., and Teitelbaum, P. (1986). Morphine subtracts subcomponents of haloperidol-isolated postural support reflexes revealing gradients of their integration. *Behav. Neurosci.* **100**, 631–46.

Pellis, S. M., Pellis, V. C., O'Brien, D. P., De La Cruz, F., and Teitelbaum, P. (1987*a*). Pharmacological subtraction of the sensory controls over grasping in rats. *Physiol. Behav.* **39**, 127–33.

Pellis, S. M., Pellis, V. C., Chesire, R. M., Rowland, N., and Teitelbaum, P. (1987). Abnormal gait sequence in locomotion after atropine treatment of catecholamine-deficient akinetic rats. *Proc. nat. Acad. Sci., USA* **84**, 8750–3.

Petree, A. D. and DeVietti, T. L. (1989). Previous experience disrupts d-amphetamine-induced stereotypic diving in rats. *Psychopharmacology* **97**, 462–5.

Rebec, G. V. and Segal, D. S. (1980). Apparent tolerance to some aspects of *l*-amphetamine stereotypy with long-term treatment. *Pharmacol. Biochem. Behav.* **13**, 793–7.

Redgrave, P., Dean P., Donohoe, T. P., and Pope, S. G. (1980). Superior colliculus lesions selectively attenuate apomorphine-induced oral stereotyping: a possible role for the nigrostriatal pathway. *Brain Res.* **196**, 541–6.

Ricaurte, G. A., Seiden, L. S., and Schuster, C. R. (1984). Further evidence that amphetamines produce long-lasting dopamine neurochemical deficits by destroying dopamine nerve fibres. *Brain Res.* **303**, 359–64.

Richter, C. P. (1957). On the phenomenon of sudden death in animals and man. *Psychosom. Med.* **29**, 191–197.

Robbins, T. W. (1981). Behavioural determinants of drug action: rate-dependency revisited. In *Theory in psychopharmacology*, Vol. 1 (ed. S. J. Cooper), pp. 1–63. Academic Press, London.

Robbins, T. W. and Sahakian, B. J. (1981). Behavioural and neurochemical determinants of stereotypy induced by drugs. In *Metabolic disorders of the nervous system* (ed. F. C. Rose), pp. 294–7. Pitman Press, London.

Sacks, O. (1976). *Awakenings*. Vintage Books, New York.

Sanberg, P. R. (1980). Haloperidol-induced catalepsy is mediated by postsynaptic dopamine receptors. *Nature* **284**, 472-3.

Sanberg, P. R., Coyle, J. T., Moran, T. H., and Kubos, K. L. (1983). Automated measurement of stereotypic behaviour in rats. *Behav. Neurosci.* **97**, 830-2.

Schallert, T., Whishaw, I. Q., Ramirez, V. D., and Teitelbaum, P. (1978a). Compulsive, abnormal walking caused by anticholinergics in akinetic, 6-hydroxydopamine-treated rats. *Science* **199**, 1461-3.

Schallert, T., Whishaw, I. Q., Ramirez, V. D., and Teitelbaum, P. (1978b). 6-Hydroxydopamine and anticholinergic drugs. *Science* **202**, 1215-17.

Schallert, T., Whishaw, I. Q., DeRyck, M., and Teitelbaum, P. (1978c). The postures of catecholamine-depletion catalepsy: their possible adaptive value in thermoregulation. *Physiol. Behav.* **21**, 817-20.

Schallert, T. DeRyck, M., Whishaw, I. Q., Ramirez, V. D., and Teitelbaum, P. (1979). Excessive bracing reactions and their control by atropine and L-Dopa in an animal analog of Parkinsonism. *Exp. Neurol.* **64**, 33-43.

Schallert, T., DeRyck, M., and Teitelbaum, P. (1980). Atropine stereotypy as a behavioural trap: A movement subsystem and EEG analysis. *J. Comp. physiol. Psychol.* **94**, 1-24.

Schiørring, E. (1971). Amphetamine induced selective stimulation of certain behaviour items with concurrent inhibition of others in an open-field test with rats. *Behaviour* **39**, 1-17.

Schiørring, E. (1979). Study of the stereotyped locomotor activity in amphetamine treated rats. *Psychopharmacology* **66**, 281-7.

Schoenfeld, R. J., Neumeyer, J. L., Dafeldecker, W., and Roffler-Tarlov, S. (1975). Comparison of structural and stereoisomers of apomorphine on stereotyped sniffing behaviour of the rat. *Eur. J. Pharmacol.* **30**, 63-8.

Segal, D. S. and Schuckit, M. A. (1983). Animal models of stimulant-induced psychosis. In *Stimulants: neurochemical, behavioural, and clinical perspectives* (ed. I. Creese), pp. 131-67. Raven Press, New York.

Segal, D. S., Weinberger, S. B., Canill, J., and McCunney, S. J. (1980). Multiple daily amphetamine administration: behavioural and neurochemical alterations. *Science* **207**, 904-7.

Szechtman, H. (1983). Peripheral sensory input directs apomorphine induced circling in rats. *Brain Res.* **264**, 332-5.

Szechtman, H., Ornstein, K., Hofstein, R., Teitelbaum, P., and Golani, I. (1980). Apomorphine induces behavioural regression: a sequence that is the opposite of neurological recovery. In *Enzymes and neurotransmitters in mental disease* (ed. E. Usdin, T. L. Sourkes, and M. B. H. Youdim), pp. 512-17. John Wiley and Sons, New York.

Szechtman, H., Ornstein, K., Teitelbaum, P., and Golani, I. (1982). Snout contact fixation, climbing and gnawing during apomorphine stereotypy in rats from two substrains. *Eur. J. Pharmacol.* **80**, 385-92.

Szechtman, H., Ornstein, K., Teitelbaum, P., and Golani, I. (1985). The morphogenesis of stereotyped behaviour induced by the dopamine receptor agonist apomorphine in the laboratory rat. *Neuroscience* **14**, 783-98.

Teitelbaum, P. (1982a). What is the 'zero condition' for motivated behaviour? In *The neural basis of feeding and reward* (ed. B. G. Hoebel and D. Novin) pp. 7-23. Haer Institute, Brunswick, Maine.

Teitelbaum, P. (1982*b*). Disconnection and antagonistic interaction of movement subsystems in motivated behaviour. In *Changing concepts of the nervous system: Proceedings of the First Institute of Neurological Sciences Symposium in Neurobiology and Learning* (ed. A. R. Morrison and P. Strick), pp. 467–78. Academic Press, New York.

Teitelbaum, P. (1986). The lateral hypothalamic double disconnection syndrome: a reappraisal and a new theory for recovery of function. In *G. Stanley Hall: essays in honor of 100 years of psychological research in America* (ed. S. H. Hulse and B. F. Green, Jr), pp. 79–125. The Johns Hopkins University Press, Baltimore, Maryland.

Teitelbaum, P. and Derks, P. (1958). The effect of amphetamine on forced drinking in the rat. *J. Comp. physiol. Psychol.* **51**, 801–10.

Teitelbaum, P., Schallert, T., DeRyck, M., Whishaw, I. Q., and Golani, I. (1980). Motor subsystems in motivated behaviour. In *Neural mechanisms of goal-directed behaviour and learning* (ed. R. F. Thompson, L. H. Hicks, and V. B. Shvyrkov), pp. 127–43. Academic Press, New York.

Teitelbaum, P., Szechtman, H., Sirkin, D. W., and Golani, I. (1982). Dimensions of movement, movement subsystems, and local reflexes in the dopaminergic systems underlying exploratory locomotion. In *Behavioural models and the analysis of drug action*. Proceedings of the 27th O H O L O Conference, Zichron Ya'acov, Israel, March 28–31 (ed. M. Y. Spiegelstein and A. Levy), pp. 357–85. Elsevier Biomedical Press, Amsterdam.

Teitelbaum, P., Schallert, T., and Whishaw, I. Q. (1983). Sources of spontaneity in motivated behaviour. In *Handbook of behavioural neurobiology* (ed. E. Satinoff and P. Teitelbaum), pp. 23–65. Plenum Publishing Corporation, New York.

Thomas, K. V. and Handley, S. L. (1978). On the mechanism of amphetamine-induced behavioural changes in the mouse. I. An observational analysis of dexamphetamine. *Arzneimittel-Forsch.* **28**, 827–33.

Ungerstedt, U. (1971). Adipsia and aphagia after 6-hydroxydopamine induced degeneration of the nigro-striatal dopamine system. *Acta physiol. scand. Suppl.* **367**, 95–122.

Vanderwolf, C. H. (1975). Neocortical and hippocampal activation in relation to behaviour: effects of atropine, eserine, phenothiazines, and amphetamine. *J. comp. physiol. psychol.* **88**, 300–23.

Voigtlander von, P. R., Losey, E. G., and Triezenberg, H. J. (1975). Increased sensitivity to dopaminergic agents after chronic neuroleptic treatment. *J. Pharmacol. exp. Ther.* **193**, 88–94.

Wolgin, D. L. (1985). Forelimb placing and hopping reflexes in haloperidol- and morphine-treated cataleptic rats. *Behav. Neurosci.* **99**, 423–35.

Yahr, M. D., Duvoisin, R. C., Schear, M. J., Barrett, R. E., and Hoehn, M. M. (1969). Treatment of parkinsonism with levodopa. *Arch. Neurol.* **21**, 343–54.

Zigmond, M. J. and Stricker, E. M. (1973). Recovery of feeding after 6-hydroxydopamine (6-O H D A) or lateral hypothalamic lesions: The role of catecholamines. *Fed. Proc.* **32**, 754.

8

Mechanisms of schedule entrainment
ALLISTON K. REID AND J.E.R. STADDON

Introduction

If hungry rats are placed on a fixed-time (FT) schedule of food delivery in which food pellets are delivered every, say, 60 seconds independent of the rat's behaviour, and if supporting apparatus such as a running wheel and a water dispenser are available, the sequence of the activities between food deliveries becomes strikingly stereotyped. Fig. 8.1 shows a second-by-second summary of an entire 45-min session for a rat on an FT 60-s schedule. Each row represents a single interfood interval, and each character or space represents one second of an activity. 'F' corresponds to 'head-in-feeder', 'D' to drinking, 'R' to wheel running, 'C' to chewing an oak block, blank spaces to unmeasured activities, and the lower case letters correspond to various inoperative levers in the apparatus. The '1' in the first column is the number of food pellets beginning the interval, and the '60' in the last column represents the duration of the interfood interval.

When data are depicted in this format, the most striking aspect is the temporal entrainment of the various activities by food presentation. With few exceptions most interfood intervals contained a relatively stereotyped temporal pattern of activities: eating the food pellet, then drinking from the water spout, running in the wheel, and finally returning to the feeder area in anticipation of the next food delivery. But there is another striking aspect of these data. Not only is drinking generally the first activity to occur after eating each pellet, the amount of drinking is much higher than that observed over the same 45-min period when all the food pellets are delivered *en masse* at the beginning of the session. There is something about the schedule of food presentation that not only entrains all, or nearly all, activities, but also induces polydipsic drinking. Excessive drinking in the absence of water deprivation in this paradigm has been termed *schedule-induced drinking* to emphasize the role of the reward schedule in the production of the augmented drinking.

The main purpose of this chapter is to identify the factors responsible for the entrainment of the temporal patterns of induced and non-induced

```
1FFFF    DDDDDDDDDDD      RRRR  FF   RR  RRRRRRR    RRRRRR   R ‡ 60
1R  FFFFDDDDDDDDDDDDDD     RRRR RRR R RRRR R R RRRR    RRRRRR ‡ 60
1 FFFFFDDDDDD RRRR     R RRR    RR RRR RFFFFFFFFFFFFFFFFFFFF ‡ 60
1     FDDDDDDDDDDD      RRRRRRRRRRR     RRRRRRRRRRRRRR  R ‡ 60
1     FDDDDD RRRRRRRRR        R FFFFFFFFFFFFFFFFFFFFFFFF ‡ 60
1   F DDDDD RRRRRRRRRR RRRR    RR RRRRR FFF FFFFFFFFFF FF ‡ 60
1FFFFFFFDDDDDD RRRRRRRR R  R RRRRRRRRR    FFFFF FFFFF FFF ‡ 60
1     FDDDDDDDDDDD    RRRRRRR   RRRRRR    RRRRRR R    FFFFF ‡ 60
1FFFFFDDDDDDDD RRRRRRRRRR RRRR     RR  RRR    FFFFFFFFFFFFF ‡ 60
1   FDDDDDDD  RRRRRRRRRR RRRRRRRR R RRRRRRR    F   FFFFFFFF ‡ 60
1   FDDDDDDDDD RR RRRRRRRRRRRRRR   RRRRR  R RRR     FF ‡ 60
1FFFFFFDDDDDDD RRRR    RRRRRRRRRRR     RRR    FFFFFFF ‡ 60
1FFFFFF DDDDDDDDD RRR  RRRRR  RRRRRRR RR   R   FF FFFFFFFF ‡ 60
1FFFFFDDDDD RRRRRRRRRRRRRRRRRRRR     R FFFFFFFFF FFF ‡ 60
1   F    DDDDDDDDDDDDD  D   C         D          ‡ 60
1    FFF              FF       R RFF   FFF FFFFFFFF ‡ 60
1FFFFF DDDDDDDDDDDDDDD RRRRRRRRRRR  RRRRRR R RR FFFFF FFF  ‡ 60
1FFFF DDDDDRRRR  RR  RRR      R RRRR    RR RR  FFFFFFF FF ‡ 60
1    FFFDDDDDDDDDDDD RRRRRRRRRRR   RRRRRRR    RRRRR R  FFFFF ‡ 60
1 FFFFF DDDDDDDDDDDD    RRRRRRRR  RRRRR RRRRRR RR FFF FFFFFFF ‡ 60
1FFFFF     R RRR             FF  F FFFFFF FFFFFFF ‡ 60
1FFFFFFDDDDDDDDDDDDDD   RRR RRRRRRRRRR R RRR    FFFFFFFFFFFF ‡ 60
1 F DD      D RRRRRRRRRRRRR   RRRRRRRRR      R R FFFFF ‡ 60
1FFFFFDDDDDD RRR   RRRRR RRRRRRRR     FFFFFFFFFFFFFFFFFF ‡ 60
1   F DDDD  RRRRR   RRRRRRRRR    FF   FFFFFFFFFFFFFFFFF ‡ 60
1FFFF DDDDD RR RRRRRRRRRRRR RRRRRRRRRRRR R    F FFFFFFFF ‡ 60
1FFFFF DDDDD RRRRRRRRRRR      RRRRRRR     R  FFFFFFFF ‡ 60
1FFFF   f  D      F      F       FFFFFFFFFFFFFFFFFFFFFFFFF ‡ 60
1FFFF DDDDDDD    RRR RRRR  RRRRRRRRRRR    RRRR    RR    FFFF ‡ 60
1FFFF   DDDDDD RRRRRRRRRRRRRRRR RRRRR    R  R FFFFFFFFFFFFFFF ‡ 60
1FFFFF DDDDDDD         C    C F     FFFFFFFFFFFFFFF ‡ 60
1   F DDDD  RRR    RRR R RRRR    RRRRRR R  R FFFFFFFFFFFFF ‡ 60
1FFFFF DDDDD RRR  RRRRRRRRRR R  R  RRR    RFFFFFFFFFFFFFFF ‡ 60
1FFFFF   DDDD       RRR  RRRRRRRR  RRRRRR R   R     FF ‡ 60
1FFFFF   DD   RRRRR RRRRR      RRRR   RR FFFFFFFFFF ‡ 60
1FFFFFFFDDDDDDD RRRR RRRRRRRR    RRRRRRR RRRRRR   RR R ‡ 60
1 FFFF   FFFF FFFFFFFFFFFF FFFFFFFFFFFFFF FFFFFFFFFFFFFFFFFF ‡ 60
1FFFFFF DDDDDDD         RRR RRRRRRRRRR    FFFFFFFF ‡ 60
1FFFFDDDDDDD  RRR   RRRRRRRR    RRRRR  RRRRR FFFFFFFFFFFFFFF ‡ 60
1      FDDDDDDDDD RRRRRRRRRRR    RRRR    R R R  R FFFFFFF ‡ 60
1FFFF DDDDDDD   RRRR  RRRRRRRR RRRR    R  R  FFFFFFFFFFF ‡ 60
1    FFFFF DDDDDDD      DDDDD   RRRRRRRRRRRRR  R RRRRR ‡ 60
1  FFFF   RRRRR  RRRRRRR RRRR   R RRRRRRR    FFFFFFFF ‡ 60
1FFFF DDDDDDDDD RRR    R RRR   RRRR FFFFFFFFFFFFFFFFFFF FF ‡ 60
```

activities in the interfood interval. We treat the observations of entrainment and elevated levels of induced activities as separate (albeit often related) phenomena, because activities can become entrained without occurring at levels above that of a massed-food baseline. There are several criteria for the classification of an activity as schedule induced or non-induced (see Falk 1969; Staddon 1977 for summaries and justifications). We will deal with three:

(1) the elevated level of induced activities relative to baseline measures;

(2) the inverted-U relation between the rates of induced activities and food delivery;

(3) the differences in the temporal distributions of the two types when they occur in the same interfood interval. That is, the induced activity occurs first in the interval, appearing food-bound, and non-induced activities seem to occur later if there is 'enough' time available.

We will not deal directly with the question of the elevated level of induced behaviour and its proper baseline measures. Historically, much emphasis has been placed on the issue of excessiveness, and Rachlin and Krasnoff (1983), Roper (1981), Timberlake (1982), and Wetherington and Brownstein (1982) discuss the measurement of the proper baseline(s) in great detail. Our emphasis is on the different temporal distributions of induced and non-induced activities.

Since Falk's (1961) discovery of schedule-induced drinking, many researchers have explored the generality of schedule induction. Schedule induction has been observed with several activities, rewards, schedules, and species (see Falk 1969, 1971; Staddon 1977 for reviews). Although several different activities have been demonstrated to be induced to elevated levels, most research has treated schedule-induced polydipsia as a paradigm for the study of schedule induction. Therefore, much more is known about induced drinking than about other induced activities, which must unavoidably bias the emphasis of this chapter.

There is little reason to believe that the induction of drinking is more important than the induction of any other activity. The intuitive idea that drinking is somehow uniquely related to eating (especially eating dry food pellets) has dominated the literature to such an extent that most explanations of schedule induction have usually assumed the existence of a (poorly defined) special relation between the induced activity and the reinforcer. For example, a widely held hypothesis regarding the causes of schedule-induced drinking is the 'motivation hypothesis' (Falk 1966*b*; Staddon 1977). This hypothesis states that drinking is induced on food schedules because of some facilitatory relation between hunger and thirst, so that increased drinking occurs with increases in drive or incentive to eat. Larger meals, higher food rates, higher food deprivation, and higher food palatability should all result in increased levels of induced drinking. It also provides an informal mechanism of how the induced activity is selected from all possibilities: drinking is most often induced on food schedules because of the special facilitatory relation between eating and drinking. Non-induced activities such as running presumably do not have the same facilitatory relation with food. Whether these relations differ qualitatively or only quantitatively remains unanswered.

Nevertheless, activities other than drinking can be induced by food schedules. For example, schedule-induced gnawing also occurs in rats, pigeons often show schedule-induced aggression, and gerbils show induced running (see Falk 1969, 1971; Staddon 1977 for reviews). It remains an open question as to whether each species has a limited number of activities capable of being induced by food schedules, and whether or not each type of reward has the ability to induce only certain activities.

It is certainly true that many activities other than induced activities become temporally entrained by periodic reward schedules. Running in Fig. 8.1 is a perfect example: it does not occur at elevated levels and, thus, should not be considered an induced activity; yet it nearly always occurs after drinking. There is little doubt that all rewards can entrain activities, although few activities may occur at levels elevated relative to some baseline measure. When a periodic reward schedule induces drinking and entrains running to a later period within the interfood interval, this entrainment demonstrates that the animal's internal state is changing in unidentified ways. After all, these behavioural transitions occur with no apparent changes in the external environment. One cannot understand the effects of even simple reward schedules until the factors responsible for the entrainment of induced and non-induced activities are identified.

Perhaps the strongest factor that determines both the amount and temporal position of schedule-induced activities is reward frequency. Reward frequency has differential effects on induced and non-induced activities. As we shall see, manipulations of the absolute frequency of reward affect these activities in a different fashion than do manipulations of relative reward frequency, and both factors may be the primary determinants of the temporal patterning observed on most reward schedules. We begin, therefore, by explaining the differential effects of manipulations of reward frequency on induced and non-induced activities.

Differential effects of reward frequency on induced and non-induced activities

Most simple schedules of reinforcement are composed of temporal periods with varying probabilities of food delivery. Often the variation is an indirect result of some aspect of the procedure, such as the low probability of food just after food delivery on fixed-ratio schedules. But some schedules explicitly control the *absolute* probability of reward over time. On fixed interval (FI) schedules, for example, the probability of reward is zero before the interval has elapsed. Even in the more complex procedures such as concurrent or multiple (Mult) schedules with more than one component, the *relative* probability of food delivery in each component is usually varied widely.

All these schedules are generally studied because of the regular patterns of operant responding they produce. However, variation in the probability of food delivery, both absolute and relative, has been repeatedly demonstrated to control the amount and distributions of schedule induced and non-induced activities (see Falk 1971; Staddon 1977, for reviews). As we will see, both classes of activities may influence the amount of operant behaviour observed on periodic schedules, either because of competition for time or perhaps because of some other behavioural interaction (Hinson and Staddon 1978; Reid and Staddon 1982).

Absolute reward rate (on simple schedules) or relative reward rate (on multiple schedules) seems to affect induced activities in at least two ways: by affecting the level of induced activities (which may, in turn, have indirect effects on other activities), and by determining the temporal distribution of induced and non-induced activities. We will deal with each of these factors in detail.

Absolute food frequency

Non-induced activities   Manipulations of reward frequency have little or no effect on the *rates* of non-induced activities, although the overall amount of each activity usually varies with the amount of time available between reward deliveries. For example, Riley *et al.* (1985) demonstrated that the rate of wheel running remained relatively constant when interpellet interval was varied, in different conditions, from 30 to 360 seconds, confirming the results of many others who have shown that running on food schedules is a non-induced activity (Penney and Schull 1977; Roper 1980; Staddon 1977; Wetherington *et al.* 1977). Similarly, Reid *et al.* (1985) manipulated the frequency of water presentation to rats and measured its effects on eight different non-induced activities, including wheel running. The rates of each of the activities were quite constant over the range of interreward times of 15 to 180 seconds.

It appears that when no induced activities occur in the interreward interval, the rate of non-induced activities is constant over a substantial range of reward frequency. However, Staddon (1977) reported that running rate *decreased* and drinking rate increased with increases in food frequency when both wheel running (non-induced) and drinking (induced) were available to rats. This observation of an inverse relation between food frequency and non-induced activities is very interesting. Perhaps the rate at which non-induced activities occur is independent of reward rate when no induced activities occur, but a decreasing function when induced activities are present—which implies that the decreasing function reflects competitive inhibition of non-induced by induced activities. To our knowledge, this hypothesis has not been explicitly tested.

Induced activities More studies have looked at the relation between schedule-induced drinking and absolute food frequency on simple schedules than any other issue concerning schedule induction. The relation between drinking rate, the amount of drinking, and food frequency is now clear. But because rate and amount of drinking are often not equivalent (and there are other ways of measuring induced drinking), the relations have historically been quite confusing. It is worthwhile, then, for us to examine both measures and their relations with food rate.

Most of the original interest in schedule-induced drinking was centred on its excess: animals drink much more than could be accounted for by any physiological, homeostatic explanation. Hence, the most appropriate measure seemed to be the amount of water consumed per session. Falk (1966a) was the first to determine the relation between the amount of water drunk (in ml per session) and fixed-interval value, ranging from 2 to 300 s. The relation was an inverted U, which he termed 'bitonic'. This bitonic relation was subsequently verified by Bond (1973, 1976), Burks (1970), Falk (1967), Flory (1971), Keehn and Colotla (1971), and others (see review in Wetherington 1979).

Hawkins *et al.* (1972) confirmed Falk's results and also proposed that the relation between drinking *rate* and food frequency is monotonically increasing with a range of FI values of 1–5 minutes. Cohen (1975) subsequently argued that the relation follows the same type of hyperbola as the single-response matching relation (Herrnstein 1970). Thus, Herrnstein's (1961, 1970) equation, originally proposed as a description of response-contingent, operant behaviour, may also be useful to quantify the relation between the rate of schedule-induced behaviour and absolute reward rate (cf. Jacquet 1972). This monotonic relation between absolute feeding and drinking rates has now been replicated by Millenson (1975), Rachlin and Krasnoff (1983), Staddon (1977), Urbain *et al.* (1979), and others (see Wetherington 1979, for a review).

After replotting Flory's (1971) data as rates, Staddon (1977) proposed that, if rats are exposed to extremely short interfood intervals, drinking rate decreases because a major proportion of the interval is taken up by eating. At high food rates, therefore, the relation between food rate and the rate of induced drinking changes from increasing to decreasing. Previous studies had used relatively long interval values and thus observed only part of the relation. Wetherington (1979) placed rats on FT schedules ranging from 15 to 480 s and confirmed that, at very high food rates, drinking rate decreases. The transformation of the bitonic relation observed with total water consumption to a monotonic relation with drinking rate is possible only when the interreinforcement interval values are greater than about 15–20 s. With high food rates, both relations are bitonic. However, the decreasing limb on the rate function may be interpreted as the result of temporal constraints imposed by eating rather than a modification of the 'motivational' factors that induce drinking.

In an attempt to quantify the bitonic relation, Wetherington (1979) showed that Herrnstein's matching relation fits the drinking data if 1 second (her estimate of the minimum time required to eat the food pellet) is subtracted from each interfood interval. The effect of this 1-s subtraction was minimal at low food rates, but at high rates it served to level off the decreasing limb, producing a hyperbolic function. Wetherington (1979) tested the feasibility of applying this modification of Herrnstein's equation. She found that Herrnstein's equation accounted for the data very well in most cases. In those cases in which it provided a poor fit, it appeared that the fit could be greatly improved by subtracting an eating time longer or shorter than 1 second per pellet.

Heyman and Bouzas (1980) proposed a very similar modification of the matching relation to account for the decreasing limb of the drinking function occurring at very high food rates. Because their model accurately accounts for all of the data on drinking rates published since then (Rachlin and Krasnoff 1983; Roper 1980; Rosellini and Burdette 1980; Shurtleff *et al.* 1983) and because no other type of model has been proposed to quantify the drinking function, we will discuss it further.

Instead of subtracting a constant eating time from each interval as Wetherington (1979) had done, Heyman and Bouzas (1980) included a fitted variable, E, in Herrnstein's (1970) matching relation

$$x = kR(x)/(R(x) + R_e) \qquad (8.1)$$

in which x represents the operant response rate, k is a fitted constant corresponding to the asymptotic rate of x, $R(x)$ is the obtained reinforcement rate, and R_e is another fitted constant which estimates the rate of all unscheduled reinforcers. Heyman and Bouzas assumed that the reinforcing strength of induced drinking varies proportionally with the food rate, and that induced drinking depends upon prior eating and is, then, constrained by time spent eating, E. Thus, in a fixed-time food schedule in which a single button press delivers water, the rate of button-pressing, B, for water is

$$B = [kW/(W + R_w)] [(T - E)/T]. \qquad (8.2)$$

Equation (8.2) states that button-pressing for water on food schedules is proportional to the reinforcing strength of drinking, W, multiplied by the proportion of the interval available to drink, $(T\text{-}E)/T$. T is the scheduled interfood time, so the reinforcing strength of drinking is proportional to the rate of food reinforcement. Heyman and Bouzas applied eq. (8.2) to their data, to those of Flory (1971), and to Allen and Kenshalo's (1976) data with rhesus monkeys. They concluded that E is relatively constant across schedules within species: around 3 seconds for rats and just over 9 seconds for monkeys.

In summary, the measured relation between drinking rate and food rate is non-monotonic. However, if drinking is truly dependent upon prior eating (discussed later), then we could consider the decreasing limb as a function of the temporal constraint of eating. This assumption allows the resulting function to be considered monotonic and well represented by the hyperbolic matching relation.

We must be aware of the difficulties inherent in the application of Herrnstein's matching equation for operant behaviour to non-contingent activities. As Heyman and Bouzas point out, there are several limitations in the use of eq. (8.2). The problems arise in its use as a explanatory model rather than as a useful modification of a hyperbolic function for curve-fitting. Eq. (8.2) describes the relation between button-pressing for water and the rate of food delivery. Additional assumptions must be made to apply it to situations in which there is no contingent response for access to the water tube. To the extent that the relation between button pressing and drinking is non-linear, or that the time taken to eat is not constant, e.g. dependent on interval value, eq. (8.2) becomes less applicable to actual drinking rates.

Cohen (1975) and Wetherington (1979) applied Herrnstein's equation directly to schedule-induced drinking. Consequently, there is no problem associated with an expressed relation between drinking and a contingent response such as button-pressing for water on a food schedule. In addition, Wetherington's model could be modified to allow the eating time to be a fitted parameter as do Heyman and Bouzas (1980). However, there are substantial problems with the interpretation of the other parameters. For example, the reinforcing strength of drinking must be in units of food rate. Wetherington reported that, with data from several studies, the asymptotic rate of drinking does not appear to be constant and is occasionally negative. She also found that R_e is also occasionally negative, which produces positively-accelerated drinking rate functions rather than negatively accelerated functions.

Studies have not directly addressed the problems associated with the application of the matching relation to schedule-induced behaviour. Its usefulness as a theory of schedule-induced behaviour is probably quite limited (Staddon 1982), but thus far it is the only quantitative model

describing the relation between the average reward rate and the average rate
of schedule-induced behaviour. Nevertheless, the model is very useful for
our purposes of describing food frequency effects. In fact, in the next section
we will see that the matching relation is exceptionally useful for the description of the main effect of manipulations of *relative* food frequency: the
allocation of induced and non-induced activities to temporal periods that
differ in the relative probability of reward.

Relative food frequency

Schedule-induced behaviour is a function not only of reward rate, but of the
stimulus properties of each schedule that signal the probability of food
delivery (cf. Alferink *et al.* 1980; Staddon 1977). It is clear that schedule-
induced activities tend to occur during periods of relatively low reward
probability on simple schedules. A schedule need not have an explicit
stimulus or temporal period signalling a lower-than-average probability of
reward—induced behaviour will also occur in periods of very low absolute
probability of reward, such as random-time food schedules with low average
food rates (Shurtleff *et al.* 1983). On simple interval and ratio schedules,
induced behaviour tends to occupy S − periods and rarely occupies the S +
periods favoured by operant behaviour. S + is a stimulus correlated with
reinforcement, S − is a stimulus correlated with non-reinforcement. The S −
hypothesis refers to the influence on induced behaviour of stimuli that
predict the probability of reward. Unfortunately, no quantitative models of
the S − hypothesis have been proposed.

Lean components of multiple schedules have, by definition, lower
probabilities of reward. Therefore, the S − hypothesis clearly predicts that
schedule-induced activities will tend to favour these lean components.
Consider the case of Alferink *et al.* (1980). They placed rats on a Mult FR-10
FR-100 schedule of food delivery and measured induced drinking. If the
immediate stimulus signalling the probability of food delivery is the most
important factor in the allocation of more induced drinking to one
component than the other, then more drinking should occur in the lean
(FR-100) component because each food delivery signals a longer time (and
more work) before the next food delivery. But if drinking is more strongly
influenced by the frequency of food delivery, then more drinking should
occur during the rich (FR-10) component. In this case, drinking occurred
almost exclusively in the FR-100 component, demonstrating that food
frequency is certainly not the only controlling factor.

The motivation hypothesis requires induced behaviour to favour the rich
components of multiple schedules, because the tendency to drink is
presumably related to eating. The motivation hypothesis is too informal to
make quantitative predictions about time allocation strategies in multiple

schedules. Matching of the relative rate of drinking with the relative food rate in each component does, however, make the precise prediction of a linear relation between relative rates, just as a strict interpretation of the motivation hypothesis informally predicts. As we will see, relativity matching may not be the best description of the time allocation strategies of schedule-induced behaviour. Nevertheless, the matching square depicted in Figs. 8.2–8.4 does provide a very useful means of examining the various ways in which induced and non-induced activities are allocated across components.

A third possible controlling factor in time allocation strategies is the dependency that induced behaviours usually show upon immediately prior reward. The postprandial pattern of drinking has been widely documented, although drinking will occur at other times in the interfood interval, usually at reduced levels (cf. Corfield-Sumner *et al.* 1977; Flory and O'Boyle 1972; McLeod and Gollub 1976; Porter and Kenshalo 1974; Rosenblith 1970; Wuttke and Innis 1972). How will induced drinking be allocated on multiple schedules that have extinction in one component? There is certainly more 'free' time for drinking to occur during extinction, but the occurrence of drinking may depend completely upon food delivery. Thus, drinking could favour the rich component because of this dependency, or it could favour the lean component (extinction) because of simpler time-allocation demands. We will return to this point in a minute.

As we shall see, the contributions of these three factors—(1) relative reward rate, (2) stimuli signaling low reward probability, and (3) the dependency that induced behaviours usually show upon immediately prior reward—to time allocation strategies are not easily determined. Often multiple schedules confound two or more of these factors, and other factors such as component duration are often even stronger determinants of the allocation of induced and non-induced activities to particular components.

Application of relativity matching to schedule-induced behaviour requires that the rate of induced behaviour in each component be determined by the equation

$$B_1/(B_1 + B_2) = R(x_1)/(R(x_1) + R(x_2)) \tag{8.3}$$

where B_i is the rate of drinking in component i, and $R(x_i)$ is the obtained food rate. Eq. (8.3) states that the relative rate of induced behaviour (the rate of induced behaviour in one component relative to the sum of the rates of induced behaviour in both components) should be equal to the relative reward rate in that component.

In contrast, an inverse relation between relative food rate and the rate of induced behaviour would be represented by antimatching, the negatively sloped line in Figs. 8.2–8.4. The antimatching relation is predicted by the S – hypothesis.

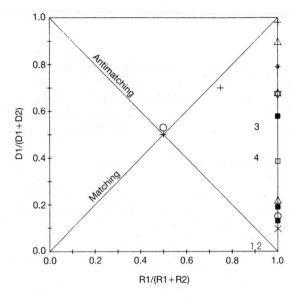

Fig. 8.2. Relative rate of drinking in rats versus relative reward rate in multiple schedules. The positively sloped line represents relatively matching, and the negatively sloped line represents antimatching. The symbols represent averaged data from different studies: Subject numbers: Alferink *et al.* (1980); asterisk: Hamm *et al.* (1981); triangles: Hamm *et al.* (1978); plus signs: Jacquet (1972); cross: Minor and Coulter (1982); star; Reid *et al.* (in prep. *a*); open square: Dougan *et al.* (1986); filled square: Dougan *et al.* (1985); open circles: wheel-running in Hinson and Staddon (1978).

There are several studies with multiple schedules that allow the determination of how rats and pigeons reallocate induced activities according to the relative frequency of reward in each component. In Fig. 8.2 we have replotted the schedule-induced drinking data from several studies with rats, and Fig. 8.3 contains the data from studies on schedule-induced aggression with pigeons.

What is the simplest time-allocation strategy that two activities, contingent responding and any other activity, might show on multiple schedules? Is the strategy the same for induced and non-induced activities? Hinson and Staddon (1978) placed rats on a multiple schedule with a constant variable interval (V I) 60-s schedule in one component and the other component contained either the same V I schedule or extinction. Rats pressed levers for milk delivery and had a running wheel available in both components. When both components contained the same V I schedules, running occurred at approximately equal rates in both. But when one

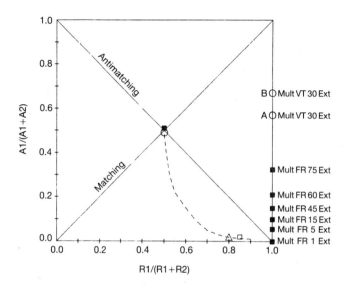

Fig. 8.3. Relative rate of aggression in pigeons versus relative reward rate in multiple schedules. The symbols represent averaged data from different studies: unfilled square: Ator (1980) triangle: Flory (1969); filled squares: Reid *et al.* (in prep. *a*; dashed line: the estimated data from Cohen and Looney (1973); circles: general activity in Buzzard and Hake (1984). The actual values of relative reward rate are often only estimates, as they were rarely specified.

component was shifted to extinction, running greatly decreased in the VI component and increased in extinction. It appears that time spent running in each component was a simple function of the level of competition between all activities: running had no strong competitor in the extinction component (it did not have to compete with lever pressing and reward-related activities) but did in the VI component. This time-allocation strategy represents anti-matching, the negatively sloped line in Fig. 8.2. Their averaged data are represented by open circles.

Perhaps the most striking result of the Hinson and Staddon study is that the availability of the running wheel was a major determinant of the amount of behavioural contrast shown by the operant lever press. Rats do not usually show stong behavioural contrast, but Hinson and Staddon argue that this is because most experiments with rats do not contain the supporting stimuli (i.e. running wheel or drinking tube) that allow the reallocation of activities that compete with lever pressing. In this case running did not occur at elevated levels, and thus was not considered a schedule-induced activity. Given that schedule-induced activities are facilitated by reinforcement schedules, they may be able to influence operant responding even more strongly than do non-induced activities. This possibility has not been directly tested

There is also reason to predict that operant responding would be influenced in opposing directions by induced activities and non-induced activities. Induced activities tend to increase (to some limit) as absolute food rate increases. Non-induced activities either decrease or are unaffected by increases in absolute food rate. Hence induced and non-induced activities should affect behaviour differently in response to changes in relative food rates—and have very different effects on the relation between relative reward (food) and response rates, on multiple schedules. Since induced activities increase with reward rate, they must increasingly compete for time with the operant response, so should limit its increase. Hence the opportunity to engage in an induced activity should reduce contrast and favour under-matching (Baum 1974) of operant responding on multiple schedules. Non-induced activities, on the other hand, show a constant or even negative relation to food rate, hence should either show no effect, or facilitate contrast (as in the Hinson and Staddon study) and tend to favour matching or overmatching of operant responding. Correspondingly, an induced activity should show a matching function similar to (but perhaps of lower slope than) the operant response, whereas a non-induced activity should show a constant or even negative (antimatching) function.

If induced and non-induced activities fall along these extremes, we might even want to define an activity as induced or non-induced by the way it behaves in multiple schedules. If activities appear to fall along a continuum between matching and antimatching (and, as we will see, they do), we might conclude that a continuum (that may eventually be quantitatively defined) between induced and non-induced activities is a more accurate description than the traditional dichotomy.

Jacquet (1972) explicitly tested the applicability of the matching relation to induced drinking in multiple schedules. Rats were placed on a Mult VI 1-min VI–X, where X was VI 1-min, VI 3-min, or Extinction (Ext). As the three 'plus signs' in Fig. 8.2 show, rats matched relative drink rates to relative food rates very closely. Possible deviations from matching (such as undermatching) could not be readily identified, unfortunately, because only three points were available.

Hamm *et al.* (1981) (represented by the asterisk in Fig. 8.2) and Hamm *et al.* (1978) (open triangles) examined the temporal allocation of induced drinking in Mult RT 30-s Ext and Mult VT 50-s Ext schedules, respectively. Both studies found that rats spent more time drinking in the food component than in extinction. Their data are replotted as relative rates in Fig. 8.2. Food delivery was not contingent upon responding in either study. Nevertheless, Reid *et al.* (in prep. *a*) (star) used a response-contingent procedure (Mult FR-X Ext) and also found more drinking in the rich (fixed ratio; FR) component; thus the contingency appears irrelevant. Because drinking favoured the rich component, each of these studies provides evidence that the relative rate of induced drinking is a positive function of the relative food rate.

Induced drinking does not always favour the rich component, however. Drinking by one rat in the Hamm *et al.* (1978) study (lower open triangle) strongly favoured the extinction component. Alferink *et al.* (1980) (represented by the rats' numbers 1–4) mentioned earlier, found that rats drank almost exclusively in the lean, FR-100, component of a Mult FR-10 FR-100 schedule. Minor and Coulter (1982) (cross) found that rats allocated about 90 per cent of the total drinking rate in the extinction component of a Mult VT-30 Ext schedule. Dougan *et al.* (1986) (open square) found that three of four rats drank more during the extinction component of a Mult VI-10 Ext schedule, although there was much variability between rats.

Parametric data are conspicuously lacking for an examination of the applicability of the relativity matching relation. With the single exception of Jacquet (1972), no studies investigating drinking on multiple schedules have looked at relative food rates in the intermediate range between 50 per cent and 100 per cent. Data from Alferink *et al.* (1980) are replotted in Fig. 8.2 as intermediate values, but, because they used fixed ratios in both components and did not publish response rates or obtained reward rates, we cannot be certain of the precise location of the points on the abscissa.

Figure 8.3 contains pigeon data replotted from multiple schedule studies investigating schedule-induced aggression. Reid *et al.* (in prep. *a*, Expt. 2) (filled squares) manipulated the ratio value on a Mult FR Ext schedule and found a systematic positive relation between the relative reward rate and the proportion of schedule-induced aggression occurring during extinction. As the ratio value was shifted from FR-1 to FR-75, induced aggression slowly shifted toward the FR component.

Although several studies have been published with pigeons on multiple ratio schedules, response rate in both components has rarely been specified (e.g. Ator 1980; Cohen and Looney 1973; Flory 1969; Knutson 1970). Thus, accurate relative rates often cannot be determined. In the study of Cohen and Looney (1973) (dashed line), the ratio value of a Mult FR-25 FR-X was manipulated parametrically. It is difficult to know how the rate of attack in the rich (FR-25) component changed with increases in the ratio requirement in the lean component, since the rates were not specified. However, the *absolute* rate of induced attack in the varied component showed an inverted-U relation with fixed-ratio value. Schedule-induced attack occurred at approximately equal rates in the two components when the schedule was Mult FR-25 FR-25 and shifted quickly to nearly 100 per cent of the attack occurring during the lean component. The dashed line in Fig. 8.3 depicts these estimated relative rates of attack.

Buzzard and Hake (1984) is the only multiple-schedule study with induced

activities other than aggression in pigeons that allows obtained rates of
induced behaviour and reward in each component to be determined. They
measured induced 'general activity' (open circles) on Mult VT-30 VT-30 and
shifted the pigeons to Mult VT-30 Ext. Induced general activity slightly
favoured the rich component, but it was never absent from the extinction
component.

Much of the confusion in the time-allocation strategies depicted in the rat
data of Fig. 8.2 can be cleared up by examining the component durations of
the various multiple schedules in the different studies. The replotted data in
Fig. 8.4 show that short component durations in multiple schedules usually
result in more induced drinking in the lean (extinction) component. As the
component duration increases, the proportion of drinking in the rich
component also increases. For example, Jacquet (1972) (plus sign) and
Dougan et al. (1985) (lower filled square) both exposed rats to Mult VI-60
Ext schedules, but the component durations differed in the two studies. The
component duration in Jacquet's (1972) multiple schedule was 600 seconds
and drinking strongly favoured the rich component, whereas the component

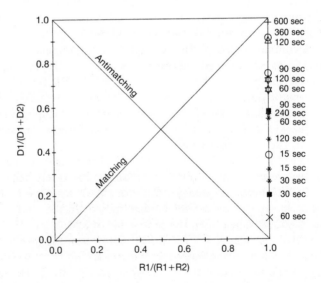

Fig. 8.4. Relative rate of drinking in rats versus relative food rate in multiple
schedules with an emphasis on the component duration. The symbols represent
averaged data from different studies: plus sign: Jacquet (1972); circles: Minor (1987,
Expt. 3); triangle: Hamm *et al.* (1978); stars: Reid *et al.* (in prep. *a*); filled squares:
Dougan *et al.* (1985); asterisks: Minor (1987, Expt. 2); cross: Minor and Coulter
(1982).

duration in Dougan *et al.* (1985) multiple schedule was 30 seconds, with drinking favouring the lean (extinction) component.

Recently, Dougan *et al.* (1985) and Minor (1987) explicitly manipulated component duration in order to determine its effect on the allocation of induced drinking. Dougan *et al.* (1985) (filled squares) exposed one group of rats to 30-s component duration and another group of rats to a 90-s component duration of a Mult VI-60 Ext. Drinking in the group with the shorter component duration strongly favoured the extinction component, whereas drinking in the group with the longer component duration slightly favoured the rich component. Minor (1987, Expt. 3) (open circles) manipulated component duration within rats over the wider range of 15–360 s in a Mult VT-30 Ext schedule, and found that the proportion of drinking in the rich component varied directly and systematically with component duration.

It really should not be surprising that component duration is a determinant of the amount of induced and non-induced behaviour allocated to different components of multiple schedules. After all, component duration is an important determinant of the rate of operant behaviour in multiple schedules (Ettinger and Staddon 1982; Hinson *et al.* 1978; Staddon 1982; Todorov 1972; Williams 1979). As component duration increases, the rate of operant behaviour in the lean component increases, and the rate of induced behaviour in that same, lean component decreases. Ettinger and Staddon (1982) and Staddon (1982) predicted that component duration should have exactly this effect on the allocation of induced behaviour due to the dynamics of behavioural competition between operant and induced activities within individual components. Early within the rich component, competition from operant behaviour is maximal, resulting in the reallocation of other activities to the less competitive periods, the lean components. As component duration is shortened, the average competitiveness of operant responding over the rich component is increased, resulting in more reallocation of induced behaviour to the lean components.

Since much of the time-allocation data in Fig. 8.2 is likely to be due, in part, to the component duration of the various multiple schedules, what effect does the relative frequency of reward actually have? In most studies with rats, the effects of relative frequency of reward are overpowered by the effects of the component duration. Available evidence with rats seems to indicate that as relative reward frequency increases, the proportion of induced drinking allocated to the lean component (extinction) increases. For example, a group of rats in the Dougan *et al.* (1985) (see Fig. 8.2, filled squares) study were exposed to Mult VI-60 Ext and to Mult VI-10 Ext schedules with constant (90 s) component durations. Induced drinking slightly favoured the rich (VI) component only when it contained a VI 60-s schedule. When it contained a VI 10-s schedule, induced drinking strongly favoured the extinction component. Nevertheless, Reid *et al.* (in prep. *a*, Expt. 1) (star) placed rats on a Mult F R Ext schedule, varied the ratio value from 1 to 60 with constant component duration, and found no effect whatsoever of ratio value. To our knowledge, no other studies with rats allow the determination of the effects of relative reward frequency without confounding component duration.

Data from studies with pigeons (Fig. 8.3) agrees with the tentative conclusions from the studies with rats. As relative reward rate increases, the proportion of induced aggression in the lean (extinction) component increases. Sufficient data are not available to determine whether or not component duration is an important factor with pigeons in their time alloca-tion strategy. Nevertheless, in the Buzzard and Hake (1984) study (see open circles in Fig. 8.3), there was a small increase in the proportion of induced general activity in the rich component when they lengthened the extinction component from 1 minute (point 'A') to 7 minutes (point 'B'). This small increase in the rich component with increases in component duration confirms the same results from the studies with rats.

Summary of reward frequency effects

In summary, the time-allocation strategy responsible for the allocation of schedule-induced activities to different components of multiple schedules is not accurately described by either the S – hypothesis or the motivation hypothesis. Reward probability or frequency is the main component of both hypotheses, and it does control behaviour. Schedule-induced behaviour on multiple schedules does not conform to relativity matching or antimatching. Rather, its allocation to rich and lean components varies along a continuum between the two extremes. The matching and antimatching relations are very useful descriptions of the complete allocation to one component or another which is occasionally observed, and accurately describe predictions from the motivation hypothesis and the S – hypothesis.

Several factors are important determinants of time allocation of induced activities in multiple schedules. The most important factor appears to be the duration of the components. As component duration increases, rats allocate more induced drinking to the richer component. This conclusion cannot be reached with pigeons, as appropriate data are unavailable.

The motivation hypothesis is not supported as a time-allocation strategy with either rats or pigeons, because, as relative reward frequency increases, induced drinking and induced aggression both increasingly favour the lean, rather than the rich, component. Early data that appeared to support the motivation hypothesis (e.g. Jacquet 1972; Hamm *et al.* 1978, 1981) typically used relatively long component durations, which may have contributed to the observation of more induced drinking in the rich component. Parametric data which vary relative reward rate with constant component duration are severely lacking. With few exceptions, published studies have used only extinction as the lean component.

The S – hypothesis is weakly supported as a time allocation strategy by available data on multiple schedules. When component duration is maintained constant, induced activities can favour either the rich or lean component, depending upon the duration of the component. Nevertheless, the observation that increases in relative reward rate result in a larger proportion of induced behaviour in the lean component is compatible with the S – hypothesis, but we must be aware that this hypothesis assumes sensitivity to the stimuli signalling low reward probability, not only behavioural control by relative reward rate. Factors other than stimulus effects could be responsible, but Minor and Coulter (1982) have successfully demonstrated that their stimulus signalling the lean component did have S – properties.

Regarding non-induced activities, available data are not nearly sufficient to identify time-allocation strategies in rats or pigeons. Only one published study (Hinson and Staddon 1978) has provided relative rates of a non-induced activity on a multiple schedule. However, their data provide us with only a single point with different reward rates, with wheel running favouring the extinction component. Neither component duration nor relative reward rate have been manipulated over a sufficient range to identify their effects on non-induced activities. Therefore, existing data are far from conclusive. It is not clear that all induced or all non-induced activities are equally sensitive to relative rates of reward or to the S – properties of schedules. Parametric data on relative rates are completely lacking for any induced or non-induced activity.

It is clear that at least three factors control the time allocation of schedule-induced activities (and perhaps non-induced activities as well): (1) reward rate (both absolute and relative); (2) component duration; and (3) stimuli that signal the probability of food delivery. Other factors are mentioned above that could also play important roles. Schedule-induced aggression has been studied most often in schedules in which the stimulus factor plays the dominant role (multiple ratio studies). Schedule-induced drinking has most often been studied in multiple schedules which allow the component duration and the relative food rate to have a dominant role (multiple interval extinction). However, each factor appears to be important with both types of induced activities, drinking and aggression. There is little reason to believe that mechanisms of time allocation differ between the various induced activities.

Non-induced activities have largely been ignored, even though they are able to influence the amount of operant behaviour, particularly in multiple schedules. Induced and non-induced activities are unlikely to follow qualitatively different strategies for time allocation. There may be quantitative differences in the sensitivity of induced and non-induced activities to any of the factors above, but current data are not sufficient to identify any differences the effects of *relative* reward rate on the two classes. *Absolute* reward rate does, however, appear to differentially affect induced and non-induced activities, producing an inverted-U relation with the rates of induced activities and typically no effect on the rates of non-induced activities.

Schedule entrainment of induced and non-induced activities

Temporal distributions in lean and rich environments

The analysis thus far has dealt with the means by which reward rate may control the overall amounts or rates of induced and non-induced activities. It refers to static measures, such as drinking rates over entire sessions or within all occurrences of particular components. Reward rate is also one of the determinants of the temporal allocation of activities to the various components of multiple and concurrent schedules. However, these analyses say nothing about the temporal properties of entrained activities *within the interreward interval*, or the means by which the various activities are entrained.

We saw an example of schedule entrainment of induced drinking and non-induced wheel running in Fig. 8.1. Running and schedule-induced drinking

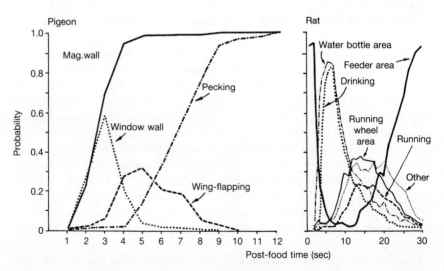

Fig. 8.5. The relative frequency of various activities as a function of post-food time for a rat (right panel) and a pigeon (left panel) on periodic food schedules. (Reprinted with permission from Staddon 1977.)

usually occupied different periods within the interfood interval on an FT
1-min food schedule. Fig. 8.5 is a similar example of schedule entrainment
that shows how the probabilities of several activities vary over the interfood
interval in pigeons on a fixed-time 12-s food schedule and in rats on a fixed-
time 30-s food schedule. The distributions in Fig. 8.5 are usually determined
by averaging across all interreward intervals, such as all rows of Fig. 5.1. Of
course, the data represented by the two figures are from different studies.

Excluding activities related to obtaining reward, the forms of the activity
distributions observed on periodic schedules depend upon whether or not an
activity is induced by the schedule and, with rats, on the amount of
supporting apparatus available. The temporal distributions of all activities
unrelated to the acquisition of reward may be multimodal, as in Fig. 8.5, or
they may be unimodal. By multimodal, we mean that the mode for each
activity occupies different periods within the interreward interval, and thus
are offset from one another. Drinking and running in Fig. 8.5 tend to occupy
different portions of the interval, and represent the distributions for induced
and non-induced activities, respectively. By unimodal, we mean that all
measured activities (other than reward-related behaviour) tend to occupy the
same temporal period within the interval, and are not offset from one
another. Table 8.1 summarizes the dependence of the form of the temporal
distributions on the occurrence of schedule induction and the availability of
supporting apparatus for rats, based on data currently available.

Table 8.1

Induced activities occur?	Amount of supporting apparatus	
	Lean environment	Rich environment
No	Unimodal	Unimodal
Yes	Unimodal	Multimodal

Non-induced activities   Unfortunately, little attention has been given to the
activity distributions of non-induced activities occurring in schedules that,
for some reason, fail to induce behaviour. The little evidence available
suggests that interreward activity distributions of non-induced activities are
always unimodal if induced activities do not occur. Unimodal distributions
occur with non-induced activities in environments containing little or no
supporting apparatus (Myerson and Christiansen 1979; Riley *et al.* 1985;
Wetherington *et al.* 1977). And, at least on water schedules, it appears that
unimodal distributions also occur with rats exposed to very rich environments in the absence of schedule-induced activities (Reid *et al.* 1985). Rats
and hamsters may engage in many activities in lean or rich environments, but

unless the schedule actually induces an activity, the activity distributions of all the non-induced activities seem to occupy approximately the same period within the interreward interval (Anderson and Shettleworth 1977; Reid *et al.* 1985).

Induced activities   Many studies have reported schedule-induced behaviour with unimodal distributions in lean environments (Allen and Kenshalo 1976; Edwards and Roper 1982; Killeen 1975; King 1974; Osborne 1978; Reberg *et al.* 1977; Reid and Dale 1983; Wetherington and Riley 1986; but see Iverson 1977 for an example of multimodal distributions in a relatively lean environment). Reid and Dale (1983) demonstrated that the form of the unimodal distribution of schedule-induced drinking was a simple inverse function of the temporal distribution of reward-related activities. At each second within the interreward interval, increases (or decreases) in the distribution of food-related activities (head-in-feeder) corresponded very closely to decreases (or increases) in the drinking distributions. This result would be expected (and trivial) if drinking and food-related activities were mutually exclusive and exhaustive, but in their experiments much time remained available for other activities.

Reid *et al.* (1985) demonstrated the same inverse relation with non-induced activities occurring in a rich environment on a periodic water schedule. All activities had essentially the same temporal distributions within the interwater interval and complemented the distribution of reward-related activities. Hence, it appears that reward and temporal control determine* the temporal distributions of reward-related activities which, in turn, determine the unimodal distributions of induced or non-induced activities. In simple periodic schedules, time spent consuming, working, or looking for reward determines the time available for all other activities, which probably have only a small impact on the amount of reward-related activities (Ator 1980; Knutson and Schrader 1975; Reid and Dale 1983; Reid and Staddon 1982; Roper 1978). We should point out that this slight impact of induced activities on reward-related activities on simple periodic schedules stands in contrast to the larger influence often shown on multiple schedules, described above.

Rats appear to require rich environments (such as the presence of a drinking tube and a running wheel while on a food schedule) for the

---

* Logically the inverse correlation between non-induced and food-related activities is consistent with several kinds of causal relations: food-related activities inhibit non-induced activities or vice versa, or both classes determined by some third factor. But there are abundant data showing that, at asymptote, the pattern of food-related activities is usually independent of the presence or absence of non-induced activities, which suggests that they determine the temporal location of non-induced activities rather than the reverse. The direction of the causal relation is even more apparent when the distribution of food-related activities varies concurrently with manipulations of food frequency, independent of the availability of other activities.

occurrence of multimodal distributions (Reid *et al.* 1985; Roper 1978; Staddon and Ayres 1975). That is, the non-induced activities observed with rats (and hamsters: cf. Anderson and Shettleworth 1977) in lean environments, such as grooming, sniffing, locomotion, etc., appear to form distributions that peak at approximately the same time in the interval. However, when rats are on a food schedule with abundant apparatus that can be manipulated (e.g. access to a drinking tube and a running wheel or an oak block), the distributions of each activity peak at substantially different times in the interval (Killeen 1975; Knutson and Schrader 1975; Reid *et al.* in prep. *b*; Roper 1978; Staddon and Ayres 1975; Wetherington and Riley 1986). Pigeons do not require such additional apparatus—their patterns of orientation and movement can be entrained to different periods within the interreward interval (Innis *et al.* 1983; Reberg *et al.* 1977).

When multimodal activity distributions are observed, the sequences of activities appear strikingly stereotyped from one interreward interval to another and even across subjects. This temporal regularity led Staddon (1977) to propose that periodic reward schedules entrain three motivational states: the *terminal* state, containing reward-related activities facilitated by the schedule (which would include head-in-feeder in Fig. 8.1 and 8.5); the *interim* state, containing the schedule-induced activities which occur shortly after reward (drinking, in both figures); and the *facultative* state, containing the non-induced activities occurring near the middle of the interreward interval which are not facilitated by the schedule, and that compete for time with interim and terminal activities (running in both figures).

Unimodal distributions imply substitutability between each of the activities that peak at the same time in the interval. That is, activities can replace one another during the same period in other interreward intervals. However, the relatively fixed sequence of activities forming multimodal distributions implies little or no substitutability. Because of the apparent regularity in the sequences of activities forming multimodal distributions and because behavioural interaction appears to be the main determinant of the form of simpler, unimodal, temporal distributions (Killeen 1979; Reid and Dale 1983; Reid and Staddon 1982; Reid *et al.* 1985), we will discuss the degree of substitutability between activities and the role it might play in the allocation of activities to various periods within the interreward interval.

Substitutability between entrained activities

How fixed is the order of entrainment on schedules when multimodal activity distributions are observed? Does the order vary from one schedule to another? Or with the types of competing activities? Unfortunately, we have more questions regarding the mechanisms of schedule entrainment than we have answers. With Staddon and Ayres' (1975) rats placed on a fixed-time 30-s food schedule (depicted in Fig. 8.5), drinking nearly always occurred earlier in the interfood interval than did running. Running usually followed drinking, but occasionally drinking and running occurred alone in an interval. Even so, drinking occupied the earlier portion of the interval and running occupied a later portion. When the drinking tube was withdrawn from the apparatus, running continued to occupy the same period, and 'other' activities occupied the period previously taken by drinking. When drinking was available but the running wheel was locked, the temporal distribution of drinking closely resembled the drinking distributions when running had been concurrently available, although drinking was slightly elevated (see also Segal 1969; Wetherington and Riley 1986). Staddon and Ayres interpreted this invariance in the temporal position of drinking and wheel running as further evidence that periodic schedules entrain three motivational states: interim, facultative, and terminal states.

In the Staddon and Ayres study, there was little evidence for substitutability between induced (interim) and non-induced (facultative) activities. Furthermore, Knutson and Schrader (1975) demonstrated invariance in the sequence and temporal positions of two induced activities, drinking and aggression, in rats. The mode of the drinking distribution always occurred earlier in the interval than aggression on fixed-interval schedules, even when the activities occurred alone in an interval. When only one activity was allowed to occur, it maintained its temporal position in the interval.

Both of these studies imply a high degree of invariance or a very low degree of substitutability between activities on periodic schedules, independent of whether both, or only one, activities are schedule-induced. However, there is also evidence of variance and substitutability between activities. For example, Killeen (1975, Expt. 5c) compared the temporal distributions of schedule-induced drinking and wood-gnawing separately and together with rats on a FT 75-s food schedule. When only drinking or only gnawing was allowed, they had similar temporal distributions. When both activities were concurrently available in the interval, gnawing occurred earlier than drinking, and both decreased substantially from their single-activity levels.In addition, Wetherington and Riley (1986) measured drinking over sessions in which the availability of a running wheel alternated each day. Drinking always preceded running (as before), but drinking was reduced over the portion of the interval when running occurred. In both of these studies, the temporal order of the activities was invariant, implying low substitutability. However, the decrease in the levels of the activities that occurred when all activities were concurrently allowed implies at least a small degree of substitutability between activities.

Occasionally, schedule-induced activities completely replace other apparently induced activities. For example, Freed and Hymowitz (1969) reported that schedule-induced drinking was spontaneously replaced by shredding of the paper liners on the floor of the apparatus. Roper (1978) reported a similar example of one activity replacing a schedule-induced activity. When rats were exposed to a FI 30-s food schedule, drinking was induced and occurred before wheel running, as in the Staddon and Ayres (1975) study reported above. However, when shifted to a FI 60-s schedule, drinking was replaced by general activity, and running retained essentially the same temporal distribution. When drinking did occur on this schedule, it retained its post-food position, occurring earlier than running but at levels far below that observed on the FT 30-s schedule.

Unfortunately, Roper (1978) gave no explanation for the replacement of drinking by general activity, other than postulating that it resulted somehow from the food rate. However, the data in Fig. 8.1 are from a FT 60-s food schedule, the same food rate as in Roper's study, yet drinking was induced. Perhaps a *change* in the reward rate was the proximal cause. This possibility is substantiated by Innis *et al.* (1983), who found increases in the variability of the sequences of entrained activities with pigeons with increases in the interfood interval of fixed-time schedules. However, it is unclear to what extent the actual sequences vary with food rate. It is difficult to compare detailed descriptions of pigeon orientation and movement to that of rats as they manipulate the available apparatus, e.g. the running wheel, a chewing block, or a drinking tube.

In summary, the sequences of entrained activities in the interreward interval appear relatively fixed when the reward rate is held constant. Increases in the duration of the interreward interval appear to increase the variability in the sequences of activities, but it is not clear whether the increase is because of an increase in the number of activities occurring in the interval (Innis *et al.* 1983) or because the actual sequence is directly affected. Few studies have directly addressed the issue of relative substitutability of induced and non-induced activities. In those that have, it is rarely clear if the altered activity distributions represent induced or non-induced activities. Nor is it clear that the activity classification is an important factor in the degree of substitutability.

Because so few studies have directly addressed the factors responsible for the sequences of activities, there are many questions and few answers. For example, what is the relation between an activity's temporal position in the interval and its resistance to displacement to other temporal periods? To what degree are entrained activities substitutable for one another, both within interreward intervals and across intervals? Does this degree depend in some systematic way upon some property of the schedule or the type of reward? More research with rich environments is needed to begin to answer these questions.

Schedule entrainment

How do reward schedules entrain activities? The motivation hypothesis (which was not supported by time allocation data on multiple schedules) suggests that the induced (interim) activities are selected from all possible activities because of their 'special' relationship with the reward. In Staddon's (1977) model which incorporates the motivation hypothesis, interim activities occur just after reward because of this special relation, and terminal activities occur prior to reward because they are reward-related activities under temporal control. The occurrence of both classes of activities are results of facilitatory relations between the schedule (and that particular type of reward) and these two motivational states controlling behavioural output. Facultative activities occur in the interval if there is enough time available for them, as they must compete for time with both interim and terminal activities. Facultative activities are not facilitated by the schedule and have no special relation with the reward. Thus, they will predominate only in very long interreward intervals, in which the facilitation of interim and terminal activities is not sufficient to occupy all the available time between rewards.

Staddon's (1977) model of schedule-entrainment makes several explicit predictions about the motivational processes involved in entrainment that have not yet been satisfactorily tested. For example, the selection of the interim activity from all possibilities depends upon the existence of a facilitatory relation between that particular type of reward and the interim (induced) activity. However, this relation has not been precisely defined. In fact, in at least some situations, the relation between the *amount* of food delivery and induced drinking is negative or bitonic (Allison and Mack 1982; Freed and Hymowitz 1972; Osborne 1978; Reid and Dale 1983; Reid and Staddon 1982, 1987).

In addition, Staddon's model predicts that periodic schedules modulate motivational states within each interreward interval. This prediction is consistent with the multimodal distributions in Figs. 8.1 and 8.5. Occasionally, however, multimodal distributions are results of averaging across intervals containing only interim behaviour or only facultative behaviour. Animals may be able to allocate the different activities to different intervals, perhaps as a net reduction of competition between activities for available time. If the precise temporal distributions are retained even when the activities occur in different intervals (a prediction supported by Knutson and Schrader 1975, and Staddon and Ayres 1975), it would be strong evidence that the temporal distributions of activities depend upon their relation with particular rewards, rather than on the overall motivational properties of the schedule, as determined by (for example) molar reinforcement rate.

However, the schedule may not modulate the tendencies to engage in induced and non-induced activities within each interreward interval. For example, Reid and Dale (1983), Reid and Staddon (1982), and Reid *et al.* (1985) demonstrated that the *unimodal* distributions of induced drinking and several non-induced activities are a by-product of the tendency to engage in reward-related activities, rather than being intrinsically motivated. The simplest mechanism of this indirect influence is disinhibition, proposed by Falk (1969) and McFarland (1970) as the mechanism responsible for the occurrence of adjunctive behaviour and displacement activities (but see Roper 1981, 1984; Roper and Crossland 1982; Roper and Posadas-Andrews 1981). There is now little doubt that the forms of observed unimodal distributions of induced and non-induced activities are determined by the shapes of the distributions of activities related to the obtainment of reward. However, the shapes of *multimodal* distributions must be determined by additional factors, since an additional factor must be responsible for the transition from the induced activity to the non-induced activity.

Can animals react to competition or temporal constraints by reallocating induced and non-induced activities across intervals? If activities that occur in a relatively fixed sequence within each interreward interval can be demonstrated to reallocate to separate intervals, then there would be less reason to believe that the schedule entrains activities by modulating their tendencies within each interval. Existing data are, again, inconclusive. Several studies have reported intervals containing only facultative or only induced activities (Anderson and Shettleworth 1977; Knutson and Schrader 1975; Roper 1978; Staddon and Ayres 1975), suggesting the ability to reallocate activities. However, these studies have also reported that the temporal distribution of each activity occurring in separate intervals is approximately the same as its distribution in intervals containing both activities; thus supporting the notion that each reward influences the time of occurrence of each activity.

What are the controlling factors of the allocation of activities within or across intervals? There seem to be several. With increases in the duration of interfood intervals (Innis *et al.* 1983), with increases in meal size (Reid and Staddon 1987), or with longer sessions (Reid and Staddon 1982), fewer intervals contain schedule-induced activities. However, at the present, there is little reason to conclude that a reduction in the percentage of intervals containing induced behaviour represents a reallocation of activities across intervals. It seems that competition for time would be a major factor for time allocation across intervals, but its influence has not been directly tested.

Summary and conclusions

We have identified several factors influencing the organization of activities on reward schedules. One factor is the differential effect of reward rate on induced and non-induced activities. The measured relation between absolute food and drinking rates is bitonic. However, the relation may be considered as a result of two factors: a facilitatory influence of food rate and a temporal constraint imposed by the requirement of food consumption, which has a major influence only at high food rates. The rates of non induced activities either decrease or are unaffected by increases in absolute food rate.

The time-allocation strategy responsible for the allocation of schedule-induced activities to different components of multiple schedules is not accurately described by either the S – hypothesis or the motivation hypothesis. Reward probability or frequency is the main component of both hypotheses, and it does control induced and non-induced activities. Schedule-induced behaviour on multiple schedules does not conform to relativity matching or antimatching. Rather, its allocation to rich and lean components varies along a continuum between the two extremes.

We have identified three factors that are important determinants of time allocation of induced activities in multiple schedules: (1) component duration; (2) relative reward rate; and (3) stimuli that signal the probability of reward. The most important factor appears to be the duration of the components. As component duration increases, rats allocate more induced drinking to the richer component.

The motivation hypothesis was not supported as a time-allocation strategy with either rats or pigeons, because as relative reward frequency increases, induced drinking and induced aggression both increasingly favour the lean, rather than the rich, component.

The S – hypothesis is weakly supported as a time allocation strategy by available data on multiple schedules. When component duration is maintained constant, induced activities can favour either the rich or lean component, depending upon the duration of the component. Nevertheless, the observation that increases in relative reward rate result in a larger proportion of induced behaviour in the lean component is compatible with the S – hypothesis.

The temporal distributions of activities within interreward intervals may be unimodal, in which all activities other than reward-related activities peak at approximately the same post-reward time, or multimodal, in which they peak at substantially different times in the interval. Unimodal distributions are observed with induced and non-induced activities, and appear to be direct results of the temporal distributions of reward-related activities.

Unimodal distributions imply a certain degree of substitutability between the activities across intervals. The sequence of activities in multimodal distributions, however, appears relatively fixed, and implies little or no substitutability between the activities in each distribution. Increases in the interreward interval appear to increase the variability in the sequences of activities, but it is not clear whether the increase is because of an increase in the number of activities occurring in the interval (Innis *et al.* 1983) or because the actual sequence is directly affected.

Because so few studies have directly addressed the factors responsible for the sequences of activities, there are many questions and few answers. For example, what is the relation between an activity's temporal position in the interval and its resistance to displacement to other temporal periods? To what degree are entrained activities substitutable for one another, both within interrreward intervals and across intervals? Does this degree depend in some systematic way upon some property of the schedule or the type of reward?

Acknowledgements

We thank Ken Steele and R. H. Ettinger for comments on an earlier version. Research supported by grants from the National Science Foundation to Duke University.

References

Alferink, L. A., Bartness, T. J., and Harder, S. (1980). Control of the temporal location of polydipsia licking in the rat. *J. exp. Anal. Behav.* **33**, 119–29.

Allen, J. D. and Kenshalo, D. R. (1976). Schedule-induced drinking as a function of interreinforcement interval in the rhesus monkey. *J. exp. Anal. Behav.* **26**, 257–67.

Allison, J. and Mack, R. (1982). Polydipsia and autoshaping: Drinking and lever pressing as substitutes for eating. *Animal Learning Behav.* **10**, 465–75.

Anderson, M. C. and Shettleworth, S. J. (1977). Behavioural adaptation to fixed-interval and fixed-time food delivery in golden hamsters. *J. exp. Anal. Behav.* **27**, 33–49.

Ator, N. A. (1980). Mirror pecking and timeout under a multiple fixed-ratio schedule of food delivery. *J. exp. Anal. Behav.* **34**, 319–28.

Baum, W. M. (1974). On two types of deviations from the matching law: bias and undermatching. *J. exp. Anal. Behav.* **22**, 231–42.

Bond, N. M. (1973). Schedule-induced polydipsia as a function of the consumatory rate. *Psychol. Rec.* **23**, 377–382.

Bond, N. M. (1976). Schedule-induced polydipsia as a function of the interval between food pellets. *Bull. Psychonomic Soc.* **7**, 139–41.

Burks, C. D. (1970). Schedule-induced polydipsia: are response-dependent procedures a limiting condition? *J. exp. Anal. Behav.* **5**, 635–40.

Buzzard, J. H. and Hake, D. F. (1984). Stimulus control of schedule-induced activity in pigeons during multiple schedules. *J. exp. Anal. Behav.* **42**, 191–210.

Cohen, I. L. (1975). The reinforcing value of schedule-induced drinking. *J. exp. Anal. Behav.* **23**, 37–44.

Cohen, P. S. and Looney, T. A. (1973). Schedule-induced mirror responding in the pigeon. *J. exp. Anal. Behav.* **19**, 395–408.

Corfield-Sumner, P. K., Blackman, D. E., and Stainer, G. (1977). Polydipsia induced in rats by second-order schedules of reinforcement. *J. exp. Anal. Behav.* **27**, 265 73.

Dougan, J.D., McSweeney, F.K., and Farmer, V.A. (1985). Some parameters of behavioural contrast and allocation of interim activities in rats. *J. exp. Anal. Behav.* **44**, 325-35.

Dougan, J.D., McSweeney, F.K., and Farmer-Dougan, V.A. (1986). Behavioural contrast in competitive and noncompetitive environments. *J. exp. Anal. Behav.* **46**, 185-97.

Edwards, L. and Roper, T.J. (1982). Schedule-induced running in gerbils. *Behav. Anal. Lett.* **2**, 205-12.

Ettinger, R.H. and Staddon, J.E.R. (1982). Behavioural competition, component duration and multiple-schedule contrast. *Behav. Anal. Lett.* **2**, 31-8.

Falk, J.L. (1961). The production of polydipsia in normal rats by an intermittent food schedule. *Science* **133**, 195-6.

Falk, J.L. (1966a). Schedule-induced polydipsia as a function of fixed interval length. *J. exp. Anal. Behav.* **9**, 37-9.

Falk, J.L. (1966b). The motivational properties of schedule-induced polydipsia. *J. exp. Anal. Behav.* **9**, 19-25.

Falk, J.L. (1967). Control of schedule-induced polydipsia: type, size, and spacing of meals. *J. exp. Anal. Behav.* **10**, 199-206.

Falk, J.L. (1969). Conditions producing psychogenic polydipsia in animals. *Ann. NY Acad. Sci.* **157**, 569-93.

Falk, J.L. (1971). The nature and determinants of adjunctive behaviour. *Physiol. Behav.* **6**, 577-88.

Flory, R.K. (1969). Attack behaviour in a multiple fixed-ratio schedule of reinforcement. *Psychonom. Sci.* **16**, 156-157.

Flory, R.K. (1971). The control of schedule-induced polydipsia: frequency and magnitude of reinforcement. *Learning Motivation* **2**, 215-27.

Flory, R.K. and O'Boyle, M. (1972). The effect of limited water availability on schedule-induced polydipsia. *Physiol. Behav.* **8**, 147-9.

Freed, E.X. and Hymowitz, N. (1969). A fortuitous observation regarding psychogenic polydipsia. *Psychol. Rep.* **24**, 224-6.

Freed, E.X. and Hymowitz, N. (1972). Effects of schedule, body weight, and magnitude of reinforcer on acquisition of schedule-induced polydipsia. *Psychol. Rep.* **31**, 95-101.

Hamm, R.J., Porter, J.H., and Oster, G.D. (1978). Compound stimulus control of operant, but not adjunctive, behaviour. *Bull. psychonom. Soc.* **12**(3), 167-70.

Hamm, R.J., Porter, J.J., and Kaempf, G.L. (1981). Stimulus generalization of schedule-induced polydipsia. *J. exp. Anal. Behav.* **36**, 93-9.

Hawkins, T.D., Schrot, J.F., Githens, S.H., and Everett, P.B. (1972). Schedule-induced polydipsia: an analysis of water and alcohol ingestion. In *Schedule effects: drugs, drinking, and aggression* (ed. R.M. Gilbert and J.D. Keehn), pp. 95-129. University of Toronto Press, Toronto.

Herrnstein, R.J. (1961). Relative and absolute strength of response as a function of frequency of reinforcement. *J. exp. Anal. Behav.* **4**, 267-72.

Herrnstein, R.J. (1970). On the law of effect. *J. exp. Anal. Behav.* **13**, 243-66.

Heyman, G. M. and Bouzas, A. (1980). Context dependent changes in the reinforcing strength of schedule-induced drinking. *J. exp. Anal. Behav.* **33**, 327-35.

Hinson, J. M., Malone, J. C., McNally, K. A., and Rowe, D. W. (1978). Effects of component length and of the transitions among components in multiple schedules. *J. exp. Anal. Behav.* **29**, 3-16.

Hinson, J. M. and Staddon, J. E. R. (1978). Behavioural competition: A mechanism for schedule interactions. *Science* **202**, 432-4.

Innis, N. K., Simmelhag-Grant, V. L., and Staddon, J. E. R. (1983). Behaviour induced by periodic food delivery: the effects of interfood interval. *J. exp. Anal. Behav.* **39**, 309-22.

Iverson, I. H. (1977). Reinforcement omission and schedule-induced drinking in a response-independent schedule in rats. *Physiol. Behav.* **18**, 535-7.

Jacquet, Y. F. (1972). Schedule-induced licking during multiple schedules. *J. exp. Anal. Behav.* **17**, 413-23.

Keehn, J. D. and Colotla, V. A. (1971). Schedule-induced drinking as a function of interpellet interval. *Psychonom. Sci.* **23**, 69-71.

Killeen, P. (1975). On the temporal control of behaviour. *Psychol. Rev.* **82**, 89-115.

Killeen, P. (1979). Arousal: its genesis, modulation, and extinction. In *Advances in analysis of behaviour, (vol. 1) Reinforcement and the organization of behaviour* (ed. M. D. Zeiler and P. Harzem), pp. 31-78. Wiley, New York.

King, G. D. (1974). Wheel running in the rat induced by a fixed-time presentation of water. *Animal Learning Behaviour* **2**, 325-8.

Knutson, J. F. (1970). Aggression during the fixed-ratio and extinction components of a multiple schedule of reinforcement. *J. exp. Anal. Behav.* **13**, 221-31.

Knutson, J. F. and Schrader, S. P. (1975). A concurrent assessment of schedule-induced aggression and schedule-induced polydipsia in the rat. *Animal Learning Behav.* **3**, 16-20.

McFarland, D. J. (1970). Adjunctive behaviour in feeding and drinking situations. *Rev. Comportement Animal* **4**, 64-73.

McLeod, D. R. and Gollub, L. R. (1976). An analysis of rats' drinking tube contacts under tandem and fixed-interval schedules of food presentation. *J. exp. Anal. Behav.* **25**, 361-70.

Millenson, J. R. (1975). The facts of schedule-induced polydipsia. *Behav. Res. Methods Instrument.* **7**, 257-9.

Minor, T. R. (1987). Stimulus and pellet induced drinking during a successive discrimination. *J. exp. Anal. Behav.* **48**, 61-80.

Minor, T. R. and Coulter, X. (1982). Associative and postprandial control of schedule-induced drinking: implications for the study of interim behaviour. *Animal Learning Behav.* **10**, 455-64.

Myerson, J. and Christiansen, B. (1979). Temporal control of eating on periodic water schedules. *Physiol. Behav.* **23**, 1-4.

Osborne, S. R. (1978). A quantitative analysis of the effects of amount of reinforcement on two response classes. *J. exp. Psychol: Animal Behav. Processes* **4**, 297-317.

Penney, J. and Schull, J. (1977). Functional differentiation of adjunctive drinking and wheel running in rats. *Animal Learning Behav.* **5**, 272-80.

Porter, J.H. and Kenshalo, D.R. (1974). Schedule-induced drinking following omission of reinforcement in the rhesus monkey. *Physiol. Behav.* **12**, 1075-7.

Rachlin, H. and Krasnoff, J. (1983). Eating and drinking: an economic analysis. *J. exp. Anal. Behav.* **39**, 385-403.

Reberg, D., Mann, B., and Innis, N.K. (1977). Superstitious behaviour for food and water in the rat. *Physiol. Behav.* **19**, 803-6.

Reid, A.K. and Dale, R.H.I. (1983). Dynamic effects of food magnitude on interim-terminal interaction. *J. exp. Anal. Behav.* **39**, 135-48.

Reid, A.K. and Staddon, J.E.R. (1982). Schedule-induced drinking: Elicitation, anticipation, or behavioural interaction? *J. exp. Anal. Behav.* **38**, 1-18.

Reid, A.K. and Staddon, J.E.R. (1987). Within-session meal-size effects on induced drinking. *J. exp. Anal. Behav.* **48**, 289-301.

Reid, A.K., Piñones, P., and Alatorre, J. (1985). Schedule induction and the temporal distributions of adjunctive behaviour on periodic water schedules. *Animal Learning Behav.* **13**, 321-6.

Reid, A.K., Gutierrez, J., and Lopez, F. (in prep. *a*). The allocation of schedule-induced activities in multiple schedules in the rat and pigeon.

Reid, A.K., Bacha, G., and Moran, C. (in prep. *b*). The organization of behaviour on periodic reward schedules.

Riley, A.L., Wetherington, C.L., Delamater, A.R., Peele, D.B., and Dacanay, R.J. (1985). The effects of variations in the interpellet interval on wheel running in the rat. *Animal Learning Behav.* **13**, 201-6.

Roper, T.J. (1978). Diversity and substitutability of adjunctive activities under fixed-internal schedules of food reinforcement. *J. exp. Anal. Behav.* **30**, 83-96.

Roper, T.J. (1980). Changes in rate of schedule-induced behaviour in rats as a function of fixed-interval schedule. *Quart. J. exp. Psychol.* **32**, 159-70.

Roper, T.J. (1981). What is meant by the term 'schedule-induced', and how general is schedule induction? *Animal Learning Behav.* **9**, 433.

Roper, T.J. (1984). Response of thirsty rats to absence of water: frustration disinhibition or compensation? *Animal Behav.* **32**, 1235-55.

Roper, T.J. and Crossland, G. (1982). Mechanisms underlying eating-drinking transitions in rats. *Animal Behav.* **30**, 602-14.

Roper, T.J. and Posadas-Andrews, A. (1981). Are schedule-induced drinking and displacement activities causally related? *Quart. J. exp. Psychol.* **33B**, 181-93.

Rosellini, R.A. and Burdette, D.R. (1980). Meal size and intermeal interval both regulate schedule-induced water intake in rats. *Animal Learning Behav.* **1**, 647-52.

Rosenblith, J.Z. (1970). Polydipsia induced in the rat by a second-order schedule. *J. exp. Anal. Behav.* **14**, 139-44.

Segal, E. (1969). The interaction of psychogenic polydipsia with wheel running in rats. *Psychonom. Sci.* **14**, 141-4.

Shurtleff, D., Delamater, A.R. and Riley, A.L. (1983). A reevaluation of the CS – Hypothesis for schedule-induced polydipsia under intermittent schedules of pellet delivery. *Animal Learning Behav.* **11**, 247-54.

Staddon, J.E.R. (1977). Schedule-induced behaviour. In *Handbook of operant behaviour* (ed. W.K. Honig and J.E.R. Staddon), pp. 125-52. Englewood Cliffs, New Jersey.

Staddon, J.E.R. (1982). Behavioural competition, contrast, and matching. In *Quantitative analysis of operant behaviour: Vol. II. Matching and maximizing accounts* (ed. R.J. Commons, R. Herrnstein, and H. Rachlin), pp. 243-61. Balinger, New York.

Staddon, J.E.R., and Ayres, S. (1975). Sequential and temporal properties of behaviour induced by a schedule of periodic food delivery. *Behaviour* 54, 26-49.

Timberlake, W. (1982). Controls and schedule-induced behaviour. *Animal Learning Behav.* 10, 535-6.

Todorov, J.C. (1972). Component duration and relative response rates in multiple schedules. *J. exp. Anal. Behav.* 17, 45-9.

Urbain, C., Poling, A., and Thompson, T. (1979). Differing effects of intermittent food delivery on interim behaviour in guinea pig and rats. *Physiol Behav.* 22, 621-5.

Wetherington, C.L. (1979). Schedule-induced drinking: rate of food delivery and Herrnstein's equation. *J. exp. Anal. Behav.* 32, 323-34.

Wetherington, C.L. (1982). Is adjunctive behaviour a third class of behaviour? *Neurosci. Biobehav. Rev.* 6, 329-50.

Wetherington, C.L. and Brownstein, A.J. (1982). Comment on Roper's discussion of the language and generality of schedule-induced behaviour. *Animal Learning Behav.* 10, 537-9.

Wetherington, C.L. and Riley, A.L. (1986). Schedule-induced polydipsia: interactions with wheel running. *Animal Learning Behav.* 14, 416-20.

Wetherington, C.L., Brownstein, A.J. and Shull, R.L. (1977). Schedule-induced running and chamber size. *Psychol. Rec.* 27, 703-13.

Williams, B.A. (1979). Contrast, component duration, and the following schedule of reinforcement. *J. exp. Psychol: animal behav. Processes* 5, 379-96.

Wuttke, W. and Innis, N.K. (1972). Drug effects upon behaviour induced by second-order schedules of reinforcement: The relevance of ethological analysis. In *Schedule effects: drugs, drinking, and aggression* (ed. R.M Gilbert and J.D. Keehn), pp. 129-47. University of Toronto Press, Toronto.

9

Stereotyped behaviour in madness and in health

C.D. FRITH and D.J. DONE

Introduction

It has long been recognized that pointless repetitive behaviour is a common component of madness. In 1701 Nehemia Grew wrote 'We see also Mad people, in whom Phancy reigns, to run upon some one action, as Reading, or Knitting of Straws, without variation'. This repetition has been particularly observed in the speech and writing of mentally deranged people. 'When lunatics attempt to write, there is a perpetual recurrence of one or two favourite ideas, intermixed with phrases which convey scarcely any meaning either separately, or in connection with the other parts. It would be a hard task for a man of common understanding, to put such rhapsodies into any intelligible form, yet patients will run their ideas in the very same track for many weeks together. . . .' (John Ferrier 1795). Such behaviour can readily be observed in schizophrenic patients today. Kraepelin (1899) listed stereotypies as one of the characteristic symptoms of dementia praecox, yet today stereotyped behaviour receives very little attention. For example, in the *Handbook of psychiatry*, Vol. III: *Psychoses of uncertain origin* (Wing and Wing 1982) Kraepelin's view of the importance of stereotyped behaviour is quoted in the introduction, but thereafter the topic is never mentioned again. This decline of interest seems to have arisen because of difficulties in defining stereotyped behaviour and hence with developing objective means for observing it. However, there also seems to have been a decline in the prevalence of some of these disorders which remains unexplained.

Problems in the definition of stereotyped behaviour

Stereotyped behaviour is one of a number of disorders of movement and action. Earlier in this century great pains were taken carefully to describe the various kinds of disorder and to distinguish one from another (e.g.

Henderson and Gillespie 1927). Although these various types of movement disorder are treated as discrete entities, it is clear that they lie along various continua. Three can readily be identified:

1. *Complexity*; this concerns the number of components involved in the movement or act and can vary from a simple finger movement to flaying of the limbs.

2. *Co-ordination*; this concerns the relationships between the agonist and antagonist muscles and might vary from the random flailing of the limbs due to a choreic twitch to a smooth 'goal-directed' movement such as dancing down the stairs backwards.

3. *Degree of conscious control*; the major distinction here is between voluntary and involuntary movements. However this distinction is not entirely clear-cut. For example, an involuntary movement such as a tic can be inhibited by an act of will, but only for a limited period. On the other hand complex co-ordinated voluntary acts may sometimes occur 'automatically' without any thought. The patient's attitude to the movement or act seems also to be taken into account. Conventionally it is considered important to discover whether the patient feels compelled to carry out the action, whether he tries to resist and feels relief when the act has finally occurred.

It is this dependence on the patient's subjective experiences of his movements or action that has made observation and classification difficult. This problem does not, of course, arise in studies of stereotyped behaviour in animals. It is also striking that the literature on stereotyped behaviour in humans is almost entirely concerned with the mentally handicapped. In this population also introspection has not been considered an appropriate source of information. In these studies stereotyped behaviour is defined simply as any purposeless movement or act that occurs repeatedly. This is the definition that we shall use in this chapter also. However, we shall extend the notion of act to cover speaking, writing, and thinking.

In psychiatric and neurological terminology the definition of stereotyped behaviour encompasses a number of different entities which we list with their usual definitions below, (see also Chapter 10, this volume, by Stoessl).

1. *Tremor*: more or less regular, rhythmic contracting of muscles and their antagonists. There are various types of tremor and it may be observed in a number of different disorders. It is commonly associated with Parkinson's disease.

2. *Tics*: sudden, brief, recurrent, inappropriate, and often irresistible movements, simple or complex, without purpose or aim. Tics have predominantly a proximal distribution and usually involve expressive musculature. They can be checked by will, but this leads to intolerable

tension. Tics are a particularly striking feature of the Gilles de la Tourette syndrome where they can take the form of involuntary obscene utterances.

3. *Tardive dyskinesia*: involuntary movements of the lips, jaws, and tongue; smacking and sucking of the lips, thrusting and rolling of the tongue, lateral jaw movements, puffing of the cheeks. Abnormal movements of this type are frequently seen in chronic schizophrenic patients and are widely believed to be the consequence of long-term treatment with dopamine-blocking drugs. However such movements have also been reported in schizophrenic patients never treated with neuroleptics (see pp. 246–7).

4. *Perseveration*: repetition of a recent movement, action, or speech in spite of the patient's effort to produce a new movement. This is distinguished from a stereotypy in that the perseveration of the action is transient and needs a stimulus. For example, a patient might be asked to write his name which he does correctly. However, when he is asked to write his address and the date he continues to write his name and does so over and over again. This is considered to be a sign of organic disease.

5. *Stereotypy*: An action, or group of actions or words monotonously repeated or a posture maintained abnormally long. It is possible that the action originally had a meaning and/or purpose, but this has largely been lost (Kläsi 1922). For example, one patient we have observed over the years used to stand near the entrance to the hospital repeatedly showing passers-by a piece of paper with her address on it and asking to be taken home. Two years later she still stands there but the piece of paper is blank and her mutterings incomprehensible. Stereotypes of posture were a classic feature of catatonic schizophrenia but are rarely seen today and more recent textbooks restrict their definition of stereotypies to active movements. The essential feature of stereotyped behaviour is that it is incessantly repeated and is inappropriate to the context.

6. *Mannerism*: a normal goal-directed behaviour which is performed in a peculiar stylized and idiosyncratic manner. For example, one of the chronic schizophrenic patients we have observed usually stops on each step of the stairs, turns round once, and touches the walls before going on to the next step.

7. *Obsessional phenomena*: repetitive, purposeless voluntary phenomena which the subject feels compelled to carry out, but does so under the influence of his or her own will. Resistance to these activities causes tension and anxiety. Any area of functioning that is under voluntary control may be involved. Motor behaviours are referred to as compulsions while thoughts are referred to as ruminations. Compulsive acts have to be distinguished

from repetitive acts consequent upon delusions. For example, a patient might believe that his or her compulsion to act emanated from some external force (delusion of passivity). Another patient might repeatedly wash him or herself because of a delusion of contamination. Neither of these phenomena would be classified as compulsive acts.

From these definitions we clearly see how difficult it is to classify the repetitive act of a chronic schizophrenic patient as a stereotypy. Over the years a stereotyped act might become so brief and fragmented that it would be indistinguishable from an involuntary movement disorder. Alternatively, in an institutional setting what was once a mannerism might become as extreme as a stereotypy. If we were unaware of the eliciting stimulus a perseverative act might be misclassified as a stereotypy. Finally, in the absence of evidence from introspection it would be difficult to distinguish a compulsive act from a stereotypy.

The position is further complicated by the conventional clinical practice of using these terms to imply something about the basis of the disorder, in particular whether it is thought to be organically based (as would be the case with perseverations and involuntary movement disorders, but not stereotypies or compulsions). This problem is discussed by Rogers (1985).

Pointless, repetitive movements in normal adults

Spontaneous stereotypies

A few minutes casual observation in a train or a canteen will reveal that normal individuals often make pointless repetitive movements. These include movements of the lips and jaw, twiddling things with the fingers, doodling, and fidgeting with the feet. This behaviour seems particularly likely to occur when the individual is bored, under stress, or trying to concentrate. It is traditional for anxious husbands to pace up and down in the maternity hospital and one of the authors of this chapter always paces up and down while trying to formulate the next paragraph he is going to write. These phenomena have received very little in the way of formal study. Asendorpf (1980) observed groups of students while resting, while waiting to perform a test, and while performing the test. He found that there was an increase in repetitive hand movements in the anticipating and testing conditions, confirming his prediction that stereotyped behaviour would increase with increasing arousal. However, these effects disappeared in another group of students who were told they were going to be observed. It is this ability to so easily stop performing stereotyped movements when they are socially inappropriate that is so strikingly absent in psychiatric patients.

Elicited stereotypies

Stereotyped behaviour can be elicited from normal subjects by giving them suitable tasks to perform. Responses in such tasks will be defined as stereotyped if (1) the responses are not determined by any relevant stimuli and (2) the responses are repetitive in the sense that only a small subset of possible responses or response sequences are emitted. In statistical terms this means that we can predict the subject's next response on the basis of his or her previous responses, but not on the basis of previous stimuli. Suitable tasks for eliciting stereotyped behaviour in this sense are variations on gambling. In these tasks there is either no stimulus on which the subject can base a response (e.g. the subject is asked explicitly to produce a random sequence) or else the stimuli occur randomly and thus provide no information upon which the subject can base a response. In these circumstances it is not surprising that the subject's behaviour tends to be stereotyped. However, the degree of stereotypy is very sensitive to instructions and to the subjects interpretation of the situation.

It is well known that human subjects are incapable of generating a totally random sequence (e.g. Slovic *et al.* 1974). Furthermore, as the number of alternatives to be randomized increases, it becomes progressively more difficult to randomize the sequence (Slak and Hirsch 1974). Slak *et al.* (1982) found that subjects asked to produce a 'completely random' sequence did indeed produce more random sequences than those asked to 'push the buttons in the order they wished'. However, both types of sequence were still far from random. The deviations from randomness observed in these kinds of experiments reflect the gambler's fallacy by which subjects reveal their ignorance of the nature of randomness. Typically, they avoid repetitions and alternations more than would occur by chance (Attneave 1959) and, in multiple alternative tasks, they incorrectly assume that all the alternatives should appear only once in a relatively short sequence. There are, however, problems with this approach. As Lopes (1982) has pointed out, the definition of randomness remains controversial and from some points of view the 'deviations' shown by normal subjects are perfectly reasonable.

A number of mechanisms have been proposed by which subjects might generate these 'random' sequences of responses. Wiegersma (1982) has reviewed these attempts and concludes that the data are best explained by a mechanism that has two principal stages. The subject first selects a suitable response to appear next in the sequence. This selection will be biased by various automatic processes such that the most likely response to be selected will be the one most recently given (perseveration) or one associated with the response recently given (association). The second component accepts or rejects this possible response by comparing it with a list of recently given responses held in short-term memory. If the subject remembers giving the response recently it will be rejected. This latter process is a deliberate strategy and results in the subject avoiding repetitions more than would occur by chance. If the subject has to divide his or her attention by doing another task at the same time then this avoidance of repetition is reduced. Wiegersma believes that it is this tendency to avoid repetitions that results in deviations from randomness rather than the subject's 'concept of randomness'. In terms of this model an increase in perseverative behaviour could either be due to an increase in the automatic tendency to perseverate or to a reduction in the extent to which the subject deliberately tries to avoid response repetitions. Wiegersma considers that the mechanism will apply not only to 'randomization' tasks, but to any task in which a sequence of responses has to be generated.

Rather than being asked explicitly to generate a random sequence a subject may be asked to guess an unpredictable outcome or solve an insoluble problem. In these tasks it is entirely a matter of chance whether a subject is correct or not and thus there is no information available to help select the response. Goodnow (1955) has shown that performance on such task depends on how the subject interprets the situation. In her experiment there were only two possible responses and the critical results were obtained when one response was much more likely to be correct than the other (either 7:3 or 9:1). In one condition the task involved finding a principle by which patterns could be matched. It was in other words a problem-solving task. The other condition was a gambling task in which the subject had to win money by selecting the 'right' key to press. Goodnow suggests that in the problem-solving situation the subject is concerned to discover a 'rule' which will lead eventually to 100 per cent success. The subject will not mind making mistakes en route to finding this rule. This strategy implies a belief that there is a rule that will lead to 100 per cent success. By contrast, in the gambling task the subject will tend to believe that there is no 'rule'. The subject will accept less than 100 per cent success as a satisfactory outcome as long as wins exceed losses. Having found a successful means of achieving wins he or she will not risk possible losses by searching for a better strategy.

These suggestions were confirmed by the observation that subjects performing the gambling task were much more likely to adopt the strategy of pressing the high winning response key every time. Thus stereotyped behaviour was more likely in the 'gambling' task than in the 'problem-solving' task, even though, formally, the tasks were identical.

From a very different starting point Schwartz (1982) made a similar observation. He demonstrated that people showed the same stereotyped behaviour that he had previously found in pigeons. He used a two-choice task in which there genuinely was a rule to be found. A reward was obtained if the two response keys were pressed four times each in any order. This means that there were 70 different response sequences which would obtain a reward. On simply being instructed to obtain as many rewards as possible people rapidly developed stereotyped behaviour in that, having found a sequence that was rewarded, they tended to produce this sequence rather than any of the other equally rewarding sequences. In these circumstances subjects were clearly adopting the gambler's strategy described by Goodnow. However, when Schwartz instructed his subject to find the rule by which reward was obtained, stereotyped behaviour did not develop since no response sequence became dominant. When searching for a rule a person will continually generate and test new hypotheses about what the rule might be. It is this spontaneous generation of new hypotheses which prevents the emergence of repetitive sequences of responses.

Conclusion

Normal adults emit stereotyped behaviours spontaneously and also in 'gambling' tasks. However, these repetitive behaviours are very sensitive to external influences and can be suppressed at will.

Pointless, repetitive movements in retarded and autistic individuals

Spontaneous stereotypies

Stereotyped behaviour is a common feature of retarded people living in institutions. In a survey by Berkson and Davenport (1962) stereotyped behaviour was observed in about two-thirds of the severely mentally retarded individuals studied. Some individuals were indulging in this behaviour for up to 50 per cent of the times they were observed. Such behaviour can raise considerable problems of management since it may either (1) be self-injurious (e.g. head banging), or (2) interfere with desired activities, particularly in the class room (e.g. manipulating objects), or (3) be very annoying (e.g. screaming, spitting). Because of these problems there is a large literature, mostly from a behaviourist point of view, on how to reduce these behaviours.

The origins of stereotyped behaviour in the retarded

Repetitive movements such as rocking are, of course, commonly observed in infants (Thelen 1979) and, to some extent, this behaviour in the mentally retarded is commensurate with their mental age. However, this clearly cannot be the whole explanation. On the basis of animal studies Ridley and Baker (1982) have proposed that stereotyped behaviour can be divided into two types having different aetiologies. The first type is a consequence of a restricted environment (cage stereotypy). Stereotyped behaviour of this kind will stop when the restrictions are removed. The second kind of stereotyped behaviour is caused by some abnormality in the central nervous system or can be induced by amphetamine, and is found together with social withdrawal and cognitive inflexibility. It does not cease when environmental restrictions are removed. Ridley and Baker suggest that this kind of stereotyped behaviour is associated with psychoses, particularly early childhood autism. These speculations suggest a number of questions about the stereotyped behaviour of different groups of retarded people. The behaviourist stance of most students of stereotyped behaviour in the retarded has meant that little attention has been paid to the differences between diagnostic categories. Nevertheless, some differences between autistic and non-autistic retarded people do emerge from the literature.

1. *Are there qualitative differences between stereotyped behaviour in autistic and non-autistic individuals?* Stereotyped behaviour is extremely frequent in autistic children and the feature 'insistence on sameness' which could be seen as a high-level stereotypy is considered characteristic of the syndrome. On this basis one might expect to see high-level stereotypies in autistic children (e.g. manipulating objects, complex finger movements, etc) rather than the rocking, and mouthing observed in other retarded people. Second, one might expect to see stereotyped behaviour even in autistic children with borderline and normal IQs whereas it would only be seen in non-autistic retarded people with low IQs. This prediction is supported by Hermelin and O'Connor (1963) who compared severely retarded autistic and non-autistic children matched for mental age. They observed that the autistic children indulged significantly more in 'self-generated' behaviour (rocking, hand and finger playing, spinning) than the non-autistic controls.

2. *Do the stereotyped behaviours of autistic children respond differently to environmental manipulations?* It is widely assumed that retarded people indulge in stereotyped behaviour in order to increase stimulation, so this is frequently called self-stimulation behaviour. This is consistent with the behaviour being a form of 'cage' stereotypy, caused by reduced stimulation from the environment. There are at least three reasons why this stimulation might be reduced: (1) the environment in a large institution is unfortunately, but typically impoverished; (2) sensory impairment will reduce stimulation from the environment. Thus children with visual and/or hearing impairments are more likely to show stereotyped behaviour (Berkson and Davenport 1962; Guess 1966); (3) cognitive and/or physical handicap will make it more difficult for a child to obtain stimulation from the environment in socially acceptable ways. Forehand and Baumeister (1971) found that the people with very low IQs (< 20) continued rocking even when restriction was removed, whereas people with IQs greater than 20 reduced rocking in these

circumstances. Presumably the people with very low I Qs were not capable of detecting the increase in environmental stimulation.

If this account of stereotyped behaviour in the non-autistic retarded is correct, then we would expect this behaviour to be reduced when environmental stimulation is increased. Young and Clements (1979) found that the complex hand movements shown by three severely retarded children were reduced when the environment was enriched by the provision of toys and encouragement to use them. On the other hand, if the hand movements were physically prevented then other stereotyped behaviour such as rocking increased. LaGrow and Repp (1984) list five studies in which provision of toys and other objects reduced stereotyped behaviour in retarded individuals. In constrast, Hutt and Hutt (1965) found that the introduction of toys increased stereotyped behaviour in six autistic children. On the basis of behavioural and psychophysiological data, Hutt and Hutt (1970) have suggested that autistic children are in a chronic state of hyper-arousal and that their stereotyped behaviours have the effect of decreasing this arousal. This is in marked contrast to the 'self-stimulation' theory of stereotypy (e.g. Young and Clements 1979) which assumes that stereotyped behaviour is essentially self-stimulation activity carried out to compensate for lack of external stimulation. These differences may well be a consequence of the different populations studied. What little evidence there is suggests that stereotyped behaviour in the non-autistic retarded is a consequence of intrinsic and extrinsic environmental restrictions whereas the same behaviour in autistic children has some other aetiology.

Elicited stereotyped behaviour

U. Frith carried out a series of experiments with autistic, retarded, and normal children using tasks analogous to Goodnow's gambling task. In one experiment the children had to guess the colour (red or black) of the next card in a shuffled pack (Frith 1970). In normal children there is a clear developmental progression in the sequence of guesses produced on such a task (Gerjuoy and Winters 1968). The youngest children perseverate, guessing the same colour every time. At age 4 to 5 this switches to an alternation of colours and at age 9–10 a relatively random sequence of guesses is observed as in Goodnow's adults (when each response was equally likely to be right). Autistic children produced more stereotyped response sequences (perseverations or alternations) than either normal children or children with Down's syndrome matched for mental age.

In other experiments Frith (1972) asked the children to make sequential patterns using either colours (stamping the pages of a booklet) or sounds (playing a xylophone). In these tasks also the autistic children produced more stereotyped sequences, using fewer of the available responses and making more rigid and repetitive patterns.

Conclusions

Stereotyped behaviour is very common in children who are retarded and/or autistic. To some extent this may be a 'normal' response to a lack of stimulation from the environment (analogous to 'cage stereotypy'). This lack of stimulation may be extrinsic (e.g. an institutional setting) or intrinsic. People who are blind, deaf, or cognitively impaired are unable to obtain as much stimulation from the environment as a person without such impairments. However autistic children seem to indulge in stereotyped behaviour more so than equally retarded children without autistic features. Thus stereotyped behaviour in autistic children may be associated with some underlying pathological process that also produces cognitive inflexibility and social withdrawal.

Stereotyped behaviour associated with organic aetiologies

Tic convulsif (Gilles de la Tourette syndrome) (see Gilroy and Meyer 1979, p. 373)

This disorder usually begins in childhood and often starts as a simple tic of the eyes, head, or face. Later this tic becomes accompanied with vocalizations such as grunting, barking, or screaming. In 60 per cent of the cases this vocalization takes the form of repetitive obscene phrases, compulsively shouted out. In addition to these very peculiar tics, patients have a compulsion to repeat or imitate words and gestures. In the words of one of Gilles de la Tourette's patients (Gilles de la Tourette 1885) 'When I listen to a speech or a lecture I am goaded by an almost irresistible need to repeat a word or the end of a phrase that has struck me'.

The aetiology of this disorder is still unknown, but there are good reasons for the belief that it reflects some organic disorder, probably in the basal ganglia (Sweet *et al.* 1973). The disorder responds to treatment with dopamine blocking drugs such as haloperidol.

Shapiro *et al.* (1974) and Sutherland *et al.* (1982) both conclude on the basis of psychological test results that patients with the Gilles de la Tourette syndrome show signs of 'brain damage'. Sutherland *et al.* found that the patients were especially impaired on tests of verbal fluency and also on tests involving memory for visually presented non-verbal material. Such deficits are shown by patients with orbitofrontal and right temporal lesions, respectively, but could also arise from lesions in subcortical areas, such as the neostriatum which project into these cortical areas.

Parkinson's disease

Apart from the characteristic tremor, patients with Parkinson's disease (PD) do not show repetitive, stereotyped movements. However, they do show perseveration on a number of psychological tests. Bowen *et al.* (1975) and Lees and Smith (1983), for example, have shown that patients with PD perform badly on the Wisconsin sorting task. In this task the subject has to classify cards according to some rule. The alternative rules are: sorting by shape, sorting by colour, or sorting by number. The subject has to discover the rule chosen by the experimenter using trial and error. When the rule has been found as indicated by a run of correct classifications the experimeter, unbeknown to the subject, switches to a new rule. The subject has to recognize that the old rule no longer works and find, once again by trial and error, the new rule. On this task patients with PD have difficulty in switching to a new rule and tend to perseverate. This behaviour clearly reflects a cognitive, rather than a motor perseveration.

Flowers and Robertson (1985) have used a simplified version of the Wisconsin task in which subjects have to pick the odd one out of three stimuli according to a rule which alternates from one trial to the next (in one rule the choice was based on shape, while in the other it was based on size). Although they were just as good as controls on the first trial, PD patients showed poor performance as soon as the alternating rules were introduced. This poor performance was not strictly due to perseveration errors since the patients did not rigidly stick to the first rule learned, but were as likely to use the second rule inappropriately when they should have been using the first. Flowers and Robertson interpret these results as showing difficulty in maintaining a 'mental set'.

These problems do not seem to be a consequence of the dementia sometimes found in PD patients since difficulties on the tasks described above can be observed in PD patients with no other signs of cognitive impairment.

As we shall see in the next section, these problems are also observed in patients with frontal lobe lesions (Flowers 1982). Morel-Maroger (1978) has compared the two groups directly using a simple task which requires the maintenance of a 'mental set'. The subject has to respond to a sign given by the experimenter by making the 'opposite' sign. For example, if the experimenter taps twice on the table the patient taps once and vice versa (Luria 1973, p. 201). Both patients with Parkinson's disease and patients with frontal lobe lesions had difficulty with such tasks. They could successfully carry out the instructions for a few trials, but then reverted to copying the experimenter. Morel-Maroger then gave L-dopa to his patients and showed that this improved the patients with PD, but not those with frontal lobe lesions.

Parkinson's disease is the consequence of damage to the nigrostriatal pathway and subsequent dopamine deficiency on the striatum. The symptoms can be reversed to some extent by treatment with L-dopa, a dopamine precursor. In view of the observation that the cortical projections of the dopamine system are to the frontal cortex, it seems reasonable that a general depletion of dopamine might lead to problems similar to those encountered after lesions of the frontal cortex.

Perseverations after frontal lobe lesions

Frontal cortex accounts for about one-third of the total cortical area and therefore it is not surprising that lesions in different parts of the frontal lobes produce different effects. Nevertheless, various kinds of perseveration seem to be a common feature of such lesions. Luria (1973, chapter 7) suggests that the perseverations become more complex with more anterior lesions.

Motor perseverations   With lesions in the premotor area patients may show simple perseverations of movement. Thus on being asked to draw a circle the patient will correctly draw a circle, but will then be unable to stop and will carry on making the movement over and over again. Similarly, if the patient is asked to tap out a rhythm of strong and weak beats (. . . . . ----- . . . . ----) he or she will only be able to produce one kind of beat (-----------). According to Luria in these cases the patient clearly has the knowledge and intention to carry out the command correctly, but is unable to execute it. When the lesion is in the dominant hemisphere the same phenomena may be observed in speech. Thus when attempting to pronounce the work 'mukha' (Russian for fly) the patient perseverates on the first syllable and says 'mu . . . m . . . mu . . . . ma'. Such problems may sometimes be observed in Broca's aphasia. The same kind of perseveration may also be observed in the writing of such patients. Liepmann (1905) called this kind of perseveration 'clonic' per-severation to distinguish it from a more complex kind which he called 'inten-tional' perseveration. In this case the patient correctly performs the first action when asked to do so, but when he or she is asked to perform another action either produces the old action or else incorporates parts of the old action in the new action. Yamadori (1981) asked aphasic patients to repeat multisyllabic words and observed these kinds of perseveration in 87 per cent of his cases. Most of these patients were suffering from Broca's aphasia. Hudson (1968) observed such perseveration in the drawing and writing of a patient with a large glioma in the left frontal lobe. Thus, having correctly drawn a cat on request, the patient also drew cats when asked to draw a house and a man.

Other frontal lobe signs   More anterior lesions produce more complex perseverations (e.g. perseverations of ideas) and what Luria calls 'inert stereotypes'. By this he seems to mean that the patient cannot regulate his responses and actions according to the actual requirements of the situation and produces a 'default' response, that is, the response most compatible with the immediate stimulus. Thus the examiner might ask the patient 'when I tap twice you tap once and when I tap once you tap twice'. The patient may be able to carry this out for one or two trials, but then defaults to imitating the examiner (echopraxia). Lhermitte (1983) has observed 'utilization behaviour' in patients with frontal lobe lesions, the presentation of objects compelling the patients to grasp and use them. Thus, if a pair of spectacles are placed in front of the patient he or she will put them on. If a second pair are presented these will be put on on top of the first pair.

Lesions in the orbital and dorsolateral regions produce problems which may all be ascribed to a lack of spontaneity which sometimes gives rise to perseveration. Failure on the Wisconsin card-sorting task (which we have described above) is a typical example of this. For example, frontal lobe patients when asked to name as many animals as they can will produce very few examples. This task does not usually elicit perseverations (i.e. repeating the same animal over and over again), but this may well be because the instructions specifically include the request not to name any animal more than once. Frontal lobe patients also perform badly on a test of design fluency. Here they are asked to draw as many different abstract designs as possible. This task elicits perseveration particularly in patients with lesions in the right frontal lobe since the designs produced tend to be very similar to one another (e.g. Jones-Gotman and Milner 1977).

Teuber (1964) has shown that patients with frontal lobe lesions also perform badly on visual search tasks. In this task the patient has to find a target object on a card which has many different objects drawn all over it in random positions. Performance of this task also depends on the ability spontaneously to generate the eye movements appropriate for the search since there is no external information which can tell the patient where to look. This task could well elicit perseverative behaviour since the patient might repeatedly look at the same part of the display which has already been searched. However, we know of no attempts to investigate this possibility.

We have examined two patients with damage to the frontal lobes on a two-choice guessing game resembling Goodnow's gambling task. This task resembles the Wisconsin sorting task in that the patient must try to find a rule which will enable him or her to predict the stimulus sequence. However, in contrast to the Wisconsin, there is no rule that actually works. As argued above, as long as the subject continues to generate and test new rules he or she will not produce stereotyped sequences of responses. One of the patients we examined with this test had a large tumour in the right frontal lobe. The other was a probable case of Pick's disease. A computer automated tomography (CAT) scan revealed bifrontal cortical atrophy which was confirmed by a brain biopsy. Both patients produced markedly stereotyped sequences characterized by alternation of the two possible responses. In one case alternations were produced for 73 per cent of the total sequence and, for the other, 88 per cent. The normal rate of alternations is less than 50 per cent.

Stereotyped behaviour associated with dementia

On the bases of the evidence presented in the preceding section we would expect stereotyped behaviour to be associated with dementia to the extent that the frontal lobes were involved in the pathological process. This is consistent with our observation of marked stereotyped behaviour in the patient with Pick's disease described above since frontal atrophy is a characteristic feature of such patients.

In contrast, patients with mild dementia of the Alzheimer type did not show stereotyped behaviour on our two-choice guessing task (Frith and Done 1983). In such patients it is the temporal lobes that are most affected while the frontal lobes are relatively spared (Gustafson *et al.* 1978). However, patients with dementias of the Alzheimer type often show perseverations (e.g. Freeman and Gathercole 1966). This may occur when a task is too difficult and the patient therefore resorts to giving one of the recent successful responses that he or she can still remember (Goldstein 1943).

Conclusions

This brief account of the various difficulties experienced by patients with frontal lobe lesions leads us to speculate that the perseverations shown by these patients are a secondary consequence of an inability spontaneously to generate new responses. In these circumstances the patient will 'default' to some other action that he or she can manage to perform. This may be the action most recently performed (i.e. a perseveration) or it may be the action most readily elicited by the current stimulus even if it is inappropriate in the circumstances (e.g. Luria's inert stereotype, Lhermitte's utilization behaviour).

While there does seem to be some resemblance, at least at the cognitive level, between the problems experienced by patients with frontal lobe lesions and those with Parkinson's disease, there is little resemblance to the picture shown by patients with the Gilles de la Tourette syndrome both with respect to the repetitive movements and the cognitive impairments. This is perhaps not surprising since the treatment for the Gilles de la Tourette syndrome is the opposite of that for Parkinson's disease, i.e. decreasing, rather than increasing the functional effects of dopamine.

Repetitive behaviour in schizophrenia

Spontaneous involuntary movement disorders

Since the syndrome was first described, observers have commented on the peculiar repetitive movements made by chronic schizophrenic patients. Kraepelin (1971) wrote of the 'spasmodic phenomena in the musculature of the face and of speech, which often appear' as being 'extremely peculiar disorders'. Bleuler (1950) wrote of patients 'performing all kinds of manipulations with their teeth . . . (with) grimaces of all kinds, (and) extraordinary movements of the tongue and lips'. There has recently been an upsurge of interest in these peculiar repetitive movements since there is evidence that they may be associated with treatment with dopamine-blocking drugs (e.g. Marsden et al. 1975). As a consequence, such movements occurring in patients with a history of exposure to dopamine blockers are often labelled 'tardive dyskinesia'. Since the vast majority of chronic schizophrenia patients these days will have received long-term treatment with neuroleptics, it is, in practice, difficult to decide whether the movement disorders are a consequence of the treatment or a late effect of the illness itself. However Kraepelin, Bleuler, and others observed such movements in patients long before neuroleptics were discovered (Rogers 1985), so it seems unlikely that drug treatment can be a sufficient explanation.

It is important to distinguish 'tardive dyskinesia' from the acute effects of neuroleptic treatment (Crane 1980). Most people given a large enough dose of a neuroleptic drug will develop parkinsonian side-effects. These will include rigidity, abnormal gait, and dystonias. However, these abnormalities usually resolve when the offending drug is withdrawn or if anticholinergic drugs are given. 'Tardive dyskinesia', in contrast, comes on later in the course of neuroleptic treatment and usually has a completely different form, affecting most commonly the orofacial region. In some people, especially the elderly, this type of abnormality may be irreversible and there is no evidence to support the efficacy of anticholinergics in their management.

The most detailed study of this phenomenon to date is that by Owens et al. (1982). For this study 1227 in-patients in a long-stay psychiatric hospital were surveyed. From these, 510 were identified who met strict criteria for the diagnosis of schizophrenia and, of these, 411 received a detailed neurological examination. In this assessment of involuntary movement disorders, stereotyped and manneristic movements were explicitly excluded on the grounds that these movements were not involuntary in the neurological sense. Fifty per cent of these patients showed involuntary movement disorders of at least moderate severity. The vast majority of these disorders involved movements in the face (85 per cent). The most common signs were choreoathetoid movements of the tongue (21 per cent), chewing (17 per cent, bon-bon (the patient moves his tongue round his cheeks as if he was sucking a sweet, 13 per cent), and puckering of the lips (12 per cent).

According to their records 47 of the patients had never been treated with neuroleptic drugs. This was because of the treatment policy practised in the part of the hospital in which the patients resided, where psychological rather than physical methods of management were emphasized. In terms of prevalence and severity of movement disorders these patients differed little from those who had been treated with neuroleptics. These results suggest that involuntary movement disorders are a late feature of the schizophrenic illness although it may well be that neuroleptic treatment can exaggerate them.

Stereotypies and perseverations

As we noted in the introduction there have been few investigations of stereotyped behaviour in schizophrenia since the intensive studies by Kraepelin and others at the beginning of this century. Kraepelin believed that stereotyped behaviour was a consequence of the weakening of volition that he considered a fundamental feature of schizophrenia. Bleuler and Fromm-Reichman, on the other hand, favoured a Freudian interpretation by which stereotyped behaviour either expressed a complex or was a defence against threatening contact. These early studies are reviewed by Jones (1965). Jones also observed 13 chronic schizophrenic patients for evidence of stereotyped behaviour. All these patients showed at least two items of stereotyped behaviour. In many cases a delusional basis could be found for the behaviour. For example, one patient believed that his ear controlled the pumping of his blood. Unless he repeatedly touched his ear the pumping would cease.

In most cases activity (e.g. work) reduced the amount of stereotyped behaviour. On the other hand, when someone approached and spoke to a patient stereotypies often increased. In these respects chronic schizophrenic patients were similar to retarded and autistic individuals.

Freeman and Gathercole (1966) studied perseveration in chronic schizo-phrenic patients and compared them with patients with organic dementia. Perseveration during performance of various psychological tests was observed frequently in both groups of patients. However, this tended to take the form of compulsive repetitions of responses in the schizophrenic patients, while the demented patients were more likely to show impairment of switching (i.e. giving responses appropriate to the first task when performing the second task). Thus the characteristic perseverative behaviour of the schizophrenic patients had repetitive and thus stereotyped features.

Repetition in speech and writing

As we noted in the introduction, the repetitive speech of lunatics was commented on at least as long ago as 1790. In the last 20 years schizophrenic language has been investigated intensively and this observation has been confirmed. It is implicit in the feature 'poverty of ideas' which Andreasen (1979) has shown to be the most characteristically schizophrenic of the various language abnormalities associated with thought disorder. For a patient to show poverty of ideas, in the absence of poverty of speech, he or she must be using a great many words to communicate very little. Thus at some level speech must be repetitive.

In a number of studies, Manschreck and his colleagues (e.g. Manschreck *et al.* 1984) have counted words and phrases in schizophrenic speech samples. A favourite measure is the 'type–token ratio' which is the number of different words in the sample divided by the total number of words in the sample and is thus a direct measure of repetition at the level of the word. This is reduced in schizophrenic speech. However, whole phrases are also more likely to be repeated. These repetitions might, of course, be quite subtle deficits which would not necessarily be noticed by a casual listener. In the more classic examples of schizophrenic speech the repetitions are deafeningly obvious since the same word or phrase is repeated hundreds of times with little regard to meaning or syntax. However, such cases are rare. The following example was collected by Allen (1983) who asked chronic schizophrenic patients to describe pictures.

While most of the schizophrenic patients in this study showed evidence of poverty of ideas, only this one patient generated such obviously abnormal speech. The picture she was describing showed a man ploughing a field in the background with two women in the foreground looking on. In the example below the repetitive phrases have been picked out in italics revealing that if these are ignored, quite a reasonable description of the picture emerges.

Some—farm houses—in a farm yard—*time*—with a horse and horseman—*time where*—going across the field as if they're ploughing the field—*time*—with ladies—or collecting crop—*time work is*—coming with another lady—*time work is*—*and where*—she's holding a book—*time*—thinking of things—*time work is*—*and time work is where*—you see her coming *time work is* on the field—*and where work is* looking towards other people *and time work is where* the lady—another lady is—looking across to the gentleman—thinking of *time with* him *and where work is*—*where* her *time is where* working *is and time* thinking of people *and where work is and where* you see the hills—going up—*and time work is*—*where* you see the—grass—*time work is*—*time work is and where* the fields are—*where* growing *is* and *where work is.*

The identical phrases concerning time and work appeared in all the descriptions given by this patient and were not distinguished by intonation.

However, she did not insert these phrases into conversation.

Similar abnormal repetition of phrases can also be found in the writings of some schizophrenic patients (e.g. Mayer-Gross *et al.* 1960, plate VI).

As might be expected direct measures of repetitiveness in speech such as the type–token ratio are found to be related to clinical ratings of thought disorder (Manschreck *et al.* 1984). In addition, repetition in speech has been found to relate to movement abnormalities, both spontaneous and elicited behaviour (Manschreck *et al.* 1981). Thus, there seems to be some connection between repetitive speech and repetitive movements.

Elicited stereotyped behaviour

In the long forgotten Zenith radio experiment, thousands of Americans tested their telepathic powers by trying to guess a sequence of random numbers. Goodfellow (1938) analysed these data and showed that the guesses were far from random. Yacorzynski (1941) then used the same technique for studying the responses of schizophrenic patients. He asked patients and normal controls to select binary patterns such as might be generated by chance. Normal people selected non-symmetric patterns containing fewer perseverations and alternations than would be expected by chance, demonstrating the 'gambler's fallacy' discussed on pp. 236–7 of this chapter. Schizophrenic patients in constrast showed the opposite deviation from randomness and selected symmetrical, stereotyped patterns, particularly strings of alternations.

A number of studies since have asked patients to generate random sequences and have obtained similar results. These are reviewed by Horne *et al.* (1982) who also conducted a study of their own. In this study, various psychiatric patients were asked to repeat numbers from 1 to 10 in a random order in time with a metronome. Schizophrenic patients produced less random sequences than depressed, alcoholic, or non-psychotic patients. Unfortunately, only a general index of departure from randomness is given in this report, so we do not know what forms the non-randomness of the schizophrenic patients took. Horne *et al.* also showed that, within the schizophrenic group, departures from randomness were associated with thinking disturbance and withdrawal. Many of the patients were tested more than once, and it was found that the randomness index changed in parallel with symptom severity. Thus, the more severe the symptoms, the less random was the patient's performance.

In all these studies the subject is explicitly asked to generate a random sequence and, thus, his or her concept of randomness must have some influence on the results. Two other studies have elicited stereotyped sequences of response from schizophrenic patients but without specifically involving the concept of randomness.

Armitage *et al.* (1964) presented subjects with a control panel containing eight green lights, each of which could be turned on by pulling one of eight levers. In a single trial the subject had to turn on each of the lights once. The end of the trial (i.e. success) was indicated by an amber light coming on. If a lever was pulled more than once in a trial, then its associated green light failed to come on. The task is thus very similar formally to that used by Schwartz (1982) discussed on pp. 237-8. With the instruction simply to pull the levers in such a way as to turn on the amber light there were no differences between the groups. The information is not given, but one would assume on the basis of Schwartz's data that all the groups produced fairly stereotyped responses. However, when subjects were told that there were many different ways to turn on the amber light and that they should try and use as many different ways as possible, differences between the groups emerged. The control patients were more flexible in their responses (i.e. less stereotyped) than the schizophrenic patients with non-psychotics intermediate. Among the schizophrenic patients the chronic patients were more stereotyped than the acute patients.

We (Frith and Done 1983) have used a two-choice guessing task analogous to Goodnow's gambling task to elicit stereotyped responses from patients. The task is equivalent to guessing the colours of successive playing cards in a shuffled pack. However, the task is presented by a microcomputer which records responses and indicates wins and losses. On each trial the subject presses a button on the left or the right to indicate where he guesses the next stimulus is going to appear. The computer indicates when he is right and displays a cumulative total of correct responses. Although the sequence of stimuli is in fact random, subjects are encouraged to try to find a rule. We found that patients with negative symptoms (poverty of speech, flattening of affect), whether chronic or acute, produced more stereotyped response sequences than normal controls or patients with affective psychoses. The sequences of the schizophrenic patients were characterized by an excess of alternations. Chronic patients with negative symptoms and cognitive impairment (defect state) were the most stereotyped of all producing sequences characterized by perseverations. We also tested a control group of demented patients (Alzheimer type) who had the same degree of cognitive impairment as the defect state schizophrenic patients. The demented patients did not produce stereotyped sequences. Thus the behaviour of the schizophrenic patients cannot solely be due to cognitive impairment.

Schizophrenic patients also show perseverative behaviour on the tasks sensitive to frontal lobe damage that we discussed on pp. 243-5. Malmo (1974) found that schizophrenic patients performed badly on the Wisconsin card-sorting task in that they had difficulty in switching to new categories. This result was confirmed by Kolb and Wishaw (1983) using patients with a

DSM-III diagnosis of schizophrenia. These patients were found to be impaired also on three other tests sensitive to frontal lobe damage. These included verbal and design fluency. On the test of design fluency schizophrenic patients tended to perseverate, producing a series of similar or even identical drawings. Thus, these patients with schizophrenia showed signs of a lack of spontaneity and perseveration similar to that shown by patients with frontal lobe damage.

Summary

Repetitive actions seem to be a consistent feature of schizophrenic behaviour. They appear in the form of spontaneous involuntary movements, stereotyped movements, and repetitive speech. Also, stereotyped behaviour is elicited when the patients are asked to perform problem-solving tasks or to generate random sequences. These different types of repetitive behaviour seem to be linked. Manschrek et al. (1981) found a relationship between repetitive speech and movement disorders and Frith and Done (1983) found a relationship between stereotyped responses in a gambling task and movement disorders. These relationships probably reflect general severity. Thus, a chronic patient with negative symptoms is more likely to show movement disorders, repetitive speech (if any), and stereotyped behaviour in guessing and problem-solving tasks. Horne et al. (1982) believe that their random-number-generating technique is an index of attention, cognitive capacity, or short-term memory, all of which terms may well be synonymous. We think it is unlikely that a rather general defect of this kind could account for this cluster of repetitive behaviours. It is difficult to see why an attention defect would cause involuntary movement disorders (although these may of course be drug-induced). Also, if the stereotyped behaviour were the result of reduction of cognitive capacity, we would expect to see it in demented patients also. We consider that these behaviours are rather specific to schizophrenia. They reflect a difficulty in spon- taneously generating new actions and (perhaps related) a difficulty in inhibiting 'default' actions based on repetition or imitation. These problems are probably a feature of chronic (Crow type II) schizophrenia rather than acute (Crow type I) schizophrenia (Crow 1980). Somehow the dopamine system seems to have a role in these behaviours. Long-term treatment with dopamine-blocking drugs may exaggerate, if not actually cause, involuntary movement disorders. On the other hand short-term treatment with these drugs ameliorates positive symptoms including thought disorder (Johnstone et al. 1978) and hence probably reduces repetition in speech. Thus, although the picture is at the moment confused and contradictory, the dopamine system is clearly implicated in the repetitive behaviours shown by schizophrenic patients.

General summary, a digression on repetition in art and life, and some pretentious conclusions

> History repeats herself, the first time as tragedy, the second time as farce.
>
>   K. Marx

It is clear from our discussion above that all kinds of people engage in repetitive, pointless behaviour. However, we wish to distinguish between normal and abnormal behaviour of this type.

Normal people will make pointless, repetitive movements, most likely when they are anxious or bored, particularly if they believe they are unseen or are unaware that they are making the movements. Once they are aware that the movements are observed, they are likely to stop since there seem to be strong social pressures against making such movements. Mentally retarded people also make such movements, but are little affected by social pressures. This especially applies to autistic people.

Why are these movements made? There is very little theorizing on this point. The most popular account depends on the notion of an optimum level of arousal or stimulation. If stimulation is lacking (or arousal is too low), the repetitive movements can supply an alternative source of stimulation and increase arousal towards an optimum level. This theory attempts to explain why repetitive movements are more common in children who are blind and/or deaf (resulting in reduced stimulation from external sources) or in children who are severely retarded (lacking the cognitive capacity for appreciating external stimulation). It also explains why a restricted environment (the cage or the institution) will elicit stereotypies.

However, there is also exactly the opposite theory which suggests that repetitive movements are made to reduce anxiety (or arousal). How this might work is not clear. We might speculate that engaging in repetitive movements uses up spare attentional capacity. This might prevent this capacity from being used to attend to distracting and irrelevant external events (thus aiding concentration) or it might prevent that capacity from being used to indulge in unwanted and distracting thoughts and apprehensions (thus combatting anxiety).

These speculations provide a framework for specifying normal circumstances in which spontaneous repetitive movements may appear, although they give no indication of what form the movements should take. On this basis we would classify the repetitive behaviour of most mentally retarded people as a normal response to their circumstances.

On the other hand, the spontaneous repetitive movements made by schizophrenic patients would be classified as abnormal because they do not respond to circumstances. In particular the patient will go on making the movements even when he or she is observed and is apparently unable to control them. It might be argued that, in their restriction to tongue, lips, and jaw, the movements made by schizophrenic patients have a different form to those made by normal and mentally retarded individuals. This proposition, we feel, has yet to be demonstrated since there are no systematically collected data on normal repetitive movements. The casual observer on the train will certainly see many peculiar facial movements. It is also interesting to note that the pointless repetitive movements engaged in when smoking or when sucking and chewing sweets (US candy) or gum are very similar to many of the components of 'tardive dyskinesia'.

Perhaps smoking and gum-chewing are commonly indulged in because they are socially acceptable behaviours which permit the participant to indulge in these particular orofacial movements. Nevertheless, even if the movements associated with 'tardive dyskinesia' can be found in normal people, they clearly form a rather small subset of possible repetitive movements. As yet, we have no explanation as to why this subset of movements rather than another is such a dominant feature of chronic schizophrenia and/or long-term treatment with neuroleptics. Of course, schizophrenic patients make many other repetitive movements as well. It may be that most of these are labelled stereotyped since they are considered to be voluntary and therefore carefully distinguished from the involuntary movements associated with 'tardive dyskinesia'. Unfortunately, these movements have not yet been systematically studied and it is not clear whether the voluntary/involuntary distinction is important in relation to schizophrenia.

The same general account can be applied to the repetitive behaviour of autistic children. Most of the movements they make (rocking, pacing, vocalizing, finger or object manipulation) can probably also be observed in normal individuals. However, autistic individuals tend to make the movements regardless of circumstances and, in particular, do not inhibit them in the presence of others. However orofacial movements do not seem to feature in their repertoire to any great extent.

People who make spontaneous repetitive movements are also likely to produce stereotyped movement sequences when performing certain tasks. As with the spontaneous movements, repetitive actions can also be elicited from normal people in certain circumstances. Once they have learned that a certain action is successful then they will repeat that response. However, if they are told to try and find a rule which determines which responses are successful, or if they are explicitly told to try and produce as wide a variety of responses as possible, then their behaviour will cease to be repetitive. Chronic schizophrenic patients, patients with frontal lobe lesions, and autistic children all have difficulty in producing such variety in their responding. They produce repetitive or perseverative behaviour in most circumstances. This seems in part to be due to a difficulty in producing novel responses spontaneously. This forces the individual to default to a normal underlying tendency to repetition.

The causes of these problems are largely unknown, but some abnormality of the dopamine system and/or the frontal cortex seems likely. The dopamine system is implicated directly or indirectly in Parkinson's disease, schizophrenia, and the Gilles de la Tourette syndrome. Perseveration behaviour is also observed in patients with frontal lobe lesions. Abnormalities in the frontal cortex have also been claimed although not definitely confirmed for schizophrenic patients on the basis of CAT and position emission tomography (PET) scans (Tanaka *et al*. 1981; Franzen and Ingram 1975). The subcortical dopamine system and the frontal cortex are of course linked in that this part of the cortex is innervated by the dopamine system (e.g. Rosvold 1972; Slopsema *et al*. 1982). Work on both these systems in animals is discussed elsewhere in this book.

One of our major themes so far has been that repetitive behaviour is normal under certain circumstances. Nevertheless, the implication has been that this is a rather primitive behaviour which is overridden by higher cognitive functions. This characterization of repetitive behaviour is clearly unjustified. Repetition is fundamental in all art forms and is an important feature of intelligent life. Repetition is obviously at the basis of dance, singing, and music, as seen particularly clearly in whirling, chanting, and drumming. However, subtle forms of repetition remain fundamental to sophisticated art forms. In music, for example, we find fugues and inversions. In the visual arts and architecture also, repetition with or without transformation is fundamental. This is particularly obvious in the art of ornament where we see repetition sometimes modified by reflection and rotation (Christie 1969; Frith 1978). Narrative arts too are repetitive (Kawin 1972) with very few plots repeatedly appearing. Some (e.g. Borges 1964) go so far as to speculate that there is only one book which every author rewrites. This, of course, is a metaphor for life. Each of us is born only to struggle through the same set of problems and then to die.

Not just in art, but wherever people impose their will upon nature, they do so by repetition, as in the vineyard or the suburban housing estate. The consequence of this is that repetition is perceived as a hallmark of intelligent behaviour. This is illustrated by the fact that, when the first pulsar was discovered, astronomers seriously considered for a time that these precisely repeating signals might emanate from an alien intelligence.

However, at the same time as repetition there is novelty. This arises both in the precise form that the repetition takes and also in what it is that is repeated. It is precisely a lack of novelty and spontaneity that distinguishes abnormal from normal repetition. It is this lack of novelty that results in the more pejorative label, perseveration.

Thus in artful repetition the response is determined neither entirely by past responses nor by current circumstances. Artful repetition includes a spontaneous and novel component that is independent of both these influences. Abnormal stereotyped behaviour, in contrast, is entirely determined by past response and/or current circumstances.

We would suggest that the frontal cortex and the dopamine system are particularly likely to be involved in the production of novel and spontaneous actions. There is much evidence that the control of movement, particularly the initiation of movement depends upon the intactness of the dopamine system within the basal ganglia (e.g. Marsden 1982; Denny-Brown and Yanagisawa 1976). The frontal cortex is believed to be concerned with planning (e.g. Luria 1973). The essence of a planned action is that it is determined by a spontaneous act of will. It anticipates rather than being caused by the future circumstances in which it will occur. Equally, planned actions are not mere repetitions of past actions. By planning we assert our will and are not the mere slaves of nature. By the conjunction of the frontal cortex and the dopamine system we are able to convert plans into actions. Thus, interferences with either or both of these systems will lead to a lack of novelty and spontaneity in action and hence to stereotyped behaviour.

Since this chapter was prepared, Nancy Lyon and her colleagues have published two papers on stereotyped responding in schizophrenic patients (Lyon *et al.* 1986; Lyon and Gerlach 1988). These results confirm that stereotyped responding can frequently be elicited in schizophrenic patients. In addition a detailed analysis of this behaviour relates it to the Lyon–Robbins theory of amphetamine-induced stereotypy (see Chapter 2, this volume).

References

Allen, H.A. (1983). Do positive and negative symptom subtypes of schizophrenia show qualitative differences in language production? *Psychol. Med.* **13**, 787–97.

Andreasen, N. (1979). Thought, language and communication disorders. *Arch. gen. Psychiat.* **36**, 1315–30.

Armitage, S.G., Brown, C.R., and Denny, M.R. (1964). Stereotypy of response in schizophrenics. *J. Clin. Psychol.* **20**, 225–30.

Asendorpf, J. (1980). Nichtreaktive Stressmessung: Bewegungs-stereotypien als Aktivierungsindikatoren. *Z. exp. angew. Psychol.* **27**, 44–58.

Attneave, F. (1959). *Applications of information theory to psychology.* Holt-Dryden, New York.

Berkson, G. and Davenport, R.K. (1962). Stereotyped movements in mental defectives: 1. Initial survey. *Am. J. ment. Deficiency* **66**, 849–52.

Bleuler, E. (1950). *Dementia Praecox or the group of schizophrenias.* (Translated by J. Zinkin.) International Universities Press, New York, (Originally published, 1911.)

Borges, J. L. (1964). The flower of Coleridge. In *Other inquisitions*. University of Texas Press, Austin, Texas,

Bowen, F. P., Kamienny, R. S., Burns, M. M., and Yahr, MD. (1975). Parkinsonism: effects of levodopa treatment on concept formation. *Neurology* **25**, 701–4.

Christie, A. H. (1969). *Pattern design*. Dover, New York.

Crane, G. E. (1980). A classification of the neurological effects of neuroleptic drugs. In *Tardive dyskinesia* (ed. W. E. Fann, R. C. Smith, J. M Davis, and E. F. Domino) pp. 187–91. Spectrum, New York.

Crow, T. J. (1980). Molecular pathology of schizophrenia: more than one disease process? *Br. med. J.* **280**, 66–8.

Denny-Brown, D. and Yanagisawa, N. (1976). The role of the basal ganglia in the initiation of movement. In *The basal ganglia* (ed. M. D. Yahr) pp. 115–49. Raven Press, New York.

Ferrier, J. (1795). *Medical histories and reflections*. Cadell and Davies, London.

Flowers, K. A. (1982). Frontal lobe signs as a component of Parkinsonism. *Behav. Brain Res.* **5**, 100–1.

Flowers, K. A. and Robertson, C. (1985). The effect of Parkinson's disease on the ability to maintain a mental set. *J. Neurol. Neurosurg. Psychiat.* **48**, 517–29.

Forehand, R. and Baumeister, A. A. (1971). Stereotyped body rocking as a function of situation, I Q and time. *J. Clin. Psychol.* **27**, 324–6.

Franzen, G. and Ingvar, D. H. (1975). Absence of activation in frontal structures during psychological testing in chronic schizophrenia. *J. Neurol. Neurosurg. Psychiat.* **30**, 1027–32.

Freeman, T. and Gathercole, C. E. (1966). Perseveration—the clinical symptoms—in chronic schizophrenia and organic dementia. *Br. J. Psychiat.* **112**, 27–32.

Frith, C. D. (1978). The subjective properties of complex visual patterns. In *Formal theories of visual perception* (eds. E. Leeuwenberg and H. Buffart) pp. 231–46. Wiley, Chichester.

Frith, C. D. and Done, D. J. (1983). Stereotyped responding by schizophrenic patients on a two-choice guessing task. *Psychol. Med.* **13**, 779–86.

Frith, U (1970). Studies in pattern detection in normal and autistic children. ii. Reproduction and production of color sequences. *J. exp. Child Psychol.* **10**, 120–35.

Frith, U. (1972). Cognitive mechanisms in childhood autism. Experiments with colour and tone sequence production. *J. Autism childh. Schizophrenia* **2**, 160–73.

Gerjuoy, I R. and Winters, J. O. (1968). Development of lateral and choice sequence preferences. In *International review of research in mental retardation*, Vol. 3 (ed. N. R. Ellis) pp. 31–63. Academic Press, London.

Gilles de la Tourette, G. (1885), Étude sur une affection nerveuse characterisée par de l'incoordination motrice accompagnée d'echolalie et coprolalie. *Arch. Neurol., Paris* **9**, 19–42, 158–200.

Gilroy, J. and Meyer, J. S (1979). *Medical neurology*, 3rd ed. Macmillan, New York.

Goldstein, K. (1943). Concerning rigidity. *Character Personality* **11**, 209–26.

Goodfellow, L. D. (1938). A psychological interpretation of the results of the Zenith Radio experiments in telepathy. *J. exp. Psychol.* **23**, 601–32.

Goodnow, J. J. (1955). Determinants of choice-distribution in two-choice situations. *Am. J.* Psychol. **68**, 106–16.

Grew, N. (1701). *Cosmologia Sacra: or a discourse of the Universe as it is the creature and kingdom of God.* Rogers *et al.*, London.

Guess, D. (1966). The influence of visual and ambulatory restrictions on stereotyped behaviour. *Am. J. ment. Deficiency* **70**, 542–7.

Gustafson, L., Hagberg, B., and Ingvar, D. H (1978). Speech disturbances in presenile dementia related to local cerebral blood flow abnormalities in the dominant hemisphere. *Brain Language* **5**, 103–18.

Henderson, D. K. and Gillespie, K. D. (1927). *Textbook of psychiatry.* Oxford University Press, Oxford.

Hermelin, B. and O'Connor, N. (1963). The response and self-generated behaviour of severely disturbed children and severely subnormal controls. *Br. J. social Clin. Psychol.* **2**, 37–43.

Horne, R. L., Evans, F. J., and Orne, M. T. (1982). Random number generation. Psychopathology, and therapeutic change. *Arch. gen. Psychiat.* **39** 680–3.

Hudson, A. J. (1968). Perseveration. *Brain* **91**, 571–82.

Hutt, C. and Hutt, S. J. (1965). Effects of environmental complexity on stereotyped behaviour of children. *Animal Behav.* **13**, 1–4.

Hutt, C. and Hutt, S. J. (1970). Stereotypies and their relation to arousal. In *Behavioural studies in psychiatry* (ed. S. J. Hutt and C. Hutt) pp. 175–204. Pergamon Press, Oxford.

Jones-Gotman, M. and Milner, B. (1977). Design fluency. *Neuropsychologia* **15**, 653–74.

Johnstone, E. C., Crow, T. J., Frith, C. D., Carney, M. W. P., and Price, J. S. (1978). Mechanisms of the antipsychotic effect in the treatment of acute schizophrenia. *Lancet* **i**, 848–57.

Jones, I. H. (1965). Observations on schizophrenic stereotypies. *Comprehens. Psychiat* **6**, 323–35.

Kawin, B. F. (1972). *Telling it again and again.* Cornell University Press, Ithaca, New York.

Kläsi, J. (1922). *Über die Bedeutung und Entstehung der Stereotypien.* Karger, Berlin.

Kolb, B. and Wishaw, I. Q. (1983). Performance of schizophrenic patients on tests sensitive to left or right frontal, temporal or parietal function in neurological patients. *J. nerv. ment. Dis.* **171**, 435–43.

Kraepelin, E. (1899). *Psychiatrie*, 6th ed. Barth, Leipzig.

Kraepelin, E. (1971). *Dementia praecox and paraphrenia.* (Translated by R. M. Barclay and G. M. Robertson.) Krieger, New York.

LaGrow, S. J. and Repp, A. C. (1984). Stereotypic responding: a review of intervention research. *Am. J. men. Deficiency* **88**, 595–609.

Lees, A. J. and Smith, E. (1983). Cognitive deficits in the early stages of Parkinson's disease. *Brain* **106**, 257–70.

Lhermitte, F. (1983). 'Utilization behaviour' and its relation to lesions of the frontal lobes. *Brain* **106**, 237–55.

Liepmann, H. (1905). *Ueber Stoerungen das Handelns bei Gehirnkranken.* Karger, Berlin.

Lopez, L L. (1982). Doing the impossible: a note on induction and the experience of randomness. *J. exp. Psychol: Learning, Memory Cognition* **8**, 626 36.

Lyon, N., Mejsholm, B., and Lyon, M. (1986). Stereotyped responding by schizophrenic outpatients: cross-cultural confirmation of perseverative switching on a two-choice guessing task. *J. Psychiat. Res.* **20**, 137–50.

Lyon, N. and Gerlach, J. (1988). Perseverative structuring of responses by schizophrenic and affective disorder patients. *J. Psychiat. Res.* **22**, 261–77.

Luria, A. R. (1973). *The working brain*. Basic Books, New York.

Malmo, H. P. (1974). On frontal lobe functions: psychiatric patient controls. *Cortex* **10**, 231–7.

Manschreck, T. C., Maher, B., and Adler, D. N. (1981). Formal thought disorder, the type–token ratio, and disturbed voluntary motor movement in schizophrenia. *Br. J. Psychiat.* **139**, 7–15.

Manschrek, T. C. Maher, B., Hoover, T., and Ames, D. (1984). The type–token ratio in schizophrenic disorders: clinical and research utility. *Psychol. Med.* **14**, 151–7.

Marsden, C. D. (1982). The mysterious motor function of the basal ganglia. *Neurology, N Y* **32**, 514–39.

Marsden, C. D., Tarsy, D., and Baldesarini, R. J. (1975). Spontaneous and drug-induced movement disorders in psychiatric patients. In *Psychiatric aspects of neurological disease* (ed. D. F. Benson and D. Blumer). Grune and Stratton, New York.

Mayer-Gross, W., Slater, E., and Roth, M. (1960). *Clinical psychiatry*. Cassell, London.

Morel-Maroger, A. (1978). Effects positifs de la L-DOPA sur une symptomatologie "marginale" observée chez les parkinsoniens. *L'Encephale* **4**, 223–31.

Owens, D. G. C., Johnstone, E. C., and Frith, C. D. (1982). Spontaneous involuntary disorders of movements. *Arch. gen. Psychiat.* **39**, 452–61.

Ridley, R. M. and Baker, H. F. (1982). Stereotypy in monkeys and humans. *Psychol. Med.* **12**, 61–72.

Rogers, D. (1985). The motor disorders of severe psychiatric illness: a conflict of paradigms. *Br. J. Psychiat.* **147**, 221–32.

Rosvold, H. C. (1972). The frontal lobe system: cortical–subcortical interrelationship. *Acta neurobiol. exp.* **32**, 125–40.

Schwartz, B. (1982). Reinforcement-induced behavioural stereotypy: how not to teach people to discover rules. *J. Exp. Psychol. General* **111**, 23–59.

Shapiro, E., Shapiro, A. K., and Clarkin, J. (1974). Clinical psychological testing in Tourette's syndrome. *J. Personality Assess.* **38**, 464–78.

Slak, S. and Hirsch, K. A. (1974). Human ability to randomise sequences as a function of information per item. *Bull. psychonom. Soc.* **4**, 29–30.

Slak, S., Shaffer, J. I., and Barone, N. C. (1982). Sequence redundancy under conditions of randomization and spontaneous activity. *Bull. psychonom. Soc.* **19**, 256–8.

Slopsema, J. S., van der Gugten, J., and de Bruin, J. P. C. (1982). Regional concentrations of noradrenaline and dopamine in the frontal cortex of the rat. *Brain Res.* **250**, 197–200.

Slovic, P., Kunreuther, H., and White, G. F. (1974). Decision processes, rationality, and judgement of natural hazards. In *Natural hazards, local, national and global* (ed. G. F. White) pp. 187–205. Oxford University Press, Oxford.

Sutherland, R. J., Kolb, B., Schoel, W.M., Wishaw, I. Q., and Davies, D. (1982). Neuropsychological assessment of children and adults with Tourette's syndrome: a comparison with learning disabilities and schizophrenia. In *Gilles de la Tourette syndrome*. (ed. A. J. Friedhoff and T. N. Chase) pp. 311–22. Raven Press, New York.

Sweet, R. D., Solomon, G., Wayne, H., Shapiro, E., and Shapiro, A. K. (1973). Neurological features of Gilles de la Tourette's syndrome. *J. Neurol. Neurosurg. Psychiat.* **36**, 1–9.

Tanaka, Y., Hazmar, H., Kawahara, R., and Kobayashi, K. (1981). Computerized tomography of the brain in schizophrenic patients. *Acta psychiat. scand.* **63**, 191–7.

Thelen, E. (1979). Rhythmical stereotypies in normal human infants. *Animal Behav.* **27**, 699–715.

Teuber, H-L. (1964). The riddle of frontal lobe function in man. In *The frontal granular cortex and behaviour* (ed. J. M. Warren and K. Akert) pp. 410–77. McGraw-Hill, New York.

Wiegersma, S. (1982). A control theory of sequential response production. *Psychol. Res.* **44**, 175–88.

Wing, J. K. and Wing, L. (1982). *Handbook of psychiatry*, Vol. 3. *Psychoses of uncertain aetiology*. Cambridge University Press, Cambridge.

Yacorzynski, G. K. (1941). Perceptual principles involved in the disintegration of a configuration formed in predicting the occurrence of patterns selected by chance. *J. exp. Psychol.* **28**, 401–6.

Yamadori, A. (1981). Verbal perseveration in aphasia. *Neuropsychologia* **19**, 591–4.

Young, R. and Clements, J. (1979). The functional significance of complex hand movement stereotypies in the severely retarded. *Br. J. ment. Subnormality* **25**, 79–87.

10

Stereotyped motor phenomena in neurological disease

A.J. STOESSL

Introduction

Stereotyped behaviour can be regarded as that which is repetitive, purposeless, and involuntary, often interfering with normal behaviour. Such behaviour is generally a consequence of disruption of the normal chemical milieu of the central nervous system and, in humans, stereotypy is usually seen as an unwanted side-effect of medications or, in the context of primary disease of the nervous system, as one of the so-called movement disorders. The taxonomy of the movement disorders is controversial and often confusing even to those well versed in neurology. One approach is to divide the disorders into those in which motor activity is either increased (hyperkinetic) or decreased (hypokinetic) or those predominantly affecting tone (i.e. the resistance to passive movement). Even this classification has its difficulties, since Parkinson's disease, for example, one of the commonest movement disorders, is characterized simultaneously by too little motor activity (bradykinesia), excessive movement (tremor), and increased muscular tone or rigidity. For the purposes of this chapter, we will first deal with primary hyperkinetic disorders, and then discuss drug-induced involuntary movements. The hyperkinetic disorders can be subclassified into tremor, chorea, tic, myoclonus, and dystonia.

Tremor

This refers to a fairly rhythmical oscillation of one or many body parts. Thus, tremor can be seen to be one type of stereotyped behaviour since it is repetitive, predictable, and rhythmic. Tremor can be present at rest, or activated by voluntary movement or by maintaining a posture against gravity.

Parkinson's disease

The most important cause of resting tremor is Parkinson's disease (PD) (Parkinson 1817). In addition to the tremor, the other cardinal features of the disorder are bradykinesia, rigidity, and postural instability. The tremor is slow (about 2–5 Hz), often attenuated by voluntary movement, and exacerbated by stress. As is often the case with movement disorders, the tremor disappears during sleep. Although a frequent source of embarrassment, the tremor is not the major cause of disability in PD, which derives rather from early impairment of fine hand co-ordination and progressive bradykinesia, leading eventually to severe immobility with loss of postural control. Thus, the patient with advanced PD stands with a fixed posture, rooted to the ground, and when motion does commence, characteristically chases his/her centre of gravity (festination). Falls are a frequent problem, especially when obstacles arise, or a change in direction is required. It has been suggested (Marsden 1982) that the basal ganglia are required for the 'motor plan', co-ordinating the execution of the component 'motor programmes'. It is the disruption of this motor plan which leads to the parkinsonian patient's curious inability to perform two motor acts simultaneously, even though the individual components may be performed without difficulty (Benecke *et al.* 1986; Schwab *et al.* 1954). Although the disabling motor features are consistent components of PD, they are not regarded as stereotyped behaviours. It is the PD tremor which is a stereotyped behaviour.

The pathological hallmark of PD is degeneration of the pigmented cells of the substantia nigra, associated with gliosis and the formation of characteristic hyaline, eosinophilic cytoplasmic inclusions (Lewy bodies) (Forno 1982). Other pigmented brainstem nuclei, notably the locus ceruleus, may be affected. The dementia of PD, which occurs in 15–20 per cent of cases (Brown and Marsden 1984) may additionally be associated with Alzheimer-type pathology, including neuritic plaques and neurofibrillary tangles (Alvord *et al.* 1975; Boller *et al.* 1980; Hakim and Mathieson 1979), as well as cell loss in the nucleus basalis of Meynert (Whitehouse *et al.* 1983).

The major biochemical abnormality of PD is dopamine deficiency, consequent upon the loss of the dopamine-producing cells of the substantia nigra (Ehringer and Hornykiewicz 1960). Since other monoamine-producing cells may be affected, deficits in noradrenalin and serotonin are also seen (Hornykiewicz 1966). Levels of a variety of peptides are depressed, including substance P (Mauborgne *et al.* 1983), cholecystokinin (Studler *et al.* 1982), the enkephalins (Taquet *et al.* 1983), neurotensin and bombesin (Bissette *et al.* 1985.) In demented parkinsonians, there is additional depression of cortical choline acetyltransfcrase (Perry *et al*. 1985) and somatostatin (Epelbaum *et al*. 1983).

The aetiology of PD is as yet undetermined. While some cases may be familial (Barbeau *et al*. 1984), this appears to be the exception rather than the rule. A recent twin study (Ward *et al*. 1983) found a very low concordance rate among the identical twins of affected probands. The high incidence of parkinsonism among the survivors of the epidemic of encephalitis lethargica led to an intensive search for a viral aetiology, but no consistent evidence of viral or immunological damage to the nervous system has been demonstrated (Elizan and Casals 1983). Many toxins, including carbon monoxide, carbon disulphide, and manganese, may result in widespread central nervous system dysfunction, of which an impure form of parkinsonism may be one manifestation. The recent demonstration of a pure form of parkinsonism in humans (Langston *et al*. 1983) and primates (Burns *et al*. 1983) exposed to the selective nigral toxin N-methyl-4-phenyl-1, 2, 3, 6-tetrahydropyridine (MPTP) has substantially narrowed the gap in the search for a plausible environmental factor in the genesis of PD. It has been suggested (Calne and Langston 1983) that PD may result from the superimposition of an environmental insult (such as MPTP or some other related compound) on the loss of dopaminergic nigral cells that is known to occur as a feature of normal ageing (McGeer *et al*. 1977).

In the late-1800s, Ordenstein, a pupil of Charcot, was treating parkinsonism with belladonna alkaloids. Since dopamine inhibits striatal cholinergic neurons, it has been postulated (McGeer *et al*. 1961) that the dopamine deficiency of PD leads to an imbalance characterized by a relative preponderance of cholinergic activity. Duvoisin (1967) provided elegant support for this hypothesis by demonstrating exacerbation of parkinsonian manifestations following physostigmine, but amelioration with anticholinergics. Although anticholinergics may help to restore the normal dopaminergic-cholinergic balance in the striatum, at least some of their beneficial effects seem to arise from inhibition of dopamine re-uptake (Coyle and Snyder 1969). Interestingly, it may be that the stereotyped element of PD, namely tremor, is most sensitive to anticholinergic treatment, whereas the non-stereotyped behaviours in PD are more sensitive to dopaminergic treatment (see below).

Most of the symptoms and signs of PD respond well to treatment with levodopa (L-dopa), which (unlike dopamine) crosses the blood–brain barrier, and is then converted to dopamine (Birkmayer and Hornykiewicz 1961; Cotzias *et al*. 1969). Peripheral side-effects, which include nausea, vomiting, postural hypotension, and cardiac arrhythmias, can largely be attenuated by the combination of lower doses of L-dopa with an extracerebral inhibitor of aromatic amino acid decarboxylase, such as carbidopa (Chase and Watanabe 1972; Rao and Calne 1973). Central nervous system side-effects of L-dopa include psychosis, loss of therapeutic efficacy, and fluctuations in disability (Marsden and Parkes 1976; see also the section on 'Levodopa', this chapter).

Loss of efficacy, fluctuations, and dyskinesias may respond in part to the addition of a dopaminomimetic, such as bromocriptine (Calne *et al.* 1974; Rascol *et al.* 1979). The advantages of dopaminomimetics may stem in part from bypassing the requirement for decarboxylation of exogenous L-dopa, and perhaps also from relatively selective actions upon the D-2 receptor.

Essential tremor

This is the other common form of tremor in neurological practice, and as suggested by the name, is of unknown aetiology. Essential tremor affects the upper limbs in the majority of cases, but other body parts, especially the head/neck and voice may be involved. Although it may occasionally be present at rest, it is more typically postural and/or action-induced (Larsen and Calne 1984).

Marsden and co-workers (1983) have classified essential tremor as a heterogeneous group of disorders consisting of four subtypes. Type I tremor is rapid (~ 10–12 Hz) and fine, and is also known as exaggerated physiological tremor. This type of tremor may be provoked by stress or stimulant medications (e.g. caffeine) in normal individuals, and is also seen as a feature of a variety of metabolic disturbances, most notably thyrotoxicosis. Type II or 'benign' essential tremor is of intermediate frequency (5–8 Hz) and amplitude. This disorder is often inherited in an autosomal dominant fashion, and may respond dramatically to alcohol and/or β-blockers. Type III or 'pathological' essential tremor is similar to Type II, but the frequency tends to be lower (2–5 Hz), the amplitude greater, and a response to alcohol and β-blockers is much less likely. Type IV tremor is that associated with other neurological diseases such as parkinsonism, dystonia, or various forms of peripheral neuropathy.

By definition, the cause of essential tremor is unknown, and there is indeed considerable controversy as to whether the underlying disturbance is in the peripheral or central nervous system. The demonstration (Young *et al.* 1975) that intra-arterial injection of the β-adrenergic antagonist propranolol fails to affect essential tremor, whereas chronic oral administration is effective, suggests a central disorder. Exact mechanisms are still poorly understood. Selective β_1-antagonists, such as atenolol or metoprolol, are slightly less effective in ameliorating tremor than the non-selective agent propranolol (Jefferson *et al.* 1979; Larsen and Teravainen 1983). However, a β_2-antagonist was relatively more ineffective than propranolol until non-selective doses were achieved (Burton *et al.* 1985). Another feature of unclear pathogenetic significance is the therapeutic benefit of non-sedative doses of drugs such as alcohol (Critchley 1949) and primidone (O'Brien *et al.* 1981).

Other action tremors

Action tremor is characterized by the onset of rhythmic, oscillating movements during wilful actions, but not at rest. While this may occur (in association with postural tremor) as a manifestation of essential tremor, it may also be a sign of central nervous system disease, particularly of the cerebellum or its connections. Tremor may then be associated with nystagmus, scanning dysarthria, and ataxia. A variety of structural, metabolic, inflammatory, and degenerative disorders beyond the scope of this review may disrupt the cerebellar circuitry.

Chorea

Chorea describes rapid, uncoordinated jerking movements of single muscles, which are generally random and flowing. Although certain choreatic disorders (notably tardive dyskinesia—see pp. 275–8 are characterized by relatively stereotypic movements, this is not generally the case for chorea caused by primary central nervous system disease, which tends to be a collection of many adventitious movements rather than a stereotyped repetition of a few selected movements.

Huntington's disease

This is the most important of the primary choreatic disorders, and is characterized by autosomal dominant inheritance with complete penetrance and dementia in addition to the movement disorder. Pathologically, the major finding is degeneration of the small and medium-sized neurons of the striatum, but cerebral cortex may also be affected (Bruyn *et al.* 1979; Forno and Jose 1973). There are depletions of striatal acetylcholine and gamma aminobutyric acid (GABA) and of the enzymes required for their synthesis, as well as substance P, angiotensin-converting enzyme, and dynorphin (Arregui *et al.* 1977; Bird and Iversen 1974; Kanazawa *et al.* 1979; Perry *et al.* 1973; Seizinger *et al.* 1986; Spokes 1980). Striatal somatostatin is increased (Aronin *et al.* 1983) and dopamine is normal or increased (Bird and Iversen 1974; Spokes 1980). Thus Huntington's disease can be regarded as the functional inverse of parkinsonism, in that it is characterized by a relative excess of dopamine compared to acetylcholine. Cholinergic agents such as physostigmine transiently ameliorate chorea, while anticholinergics exacerbate the movements (Klawans and Rubovits 1972). Direct or indirect GABA-ergic agents have not resulted in sustained benefit (Perry *et al.* 1982; Shoulson *et al.* 1975, 1976).

While the end-stages of HD may be associated with non-specific rigidity, some patients, typically those with juvenile onset, experience the parkinson-like symptoms of bradykinesia and rigidity as the major manifestations of the disorder, and chorea may be minimal or absent. In such patients, symptoms may respond to L-dopa (Barbeau 1969; Schenk and Leijnse-Ybema 1974). Recent evidence from positron emission tomography (PET) using the L-dopa analogue 6-fluorodopa (6-FD) suggests that dopamine synthesis is impaired in patients with rigid HD, as opposed to those with chorea, in whom 6-FD uptake was normal (Stoessl *et al.* 1986 *b*).

Since the symptoms of Huntington's disease do not usually appear until the end of the third decade or the fourth decade of life, most patients have already had their families before realizing that they are affected. Thus, the ability to predict the subsequent development of the disease would have major implications for its eventual eradication, and the prevention of untold suffering. In this regard, two unrelated techniques may prove valuable. It is now known that the gene for Huntington's disease is located on the short arm of the fourth chromosome and is closely linked to the G8 marker (Gusella *et al.* 1983). Thus, in some families of appropriate structure, in whom enough members are available for testing, it may be possible to predict with 95 per cent certainty which individuals are presymptomatic heterozygotes for the Huntington gene. Positron emission tomography (PET) studies have revealed caudate glucose hypometabolism in Huntington's disease (Kuhl *et al.* 1982) and this is evident even in subjects without radiological evidence of atrophy (Hayden *et al.* 1986). When subjects at risk for Huntington's disease on the basis of a positive family history undergo both DNA analysis and PET scanning, those individuals whose DNA patterns suggest a high likelihood that they will develop the disease also show either absolute or relative caudate glucose hypometabolism (Hayden *et al.* 1987).

Other choreatic disorders

Chorea may occur in a variety of other primary disorders of the nervous system, including benign hereditary chorea, Wilson's disease, and hereditary dentatorubralpallidoluysian atrophy. Chorea may also be seen in association with tics and/or parkinsonism, as part of a systemic disorder characterized by peripheral blood acanthocytosis (Kito *et al.* 1980; Spitz *et al.* 1985). Immunological damage to the striatum, occurring after rheumatic fever or as a consequence of systemic lupus erythematosus, may also result in chorea. Finally, a variety of hormonal alterations, including pregnancy, use of oestrogen-containing preparations, and thyrotoxicosis, may be complicated by a choreiform disorder. All of these forms of chorea have consistent hyperkinetic movements but, due to their great variety, are not usually classified as stereotyped behaviours.

Tic

The term tic usually refers to 'motor tics' which are brief, rapid movements that are often stereotyped in appearance. Although the particular movements may vary both within and between patients, facial blinking and grimacing are common manifestations, as are shoulder shrugging and other proximal muscle contractions (Jankovic and Fahn 1986; Sweet *et al*. 1973). Another type of tic is a 'vocal tic' which is a stereotyped involuntary vocalization. Involuntary vocalizations are seen as part of the classical picture of the Gilles de la Tourette syndrome, which is a childhood disorder of both motor and vocal tics. Vocal tics in the Gilles de la Tourette syndrome can range from simple throat clearing, sniffing, barking, and grunting to the more colourful utterance of obscenities (coprolalia) that is classically associated with this syndrome.

The Gilles de la Tourette syndrome can also be associated with a large number of much more complex stereotypies (e.g. squatting, skipping, facial wiping), as well as echolalia (repetition of words or phrases), echopraxia (mimicking of gestures), and copropraxia (obscene gestures). As such, the Gilles de la Tourette syndrome may be one of the neurological disorders richest in varieties of stereotyped behaviours. Some of the most important clinical features which characterize tics and behavioural stereotypies in this syndrome are (1) the sensation of an irresistible urge to allow the movements to be expressed, and (2) the ability voluntarily though temporarily, to suppress the movements. Such voluntary suppression is generally followed by mounting tension and rebound exaggeration.

Tic disorders usually have their onset in childhood, but considerable variation occurs. Such disorders include transient tic of childhood, chronic simple tic, and the Gilles de la Tourette syndrome. The course of tic disorders is typically characterized by waxing and waning severity, often with periods of spontaneous remission. These features make short-term therapeutic trials difficult to evaluate. A family history is often present (Eldridge *et al*. 1977; Pauls and Leckman 1986), as may be a history of birth trauma (Sweet *et al*. 1973).

Although there has been much controversy over the years as to whether tics are 'organic' or 'psychogenic' in origin, few people would argue in favour of the latter point of view today. Sweet and co-workers (1973) found a high incidence of left-handedness and of 'soft' neurological signs and asymmetrics in patients with the Gilles de la Tourette syndrome, and suggested that these may reflect birth injury (although some of the 'soft' signs might have been related to medication, and, in contrast to many individuals with asymmetric motor impairment following birth trauma, there were no discrepancies in limb size, nor was there any evidence of delayed development). Perhaps some of the most compelling evidence in favour of organicity are the observations that (1) tics persist during all stages of sleep (Glaze *et al.* 1983) and (2) tics are not preceded by a '*Bereitschaft*' or 'readiness' potential on the EEG (Obeso *et al.* 1981). In fact, although non-specific EEG abnormalities, including paroxysmal activity, occur with increased incidence in the Gilles de la Tourette syndrome, the latter is not temporally related to the tics. This finding, and the persistence of tics during sleep, suggest a subcortical origin.

It has been suggested that a number of psychological abnormalities may be associated with Gilles de la Tourette's syndrome. To a certain extent, these may reflect the response to living with a chronic, socially embarrassing disorder. Two specific abnormalities, however, deserve further comment. The first of these is attention deficit disorder (also loosely referred to as 'hyperactivity' syndrome in children). While an association between the two disorders is said to exist, a recent study fails to support a genetic relationship. Pauls *et al.* (1986*a*) studied individuals with Tourette's syndrome and those suffering from Tourette's syndrome plus attention deficit disorder. The frequency of Tourette's syndrome among relatives of probands in both groups was virtually identical, but the rate of attention deficit disorder was much greater (approximately eight times higher) in relatives of probands in the latter group. In families where the proband had both disorders, the traits segregated independently.

A clearer relationship exists between Tourette's syndrome and obsessive–compulsive disorder. An obsession is a compelling thought, which may lead to the expression of compulsion, which is a form of stereotyped, often ritualistic behaviour. The obsession may be associated with a great deal of inner tension and anxiety, which can be relieved by the performance of the compulsion. The analogy to tic disorders, particularly more complex ritua-listic tics, is clear. Indeed, in contrast to their findings concerning the relationship between Tourette's syndrome and attention deficit disorder, Pauls *et al.* (1986*b*) found evidence of a genetic link between tic and obsessive–compulsive disorder. Furthermore, other evidence suggests that basal ganglia dysfunction may cause obsessive–compulsive behaviour (Weilburg *et al.* 1989).

Pathological studies in the Gilles de la Tourette syndrome are sparse. A review by Richardson (1982) revealed only two cases. In one, there were no abnormalities. In the second, there was an increase in the packing density of small striatal neurons. In a very recent study of a single case, Haber *et al.* (1986) found multiple tiny cerebral and cerebellar embolic infarcts thought to be unrelated to the movement disorder. Immunocytochemical studies however revealed a profound loss of dynorphin-like immunoreactivity in the pallidum, while substance P and encephalin-like immunoreactivity were normal.

A single underlying biochemical abnormality in tic has not yet been identified. The beneficial response to dopamine receptor blockade (Shapiro *et al*. 1973) or dopamine depletion (Jankovic *et al*. 1984) have suggested a state of excess dopaminergic activity. The therapeutic efficacy of D-2 selective dopamine antagonists may even suggest that the Gilles de la Tourette syndrome is associated with functional dopaminergic hyperactivity (Uhr *et al*. 1986). This is also supported by the induction and/or exacerbation of tics by indirect dopamine agonists, such as methylphenidate (Denckla *et al*. 1976), and by the development of the Gilles de la Tourette syndrome as a manifestation of tardive dyskinesia (Klawans *et al*. 1978; Stahl 1980). Biochemical studies of cerebrospinal fluid (CSF) have revealed decreased dopamine turnover in the Gilles de la Tourette syndrome (Butler *et al*. 1979; Cohen *et al*. 1978) and it has been suggested (Butler *et al*. 1979) that this reflects feedback inhibition due to receptor supersensitivity. A recent study of dopamine receptors in the Gilles de la Tourette syndrome using positron emission tomography and C-N-methylspiperone (Singer *et al*. 1984) failed to demonstrate any abnormalities.

Other transmitter systems have been implicated in the Gilles de la Tourette syndrome. Since imbalance of striatal dopaminergic and cholinergic activity appears to be important in PD and Huntington's disease, Stahl and Berger (1980, 1981) hypothesized that there may be a relative cholinergic deficit in patients with tic. They found a definite improvement of symptoms in the Gilles de la Tourette syndrome after intravenous physostigmine in their patients. Similarly, Barbeau (1980) found lecithin to be beneficial. In contrast, however, Tanner and her colleagues (1980) found that scopolamine abated tics, while physostigmine resulted in an exacerbation. In open studies, Cohen and co-workers (1979, 1980) found that the α_2-agonist clonidine ameliorated the Gilles de la Tourette syndrome. Although this might suggest that elevated noradrenergic activity is important in the genesis of tics, no consistent abnormalities of plasma or CSF methoxyhydroxyphenylglycol (MHPG), the major metabolite of noradrenalin, have been reported. A more recent placebo-controlled, double-blind study found evidence of subjective, but not objective improvement, following clonidine (Goetz *et al*. 1986).

The stereotyped head-shakes induced by serotonergic agents (Curzon, Chapter 6, this volume; Handley and Singh 1986), which are thought to be mediated by 5-HT_2 receptors, are reminiscent of some aspects of tic disorders, and some aspects of myoclonic disorders in man (see below). Clonidine may also inhibit brainstem serotonergic neurons (Svensson *et al*. 1975) and this has indeed been suggested as a possible mechanism of action in tic (Cohen *et al*. 1980). CSF studies reveal that serotonin turnover is decreased, however (Cohen *et al*. 1978; Butler *et al*. 1979) and the PET study cited above (Singer *et al*. 1984) would suggest that this is not due to

5-HT$_2$-receptor supersensitivity. Indeed, Van Woert and his colleagues (1977) found that the serotonin precursor L-5-hydroxytrytophan was effective in reducing tic in some patients, as they did for postanoxic myoclonus.

Finally, it should be noted that tic may occur as a manifestation of other neurological disease, including trauma (Fahn 1982), post-encephalitic parkinsonism, stroke and carbon monoxide intoxication (Sacks 1982), and neuroacanthocytosis (Spitz *et al.* 1985).

Myoclonus

Myoclonus refers to sudden, brief, shock-like muscle contractions of central origin. Many elements of myoclonic disorders have stereotyped behavioural features including rhythmic, stimulus-linked, repetitive, reproducible, and recurrent characteristics in some patients. The nosology and classification of this exceedingly complex group of disorders have been the subject of recent extensive reviews (Fahn *et al.* 1986; Marsden *et al.* 1982*a*). The muscular contractions may be focal, segmental, multifocal, or generalized, and they may be rhythmic, oscillatory, or arrhythmic in nature. The movements may be highly stimulus-sensitive, and may be provoked by motor activity. Myoclonus may occur as a physiological event (e.g. on falling asleep) or as an isolated neurological disorder of unknown aetiology (essential myoclonus). A variety of epileptic disorders are characterized by myoclonus, as are a host of degenerative and infectious diseases of the nervous system. Myoclonus is a frequent sign of toxic or metabolic encephalopathies, and may also result from hypoxia (the Lance–Adams syndrome), trauma, or stroke.

Obviously, the wide variety of disorders accompanied by myoclonus render the identification of a single underlying pathological substrate impossible. Indirect evidence suggests that a number of pharmacological alterations may produce or alleviate myoclonus. Post-hypoxic intention myoclonus (Lance and Adams 1963) responds well to the serotonin precursor, L-5-hydroxytryptophan (L-5-HTP) (Van Woert *et al.* 1977) and is associated with CSF evidence of decreased serotonin turnover (Chadwick *et al.* 1977). Lisuride is beneficial in cortical reflex myoclonus (Obeso *et al.* 1983*b*) and this may be related to its action on serotonin or DA receptors. On the other hand, L-dopa can induce myoclonus, and, since this is blocked by methysergide, it is probably mediated via serotonergic mechanisms (Klawans *et al.* 1975).

In guinea-pigs, L-5-HTP induces myoclonus, which is blocked by the serotonin antagonists methysergide and cyproheptadine (Klawans *et al.* 1973). This is blocked acutely by co-administration of dopaminergic agents (Weiner *et al.* 1979) although chronic L-dopa therapy renders animals supersensitive to 5-HTP myoclonus (Carvey *et al.* 1983). Stimulus-sensitive myoclonus can also be produced in rodents following administration of p,p'-DDT[1,1,1-trichloro-2,2-*bis* (p-chlorephenylethane] (Chung Hwang and Van Woert 1978). This is attenuated by 5-HT agonists or re-uptake blockers, and is exacerbated by 5-HT antagonists. This form of myoclonus is inhibited by intracerebroventricular glycine (Truong *et al.* 1986).

In humans, a variety of other drugs may be useful in the treatment of myoclonus. Of particular note are valproic acid (Van Woert and Chung 1986) and clonazepam (Jenner *et al.* 1986). Although an indirect action of these drugs on serotonergic mechanisms is not entirely excluded, it seems more likely that they mediate their effects by facilitating GABA-ergic inhibition. The nootropic agent, piracetam, may be effective in some patients with cortical reflex myoclonus or in Lance–Adams syndrome (Fahn *et al.* 1986), but the mechanism of action is not understood.

Dystonia

Another set of abnormal movements, namely the dystonias, exhibits certain stereotyped clinical features. Dystonia describes the sustained assumption of an abnormal posture. Thus, in the advanced stages of so-called 'torsion dystonia', the affected body parts may appear to be permanently twisted into bizarre deformities, although in the earlier stages of the disease, prior to the onset of flexion contractures, the abnormalities will abate or disappear during sleep. Dystonic movements are not always fixed, however. They may be jerky, as in 'spasmodic' torticollis, or slow and writhing. Dystonia may commonly be associated with essential tremor (Couch 1976) and less frequently with myoclonus (Obeso *et al.* 1983*a*). The dystonias are classified according to clinical distribution as focal (affecting a single body part), segmental (affecting two contiguous body parts), or generalized (Fahn and Eldridge 1976). In addition, the disorder may be primary or secondary to a diverse range of underlying neurological disease. Primary dystonia may be sporadic or hereditary, and inheritance may be autosomal dominant or recessive (Eldridge 1970).

In most cases, the cause of dystonia is unknown. Pathological studies of generalized dystonia have been sparse and largely unrewarding (Zeman and Dyken 1968). In a few cases of torticollis, post-mortem studies have revealed minor inflammatory and degenerative changes affecting the basal ganglia (Alpers and Drayer 1937; Foerster 1933; Grinker and Walker 1933). In Meige syndrome, a segmental dystonia characterized by blepharospasm and oromandibular dyskinesias, pathological study of a single case revealed focal striatal degeneration (Altrocchi and Forno 1983). Blepharospasm has also been associated with lesions of the upper brainstem (Jankovic and Patel 1983) and striatum (Keane and Young 1985). In patients with symptomatic hemidystonia, the lesion is in the basal ganglia and/or thalamus (Marsden *et al.* 1985) and may be even more discretely localized to the putamen (Burton *et al.* 1984).

From an electrophysiological point of view, dystonia is characterized by an abnormal attenuation of reciprocal inhibition, suggesting a defect in presynaptic inhibition at the spinal level (Rothwell *et al.* 1983). In patients with blepharospasm, both the early and late phases of the blink reflex are of increased amplitude and duration, suggesting that in these patients, brainstem inhibition is impaired (Berardelli *et al.* 1985; Tolosa and Montserrat 1985). A recent study using surface electromyographic recording of affected muscle activity indicates that in torticollis, as in tic, the abnormal movements persist in all stages of sleep, although the amplitude is so attenuated that they may not be perceptible to the naked eye (Forgach *et al.* 1986). This observation surely places the final nail in the coffin of long-standing arguments that the disease has an hysterical basis, at least in the great majority of cases, and lends further support to the view that the abnormal movements are subcortical in origin. Finally, PET studies indicate that, although there is no abnormality of regional cerebral glucose metabolism in patients with torticollis, normal patterns of metabolic coupling between subregions of the basal ganglia and the thalamus are disrupted (Stoessl *et al.* 1986*a*).

The biochemical and pharmacological substrate of the dystonias remains among the most perplexing problems of all neurological disease. Some CSF studies have indicated diminished levels of MHPG in the ventricular fluid of patients with childhood-onset dystonia (Wolfson *et al.* 1983), but the controls were not strictly comparable. Hornykiewicz and co-workers (1986) have recently reported detailed post-mortem analysis of the brains of two individuals who had childhood-onset dystonia. No significant histological abnormalities were detected, but there were complex regional alterations in adrenalin, serotonin, and dopamine, while GABA, glutamate, and choline acetyltransferase were normal. An underlying abnormality of noradrenergic transmission derives further support from the finding of elevated noradrenalin levels in the cerebellum of the mutant dystonic rat (Lorden *et al.* 1984).

Pharmacological treatment of dystonia patients is often ineffective. However, the most consistent benefit is seen with high-dose anticholinergic therapy (Fahn 1983). Dopamine-active drugs produce a variety of seemingly paradoxical effects. On the one hand, neuroleptics may precipitate dystonia acutely (Rupniak *et al.* 1986), and some dystonia patients may respond to treatment with L-dopa (Segawa *et al.* 1976) or dopamine agonists (Lees *et al.* 1976; Micheli *et al.* 1982; Quinn *et al.* 1985; Stahl and Berger 1982). All of this suggests an underlying state of dopamine deficiency in dystonia. On the other hand, however, chronic neuroleptic use may result in tardive dystonia, suggesting dopamine receptor supersensitivity (see pp. 275–8), and some dystonic patients respond best to dopaminergic blockade (Gilbert 1972) or depletion (Swash *et al.* 1972), or a combination thereof (Marsden *et al.* 1984). PET studies of dopamine metabolism in dystonia have yielded similarly confusing results (Martin *et al.* 1987). Finally, some patients respond to benzodiazepines, and this suggests that GABA-ergic mechanisms may be important, perhaps at a spinal level. The role of peptides in dystonia is simply not known.

Even when we have a firmer understanding of the neurochemical imbalance underlying this probably heterogeneous group of disorders, many clinical observations will remain equally mystifying. By what mechanism does peripheral trauma precipitate dystonia in the affected limb (Schott 1986)? Why do some patients with action dystonia suffer from impairment only during the performance of highly specific tasks needed for their occupation—e.g. the radio broadcaster with spasmodic dysphonia or the stenographer with writer's cramp (see Sheehy and Marsden 1982)? Clearly, this is an area of neurology begging for many more answers.

Drug-induced movement disorders

Many medications can induce involuntary stereotyped movements. By far the most important, however, both statistically and in terms of suffering, are those resulting from L-dopa, direct and indirect dopamine agonists, and the neuroleptics.

Levodopa (L-dopa)

This drug is the mainstay of treatment for parkinsonism. It must therefore be borne in mind that a number of the therapeutic complications may reflect the interactions between medication effect and the underlying disease process itself. Thus, freezing, kinesia paradoxica (the sudden, transient increase in mobility associated with anxiety or fear), sleep benefit, fatiguability, and emotion-dependent fluctuations were all well recognized before the introduction of L-dopa (Marsden *et al.* 1982*b*). Even dyskinesias were known to occur occasionally in parkinsonian patients who never received L-dopa. Conversely, L-dopa given to normal individuals does not produce involuntary movements, unless very high doses are given, suggesting that many of the toxic effects require for their expression the substrate of a diseased brain, perhaps one in which dopamine receptors are supersensitive (Lee *et al.* 1978). In the early stages of L-dopa therapy, most parkinsonians derive significant benefit within 15–60 min of taking the drug, lasting for approximately 4 hours. With multiple daily doses, a fairly smooth response is then obtained. As disease progresses, the duration of benefit diminishes, and end-of-dose deterioration occurs. This may initially respond to more frequent administration of lower doses of medication, but eventually, drug-resistant 'off' periods develop, and patients may be faced with the choice of dangerous immobility on the one hand, or disabling dyskinesias on the other, with rapid fluctuations between the two states, often seemingly unrelated to dosage schedule, at least on cursory analysis (Marsden and Parkes 1976).

The involuntary movements seen in L-dopa-treated parkinsonism may mimic all variety of spontaneously occurring movement disorders (Barbeau *et al*. 1971). Most common are choreiform movements, which preferentially affect the orofacial musculature, although the limbs may be affected, particularly during ambulation. Dystonic movements may occur ranging from blepharospasm and torticollis to severe generalized muscle contractions (Parkes *et al*. 1976). Ballism, an extreme form of chorea with wild, flailing movements, may be seen, as may myoclonus (Klawans *et al*. 1975).

In most cases, dyskinesias occur when maximum mobility has been reached, and plasma dopa levels are high ('peak-dose' dyskinesias) (Muenter *et al*. 1977). In a smaller percentage of patients, dyskinesias occur following a dose of L-dopa, but prior to clinical improvement, and again as mobility declines and parkinsonian features return ('diphasic' or 'D-I-D' dyskinesias; Muenter *et al*. 1977). Finally, 'early morning' dystonia occurs prior to the first daily dose of L-dopa and resolves over 1–2 hours after medication, but disappears entirely if L-dopa is withdrawn for several days (Melamed 1979). These abnormal movements induced by L-dopa are all relatively stereotyped, and consistent within a given individual patient.

The pathophysiology of fluctuations in disability is poorly understood. Peak-dose dyskinesias seem to be clearly related to dopamine excess. Since dyskinesias are less of a problem with dopamine agonists, such as bromocriptine, which are more selective for D-2 receptors, it has been suggested that the dyskinesias may result from D-1 stimulation (Calne 1982). Fluctuations from immobility to dyskinesia may be partially explained by pharmacokinetic alterations in L-dopa bioavailability, since these can be largely dampened by continuous intravenous infusion of L-dopa (Hardie *et al*. 1984; Nutt *et al*. 1984; Quinn *et al*. 1984) or of the dopamine agonist, lisuride (Obeso *et al*. 1986). However, there remain patients whose fluctuations are truly independent of dose schedule. Fahn (1974) has suggested that, in these individuals, sudden deterioration may be related to rapid conformational changes in dopamine receptor proteins, but patients are still able to respond to exogenously administered apomorphine when 'off', suggesting that receptor mechanisms are intact (Stibe *et al.* 1988). 3 O-methyl-dopa, formed from L-dopa by the ubiquitous action of catechol-O-methyl-transferase (COMT) may compete with L-dopa for transport across the blood–brain barrier and result in deterioration, but the mechanism for its purported contribution to the genesis of dyskinesias is unclear (Rivera-Calimlim *et al.* 1977).

Dopamine agonists

Direct agonists such as bromocriptine may result in dyskinesias, but this is generally less of a problem than with L-dopa (Parkes 1979; Calne 1982). Preferential activation of D-2 receptors has been suggested as an explanation.

Indirect agonists, such as amphetamine and cocaine, may result in choreo-athetoid movements and ataxia. Although the involuntary movements are maximal immediately following drug ingestion, they may persist in a milder form even years after drug use has stopped (Lundh and Tunving 1981). In addition to the more primitive involuntary movements noted above, complex stereotyped behaviours may be seen, such as continual picking at the skin ('cocaine bugs'), or repetitive buttoning and unbuttoning of clothes. Such repetitive, purposeless behaviour is also known as pundning (Randrup and Munkvad 1967). These stereotyped behaviours are usually seen in amphetamine or cocaine addicts while taking a euphoriant or toxic dose of drug. Such phenomena are reminiscent of various spontaneous stereotyped behaviours observed in patients with schizophrenia or autism, or as a component of complex partial seizures. As noted before, other indirect dopaminergic agents such as methylphenidate (Denckla *et al.* 1976) and cocaine (Mesulam 1986) may result in tic.

Neuroleptics

Short-term effects   It has been recognized for many years that dopamine receptor antagonists and dopamine-depleting agents may result in parkinsonism, which is usually rapidly reversible upon withdrawal of the offending agent, but may persist for weeks. Neuroleptics may also precipitate acute dyskinesias and dystonic reactions in man and non-human primates (see Rupniak *et al.* 1986). Both parkinsonism and dystonia induced by neuroleptics respond to anticholinergic treatment, but the pathophysio-logy of the latter disorder is nevertheless unclear. Pre-treatment with dopamine-depleting agents may prevent the development of acute neurolep-tic-induced dystonia in baboons (Meldrum *et al.* 1977) and acute neurolep-tic-induced receptor supersensitivity and enhanced dopamine turnover outlast the effects of receptor blockade (Kolbe *et al.* 1981). This has led to the suggestion that even acute dystonia resulting from neuroleptics may derive from a state of excessive dopaminergic activity.

Another poorly understood short-term effect of neuroleptics is akathisia. This refers to a restlessness, or inability to remain seated still. A number of stereotyped behaviours are associated with this subjective sense of restlessness and the affected individual may exhibit pacing, fidgety movements or may simply experience the urge to move. It is likely, therefore, that the syndrome represents both a movement disorder and a state of psychic unrest (Stahl 1985). That it is a manifestation of relative hypodopaminergic-hypercholinergic imbalance seems likely, given the beneficial response to anticholinergics and its occurrence in patients with idiopathic Parkinson's disease (Lang and Johnson 1986).

Chronic effects: tardive dyskinesia   This group of disorders represents a common and serious adverse effect of neuroleptic therapy. The prevalence is about 10–20 per cent (Baldessarini 1985; Casey 1985; Kane *et al*. 1982). A number of clinical variants occur, and are frequently compared to the spontaneously occurring choreiform disorders discussed above. However, in tardive dyskinesia the movements within a given patient may be more stereotyped than in spontaneous chorea, as the former generally involve a smaller collection of movements. Also, movements in tardive dyskinesia are frequently uncovered or exacerbated in a stereotyped manner by voluntary movements in unaffected parts of the body. The commonest variant is orofacial dyskinesia or the buccal–lingual masticatory syndrome, consisting of involuntary tongue protrusions, lip-smacking, chewing, and related movements. This may be associated with choreiform movements of the limbs. A combination of truncal and lower extremity involvement may lead to bizarre postures and gait. All of these manifestations are reminiscent of, but many investigators feel not identical to, those of Huntington's disease. Other differential diagnoses include senile chorea (characterized by late-onset chorea with no dementia) and the spontaneous oral masticatory syndrome (Klawans and Barr 1982). Dystonia may also occur as a manifestation of tardive dyskinesia. This complication generally affects younger patients, and is often associated with a poor prognosis (Burke *et al*. 1982). As previously noted, tic may occur following long-term neuroleptics (Klawans *et al*. 1978; Stahl 1980). Finally, subjective restlessness after cessation of neuroleptics has been termed 'tardive akathisia' (Barnes and Braude 1985; Weiner and Luby 1983). In children, discontinuation of neuroleptics is not uncommonly complicated by a transient generalized choreiform disorder. Some investigators prefer to separate this 'withdrawal emergent' syndrome from the tardive dyskinesias.

By convention, tardive dyskinesia refers to those movement disorders

arising during or following neuroleptic therapy of at least 3 months dura
tion. An underlying disorder providing an alternate explanation for the
involuntary movements must be excluded. One complicating issue is the
well-described occurrence of involuntary movements in unmedicated
schizophrenics (Crow *et al*. 1982; Frith and Done, Chapter 9, this volume;
Lees 1986). This has even led to suggestions that tardive dyskinesia may be a
manifestation of schizophrenia or of a subtype of schizophrenia, called Type
II syndrome (Crow *et al*. 1982), rather than a complication of neuroleptic
use. However, most experts would agree that, while tics and more complex stereotypies may occur in schizophrenia, spontaneous choreiform
movements are quite rare (Jenner and Marsden 1983; Lees 1985; Mackay
1982). Earlier descriptions of chorea may reflect failure to diagnose other
conditions characterized by both psychosis and involuntary movements,
notably Huntington's disease, encephalitis, and syphilis. Finally, classical
tardive dyskinesia can occur in non-psychotic patients treated with neuroleptics (Klawans *et al*. 1974; Orme and Tallis 1984). Thus, the link with
neuroleptics appears incontrovertible.

Risk factors for the development of tardive dyskinesia are not well
established. There is general agreement that the incidence increases with
advancing age, and probably with duration of neuroleptic therapy. Females
seem to be more prone to develop tardive dyskinesia, and Waddington and
co-workers (1985) have suggested that tardive dyskinesia is more likely
to occur in schizophrenics with intellectual impairment and 'negative'
symptoms. Somewhat surprisingly, interruption of neuroleptic therapy
(drug holiday) seems to increase the risk of developing tardive dyskinesia
(Jeste *et al*. 1979).

The pathogenesis of tardive dyskinesia is also unclear. Christensen *et al*.
(1970) examined the brains of 28 patients with dyskinesias (neuroleptic-
induced in only 21 cases) and compared the findings with those in 28
'control' brains. The control group consisted of an identical make-up
of schizophrenics, senile dements, and 'other organic psychoses', and
contained 19 subjects who had received neuroleptics. The most consistent
difference between the two groups was a significantly higher incidence of
nigral degeneration and midbrain–brainstem gliosis in the patients with
dyskinesia. Since tardive dyskinesia may be indistinguishable from L-dopa-
induced dyskinesias, it has been assumed that the disorder reflects excessive
dopaminergic stimulation, likely due to neuroleptic-induced receptor supersensitivity (Burt *et al*. 1977). Although chronic neuroleptics in animals may
produce spontaneous dyskinesias (see Goetz and Klawans 1982; Gunne and
Haggstrom 1985), their relationship to tardive dyskinesia is imperfect. It is
clear, however, that the increased D-2 receptor binding seen in chronic
neuroleptic treatment is associated with increased behavioural sensitivity to

the effects of amphetamine and apomorphine (Goetz and Klawans 1982). Further clinical support for dopaminergic excess derives from the exacerbation of tardive dyskinesia by dopaminergic agents, and its amelioration by dopaminergic blockade or depletion (Gerlach *et al*. 1974); Jenner and Marsden 1983; Kazamatsuri *et al*. 1972). In a situation analogous to Huntington's disease and converse to parkinsonism, symptoms may also respond to cholinergic agents (Davis *et al*. 1976; Fann *et al*. 1974; Gerlach *et al*. 1974; Stahl *et al*. 1982).

There are a number of problems with the DA receptor supersensitivity model of tardive dyskinesia which have been reviewed by Fibiger and Lloyd (1984). First, tardive dyskinesia by definition develops months to years after the initiation of neuroleptic therapy, whereas increased receptor binding occurs within 2–3 weeks. Secondly, tardive dyskinesia often persists for a long time after neuroleptics are discontinued, while receptor binding returns rapidly to normal. Third, while receptor supersensitivity is invariant, the development of tardive dyskinesia is not, and, finally, receptor supersensitivity does not account for the anatomical distribution of the abnormal movements. Indeed chronic neuroleptic therapy in animals induces degeneration in the striatum (Pakkenberg and Nilakantan 1973) which is concentrated in the ventrolateral region, the area concerned with innervation of oral musculature (Nielsen and Lyon 1978). Although many striatal interneurons are cholinergic (thus perhaps accounting for the beneficial response to cholinergic agents in tardive dyskinesia), the majority of the projecting neurons from the striatum are GABA-ergic, and chronic neuroleptic treatment in animals is associated with depletion of pallidal and nigral glumatic acid decarboxylase (Gunne and Haggstrom 1983; Gunne *et al*. 1984). Fibiger and Lloyd postulate that the critical abnormality in tardive dyskinesia is GABA deficiency. Since GABA-ergic neurons normally decline with age (McGeer and McGeer 1976), this would explain the increased risk of tardive dyskinesia in older patients. Additional clinical support for a critical role of GABA comes from the beneficial response to GABA-ergic agents, such as benzodiazepines (Sedman 1976), muscimol (Tamminga *et al*. 1979), and gamma-vinyl-GABA (Stahl *et al*. 1985; Tell *et al*. 1981).

The peptide cholecystokinin (CCK) is known to co-exist with dopamine in mesolimbic neurons and interactions between the two transmitters may be important in the pathogenesis of schizophrenia (Phillips *et al*. 1986). A recent study has demonstrated amelioration of tardive dyskinesia in patients treated with ceruletide, a CCK analogue (Nishikawa *et al*. 1986). CCK also suppresses the vacuous chewing mouth movements that develop in rats treated with long term neuroleptics (Stoessl *et al*. 1989). Finally, it has been suggested that chronic neuroleptics may foster free radical-induced damage to striatal neurons, perhaps by increasing dopamine turnover, and that this is in some way related to the development of tardive dyskinesia (Cadet et al. 1986).

Summary

A number of disorders characterized by involuntary movements have been discussed. The common pharmacological thread tying them together seems to be an imbalance among neurotransmitters, frequently involving the monoamines, acetylcholine, and/or GABA. It is now clear, however, that traditional models of imbalance between two neurotransmitters are overly simplistic. In the future, post-mortem studies will need to examine simultaneously the levels of multiple transmitters and assess receptor status using autoradiography, so that topographical details are preserved. Furthermore, it is now increasingly important that such studies are meticulously correlated with detailed clinical assessments, including the documentation of cognitive and emotional state. Too often in the past, failure to obtain such information has resulted in overly simplistic and occasionally incorrect conclusions regarding the biochemical substrates of abnormal motor function. Areas of particular interest will include disease-related alterations in peptide transmitters, interactions between different transmitter systems, and the role of excitatory amino acids in initiating or perpetuating the neuronal degeneration associated with some of these disorders.

Whilst detailed pathological assessment is important, the ability to determine dynamic changes in transmitter and/or receptor function *in vivo* would avoid the pitfalls of post-mortem delay, non-specific agonal changes, and end-stage disease. Positron emission tomography is a promising tool to this end. There have already been dramatic improvements in spatial resolution and in the variety of isotopically labelled drugs available. Further attention is now needed in the development, validation, and rigorous application of tracer kinetic models, so that quantitative data can be reliably extracted.

As better neurochemical documentation emerges, so too will the realization that many of the disease labels discussed here are nothing but descriptive terms. The dystonias are an undoubted example of a heterogeneous group of disorders. In the future, classification of such disorders may well be based on biochemical as well as clinical parameters.

Finally, better animal models of human disease are needed. 6-hydroxy-dopamine causes toxic damage to catecholamine-containing pathways, and has provided a good basis for research into Parkinson's disease. This has now largely been superseded by the MPTP model which is more selective and which has the added advantage of fitting in with speculation regarding environmental aetiologies. Still, subtle differences from the idiopathic disease do exist. While excitotoxic damage to the striatum may resemble the pathological and biochemical hallmarks of Huntington's disease, it does not result in the chief behavioural manifestation, chorea (at least not spontaneously). The relationship between animal behaviour induced by serotonin and human disease is similarly not straightforward. Thus, tremor in humans is, if anything, associated with β-adrenergic imbalance and is not typically known to result from serotonergic excess (although adequate documentation is unavailable). Similarly, in humans, many myoclonic disorders are actually ameliorated by serotonergic therapy, which would initiate myoclonus in guinea-pigs. There is no accepted model for tic disorders (although head twitches are one possibility) and the mutant dystonic rat is still incompletely characterized, but may offer important clues in a group of diseases notable for a lack of readily identifiable pathology. Exploitation of all these avenues is urgently needed to allow the pharmacological delineation of these disorders that will form the cornerstone of rational therapy.

Appendix—glossary of terms

Acanthocytosis: a disorder of red blood cell membranes, resulting in 'spur-shaped' cells.

Akathisia: motor and psychic restlessness; inability to remain seated still.

Arrhythmia: any disturbance of cardiac rhythm, including irregularities and additional beats.

Ataxia: abnormalities in the rate, range, force and direction of voluntary movement.

Ballism: rapid, wild flailing movements; an extreme form of chorea.

Blepharospasm: involuntary contraction of the eyelids.

Bradykinesia: slowing and hesitancy of voluntary movement.

Chorea: rapid, uncoordinated jerk-like contractions of single muscles.

Dysarthria: distorted articulation of speech (i.e. implying weakness or incoordination of the muscles of the lips and tongue). Scanning dysarthria refers to a monotonous staccato quality of speech, typical of cerebellar disorders.

Dyskinesias: a nonspecific term referring to any irregular hyperkinetic involuntary movements—as in drug-induced or tardive dyskinesias.

Dysphonia: a disorder of voice production, implying an abnormality of the contraction of the vocal cords or pharyngeal muscles.

Dystonia: the sustained assumption of an abnormal position due to involuntary muscle contraction

Festination: the characteristic (but not universal) gait of Parkinson's disease giving the impression that the patient is 'chasing his/her centre of gravity'.

Freezing: transient attacks of immobility of very sudden onset, in Parkinson's disease. Does *not* refer to more sustained periods of akinesia.

Lupus erythematosus: a multisystem inflammatory disorder, thought to be of autoimmune origin, particularly affecting the skin, internal membranes, and blood vessels.

Myoclonus: sudden, brief, shock-like muscle contractions.

Nystagmus: rapid, fine, involuntary movements of the eyes. Often a sign of brainstem or cerebellar dysfunction.

Thyrotoxicosis: disorder resulting from excess circulating thyroid hormone, either due to thyroid disease or to administration of exogenous thyroxine.

Tic: brief, rapid, and stereotypic muscle contractions that can be voluntarily suppressed, and are associated with an 'urge to move'.

Tone: the resistance to passive movement.

Torticollis: a form of focal dystonia, characterized by involuntary contraction of the neck muscles, 'wry neck'.

Tremor: fairly regular, rhythmical oscillation of a body part.

Acknowledgement

A. J. Stoessl was a Canadian MRC Fellow during the preparation of this chapter. The author is grateful to Dr S. M. Stahl for helpful comments on the manuscript.

References

Alpers, B. J. and Drayer, C. S. (1937). The organic background of some cases of spasmodic torticollis: report of case with autopsy. *Am. J. med. Sci.* **193**, 378–84.
Altrocchi, P. H. and Forno, L. S. (1983). Spontaneous oral-facial dyskinesia: neuropathology of a case. *Neurology* **33**, 802–5.
Alvord, E. C., Forno, L. S., Kusske, J. A., Kauffman, R. J., Rhodes, B., and Goetowski, C. R. (1975). The pathology of parkinsonism: a comparison of degenerations in cerebral cortex and brainstem. *Adv. Neurol.* **5**, 175–93.

Aronin, N., Cooper, P.E., Lorenz, L.J., Bird, E.D., Sagar, S.M., Leeman, S.E., and Martin, J.B. (1983). Somatostatin is increased in the basal ganglia in Huntington disease. *Ann. Neurol.* **13**, 519–26.

Arregui, A., Bennett J.P., Bird, E.D., Yamamura, H.I., Iversen, L.L., and Snyder, S.H. (1977). Huntington's chorea: selective depletion of activity of angiotensin converting enzyme in the corpus striatum. *Ann. Neurol.* **2**, 294–8.

Baldessarini, R.J. (1985). Clinical and epidemiological aspect's of tardive dyskinesia. *J. clin. Psychiat.* **46**(4), 8–13.

Barbeau, A. (1969). L-Dopa and juvenile Huntington's disease. *Lancet* **ii**, 1066.

Barbeau, A. (1980). Cholinergic treatment in the Tourette syndrome. *N. Engl. J. Med.* **302**, 1310–11.

Barbeau, A., Mars, H., and Gillo-Joffroy, J. (1971). Adverse clinical side effects of levodopa therapy. In *Recent advances in Parkinson's disease* (ed. F.H.M. Dowell and C.H. Markham), pp. 204–37. F.A. Davis, Philadelphia.

Barbeau, A., Roy, M., and Boyer, L. (1984). Genetic studies in Parkinson's disease. *Adv. Neurol.* **40**, 333–40.

Barnes, T.R.E. and Braude, W.M. (1985). Akathisia variants and tardive dyskinesia. *Arch. gen. Psychiat.* **42**, 874–8.

Benecke, R., Rothwell, J.C., Dick, J.P.R., Day, B.L., and Marsden, C.D. (1986). Performance of simultaneous movements in patients with Parkinson's disease. *Brain* **109**, 739–57.

Berardelli, A., Rothwell, J.C., Day, B.L., and Marsden, C.D. (1985). Pathophysiology of blepharospasm and oromandibular dystonia. *Brain* **108**, 543–608.

Bird, E.D. and Iversen, L.L. (1974). Huntington's chorea: post-mortem measurement of glutamic acid decarboxylase, choline acetyltransferase and dopamine in basal ganglia. *Brain* **97**, 457–72.

Birkmayer, W. and Hornykiewicz, O. (1961). Der L-Dioxy-phenylalanin (= L-DOPA)—Effekt bei der Parkinson-Akinese. *Wiener Klin. Wochenschr.* **73**, 787–8.

Bissette, G., Nemeroff, C.B., Decker, M.W., Kizer, B., Agid, Y., and Javoy-Agid, F. (1985). Alterations in regional brain concentrations of neurotensin and bombesin in Parkinson's disease. *Ann. Neurol.* **17**, 324–8.

Boller, F., Mizutani, T., Roessman, V., and Gambetti, P. (1980). Parkinson's disease, dementia, and Alzheimer disease: clinicopathological correlations. *Ann. Neurol.* **7**, 329–35.

Brown, R.G. and Marsden, C.D. (1984). How common is dementia in Parkinson's disease. *Lancet* **ii**, 1262–5.

Bruyn, G.W., Bots, G.T.A.M., and Dom, R. (1979). Huntington's chorea: current neuropathological status. *Adv. Neurol.* **23**, 83–94.

Burke, R.E., Fahn, S., Jankovic, J., Marsden, C.D., Lang, A.E., Gollomp, S., and Ilson, J. (1982). Tardive dystonia: late-onset and persistent dystonia caused by antipsychotic drugs. *Neurology* **32**, 1335–41.

Burns, R.S., Chiueh, C.C., Markey, S.P., Ebert, M.H., Jacobowitz, D.M., and Kopin, I.J. (1983). A primate model of parkinsonism: selective destruction of dopaminergic neurons in the pars compacta of the substantia nigra by N-methyl-4-phenyl-1, 2, 3, 6-tetrahydropyridine (MPTP). *Proc. nat. Acad. Sci.,* *USA* **80**, 4546-50.

Burt, D. R., Creese, I., and Snyder, S. H. (1977). Anti-schizophrenic drugs: chronic treatment elevates dopamine receptor binding in brain. *Science* **196**, 326-8.

Burton, K., Farrell, K., Li, D., and Calne, D. B. (1984). Lesions of the putamen and dystonia: CT and magnetic resonance imaging. *Neurology* **34**, 962-5.

Burton, K., Beckman, J. H., Ong, U. C., Rangno, R. E., Mak, E., and Calne, D. B. (1985). Beta-adrenergic receptors and essential tremor: results with L1 32-468, a selective beta-2 receptor antagonist. *Neurology* **35**, (Suppl. 1), 111.

Butler, I. J., Koslow, S. H., Seifert, W. E., Caprioli, R. M., and Singer, H. S. (1979). Biogenic amine metabolism in Tourette syndrome. *Ann. Neurol.* **6**, 37-9.

Cadet, J. L., Lohr, J. B., and Jeste, D. V. (1986). Free radicals and tardive dyskinesia. *Trends Neurosci.* **9**, 107-8.

Calne, D. B. (1982). Dopamine receptor agonists in the treatment of basal ganglia disorders. *Semin. Neurol.* **2**, 359-64.

Calne, D. B. and Langston, J. W. (1983). Aetiology of Parkinson's disease. *Lancet* ii, 1457-9.

Calne, D. B., Teychenne, P. F., Claveria, L. E., Eastman, R., Greenacre, J. K., and Petrie, A. (1974). Bromocriptine in parkinsonism. *Br. med. J.* **4**, 442-4.

Carvey, P. M., Goetz, C. G., and Klawans, H. L. (1983). The effect of chronic levodopa treatment on stereotypic and myoclonic jumping behaviour in the guinea pig. *Neurology* **33** (Suppl. 2), 67.

Casey, D. E. (1985). Spontaneous and tardive dyskinesias: clinical and laboratory studies. *J. clin. Psychiat.* **46**(4), 42-7.

Chadwick, D., Hallett, M., Harris, R., Jenner, P., Reynolds, E. H., and Marsden, C. D. (1977). Clinical, biochemical, and physiological features distinguishing myoclonus responsive to 5-hydroxytryptophan, tryptophan with a monoamine oxidase inhibitor, and clonazepam. *Brain* **100**, 455-87.

Chase, T. N. and Watanabe, A. M. (1972). Methyldopahydrazine as an adjunct to L-dopa therapy in parkinsonism. *Neurology* **22**, 384-92.

Christensen, E., Moller, J. E., and Faurbye, A. (1970). Neuropathological investigation of 28 brains from patients dying with dyskinesia. *Acta psychiat. scand.* **46**, 14-23.

Chung Hwang, E. and Van Woert, M. H. (1978). p,p'-DDT-induced neurotoxic syndrome: experimental myoclonus. *Neurology* **28**, 1020-5.

Cohen, D. J., Shaywitz, B. A., Caparulo, B., Young, J. G., and Bowers, M. B. (1978). Chronic multiple tics of Gilles de la Tourette's disease. Acid monoamine metabolites after probenecid administration. *Arch. gen. Psychiat.* **35**, 245-50.

Cohen, D. J., Nathanson, J. A., Young, J. G., and Shaywitz, B. A. (1979). Clonidine in Tourette's syndrome. *Lancet* ii, 551-3.

Cohen, D. J., Detlor, J., Young, J. G., and Shaywitz, B. A. (1980). Clonidine ameliorates Gilles de la Tourette syndrome. *Arch. gen. Psychiat.* **37**, 1350-7.

Cotzias, G. C., Papavasiliou, P. S., and Gellene, R. (1969). Modification of parkinsonism—chronic treatment with L-DOPA. *N. Engl. J. Med.* **280**, 337-45.

Couch, J. R. (1976). Dystonia and tremor in spasmodic torticollis. *Adv. Neurol* **14**, 245-58.

Coyle, J.T. and Snyder, S.H. (1969). Antiparkinsonian drugs: inhibition of dopamine uptake in the corpus striatum as a possible mechanism of action. *Science* 166, 899-901.

Critchley, M. (1949). Observations on essential (heredofamilial) tremor. *Brain* 72 113-39.

Crow, T.J., Cross, A.J., Johnstone, E.C., Owen, F., Owens, D.G.C., and Waddington, J.L. (1982). Abnormal involuntary movements in schizophrenia: are they related to the disease process or its treatment? Are they associated with changes in dopamine receptors? *J. clin. Psychopharmacol.* 2, 336-40.

Davis, K.L., Hollister, L.E., Barchas, J.D., and Berger, P.A. (1976). Choline in tardive dyskinesia and Huntington's disease. *Life Sci.* 19, 1507-16.

Denckla, M.B., Bemporad, J.R., and Mackay, M.C. (1976). Tics following methylphenidate administration. A report of 20 cases. *J. Am. med. Ass.* 235, 1349-51.

Duvoisin, R.C. (1967). Cholinergic-anticholinergic antagonism in parkinsonism. *Arch. Neurol.* 17, 124-36.

Ehringer, H. and Hornykiewicz, O. (1960). Verteilung von Noradrenalin und Dopamin (3-Hydroxytyramin) im Gehirn des Menschen und ihr Verhalten bei Erkrankungen des extrapyramidalen Systems. *Klin. Wochenschr.* 38, 1238-9.

Eldridge, R. (1970). The torsion dystonias: literature review and genetic and clinical studies. *Neurology* 20, 1-78.

Eldridge, R., Sweet, R., Lake, R., Ziegler, M., and Shapiro, A.K. (1977). Gilles de la Tourettes syndrome: clinical genetic, psychologic and biochemical aspects in 21 selected cases. *Neurology* 27, 115-24.

Elizan, T.S. and Casals, J. (1983). The viral hypothesis in parkinsonism. *J. Neurol. Trans. Suppl.* 19, 75-88.

Epelbaum, J., Ruberg, M., Moyse, E., Javoy-Agid, F., Dubois, B., and Agid, Y. (1983). Somatostatin and dementia in Parkinson's disease. *Brain Res.* 278, 376-9.

Fahn, S. (1974). 'On-off' phenomenon with levodopa therapy in parkinsonism: clinical and pharmacologic correlations and the effect of intramuscular pyridoxine. *Neurology* 24, 431-41.

Fahn, S. (1982). A case of post-traumatic tic syndrome. *Adv. Neurol.* 35, 349-50.

Fahn, S. (1983). High dose anticholinergic therapy in dystonia. *Neurology* 33, 1255-61.

Fahn, S. (1986). New drugs for posthypoxic action myoclonus: observations from a well-studied case. *Adv. Neurol.*43, 197-9.

Fahn, S. and Eldridge, R. (1976). Definition of dystonia and classification of the dystonic states. *Adv. Neurol.* 14, 1-5.

Fahn, S., Marsden, C.D., and Van Woert, M. (Eds.) (1986). Myoclonus. *Adv. Neurol.* Vol. 43. Raven Press, New York.

Fann, W.E., Lake, C.R., Gerber, C.J., and McKenzie, G.M. (1974). Cholinergic suppression of tardive dyskinesia. *Psychopharmacologia* 37, 101-7.

Fibiger, H.C., and Lloyd, K.G. (1984). Neurobiological substrates of tardive dyskinesia: the GABA hypothesis. *Trends Neurosci.* 7, 462-4.

Foerster, O. (1933). Mobile spasm of the neck muscles and its pathological basis. *J. comp. Neurol.* 58, 725-35.

Forgach, L., Eisen, A., Fleetham, J., and Calne, D.B. (1986). Studies on dystonic torticollis during sleep. *Neurology* 36, (Suppl. 1), 120.

Forno, L.S. (1982). Pathology of Parkinson's disease. In *Movement disorders* (ed. C.D. Marsden and S. Fahn), pp. 25–40, Butterworths, London.

Forno, L.S. and Jose, C. (1973). Huntington's chorea: a pathological study. *Adv. Neurol.* 1, 453–70.

Gerlach, J., Reisby, N., and Randrup, A. (1974). Dopaminergic hypersensitivity and cholinergic hypofunction in the pathophysiology of tardive dyskinesia. *Psychopharmacologia* 34, 21–35.

Gilbert, G.J. (1972). The medical treatment of spasmodic torticollis. *Arch. Neurol.* 27, 503–6.

Glaze, D.G., Frost, J.D., and Jankovic, J. (1983). Gilles de la Tourette's syndrome. Disorder of arousal. *Neurology* 33, 586–92.

Goetz, C.G. and Klawans, H.L. (1982). Controversies in animal models of tardive dyskinesia. In *Movement disorders* (ed. C.D. Marsden and S. Fahn), pp. 263–76, Butterworths, London.

Goetz, C.G., Tanner, C.M., Wilson, R.S., Carroll, S., and Shannon, K.M. (1986). Clonidine in Tourette's syndrome: double-blind objective study. *Ann. Neurol.* 20, 151.

Grinker, R.R. and Walker, A.E. (1983). The pathology of spasmodic torticollis with a note on respiratory failure from anesthesia in chronic encephalitis. *J. nerv. ment. Dis.* 78, 630–7.

Gunne, L.M. and Haggstrom, J.E. (1983). Reduction of nigral acid decarboxylase in rats with neuroleptic-induced acid dyskinesia. *Psychopharmacology* 81, 191–4.

Gunne, L.M. and Haggstrom, J.E. (1985). Experimental tardive dyskinesia. *J. clin. Psychiat.* 46(4), 48–50.

Gunne, L.M., Haggstrom, J.E., and Sjoquist, B. (1984). Association with persistent neuroleptic-induced dyskinesia of regional changes in brain GABA synthesis. *Nature* 309, 347–9.

Gusella, J.F., Wexler, N.S., Conneally, P.M.. Naylor, S.L., Anderson, M.A., Tanzi, R.E., Watkins, P.C., Ottina, K., Wallace, M.R., Sakaguchi, A.Y., Young, A.B., Shoulson, I., Bonilla, E., and Martin, J.B. (1983). A polymorphic DNA marker genetically linked to Huntington's disease. *Nature* 306, 234–8.

Haber, S.N., Kowall, N.W., Vonsattel, J.P., Bird, E.D., and Richardson, E.P. (1986). Gilles de la Tourette's syndrome. A postmortem neuropathological and immunohistochemical study. *J. neurol. Sci.* 75, 225–41.

Hakim, A.J. and Mathieson, G. (1979). Dementia in Parkinson disease: a neuropathological study. *Neurology* 29, 1209–14.

Handley, S.L. and Singh, L. (1986). Neurotransmitters and shaking behaviour—more than a 'gut-bath' for the brain? *Trends pharmacol. Sci.* 7, 324–8.

Hardie, R.J., Lees, A.J., and Stern, G.M. (1984). On–off fluctuations in Parkinson's disease. A clinical and neuropharmacological study. *Brain* 107, 487–506.

Hayden, M.R., Martin, W.R.W., Stoessl, A.J., Clark, C., Hollenberg, S., Adam, M.J., Amman, W., Harrop, R., Rogers, J., Ruth, T., Sayre, C., and Pate, B.D.

(1986). Positron emission tomography in the early diagnosis of Huntington's disease. *Neurology* **36**, 888-94.

Hayden, M. R., Hewitt, J., Stoessl, A. J., Clark, C., Ammann, W., and Martin, W. (1987). The combined use of positron emission tomography and DNA polymorphisms for preclinical detection of Huntington disease. *Neurology* **37**, 1441-47.

Hornykiewicz, O. (1966). Dopamine (3-hydroxytyramine) and brain function. *Pharmacol. Rev.* **18**, 925-64.

Hornykiewicz, O., Kish, S. J., Becker, L. E., Farley, I., and Shannak, K. (1986). Brain neurotransmitters in dystonia musculorum deformans. *N. Engl. J. Med.* **315**, 347-53.

Jankovic, J. and Fahn, S. (1986). The phenomenology of tics. *Movement Disorders* **1**, 17-26.

Jankovic, J. J. and Patel, S. C. (1983). Blepharospasm associated with brainstem lesions. *Neurology* **33**, 1237-40.

Jankovic, J., Glaze, D. G., and Frost, J. D. (1984). Effect of tetrabenazine on tics and sleep of Gilles de la Tourette's syndrome. *Neurology* **34**, 688-92.

Jefferson, D., Jenner, P., and Marsden, C. D. (1979). Beta-adrenoreceptor antagonists in essential tremor. *J. Neurol. Neurosurg. Psychiat.* **42**, 904-9.

Jenner, P. and Marsden, C. D. (1983). Neuroleptics and tardive dyskinesia. In *Neuroleptics: neurochemical, behavioural and clinical perspectives.* (ed. J. T. Coyle and S. J. Ennal), pp. 223-54. Raven, Press, New York.

Jenner, P., Pratt, J. A., and Marsden, C. D. (1986). Mechanism of action of clonazepam in myoclonus in relation to effects on GABA and 5-HT. *Adv. Neurol.* **43**, 629-43.

Jeste, D. V., Potkin, S. G., Sinha, S., Feder, S., and Wyatt, R. J. (1979). Tardive dyskinesia-reversible and persistent. *Arch. gen. Psychiat.* **36**, 585-90.

Kanazawa, I., Bird, E. D., Gale, J. S., Iversen, L. L., Jessell, J. M., Muramoto, O, Spokes, E. G., and Sutoo, D. (1979). Substance P: decrease in substantia nigra and globus pallidus in Huntington's disease. *Adv. Neurol.* **23**, 495-504.

Kane, J. M., Woerner, M., Weinhold, P., Wegner, J., and Kinon, B. (1982). A prospective study of tardive dyskinesia development: preliminary results. *J. clin. Psychopharmacol.* **2**, 345-347.

Kazamatsuri, H., Chien, C. P., and Cole, J. O. (1972). Treatment of tardive dyskinesia. 1. Clinical efficacy of a dopamine-depleting agent, tetrabenazine. *Arch. gen. Psychiat.* **27**, 95-9.

Keane, J. R. and Young, J. A. (1985). Blepharospasm with bilateral basal ganglia infarction. *Arch. Neurol.* **42**, 1206-8.

Kito, S., Hoga, E., Hiroshige, Y., Matsumoto, N., and Miwa, S. (1980). A pedigree of amyotrophic chorea with acanthocytosis. *Arch. Neurol.* **37**, 514-17.

Klawans, H. L. and Barr, A. N. (1982). Prevalence of spontaneous lingual-facial-buccal dyskinesias in the elderly. *Neurology* **32**, 558-9.

Klawans, H. L. and Rubovits, R. (1972). Central cholinergic-anticholinergic antagonism in Huntington's chorea. *Neurology* **22**, 107-16.

Klawans, H. L., Goetz, C., and Weiner, W. J. (1973). 5-hydroxytryptophan-induced myoclonus in guinea pigs and the possible role of serotonin in infantile myoclonus. *Neurology* **23**, 1234-40.

Klawans, H. L., Bergen, D., Bruyn, G. W., and Paulson, G. W. (1974). Neuroleptic-induced tardive dyskinesias in non-psychotic patients. *Arch. Neurol.* **30**, 338–9.

Klawans, H. L., Goetz, C., and Bergen, D. (1975). Levodopa-induced myoclonus. *Arch. Neurol.* **32**, 331–4.

Klawans, H. L., Falk, D. K., Nausieda, P. A., and Weiner, W. J. (1978). Gilles de la Tourette syndrome after long-term chlorpromazine therapy. *Neurology* **28**, 1064–8.

Kolbe, H., Clow, A., Jenner, P., and Marsden, C. D. (1981). Neuroleptic induced acute dystonic reactions may be due to enhanced dopamine release onto supersensitive postsynaptic receptors. *Neurology* **31**, 434–9.

Kuhl, D E., Phelps, M. E., Markham, C. H., Metler, E. J., Riegge, W. H., and Winter, J. (1982). Cerebral metabolism and atrophy in Huntington's disease determined by ^{18}FDG and computed tomographic scan. *Ann. Neurol.* **12**, 425–34.

Lance, J. W. and Adams, R. D. (1963). The syndrome of intention or action myoclonus as a sequel to hypoxic encephalopathy. *Brain* **86**, 111–36.

Lang, A. E. and Johnson, K. (1986). Akathisia in idiopathic Parkinson's disease. *Neurology* **36**, (Suppl. 1), 215–16.

Langston, J. W., Ballard, P., Tetrud, J. W., and Irwin, I. (1983). Chronic parkinsonism in humans due to a byproduct of meperidine-analog synthesis. *Science* **219**, 979–80.

Larsen, T. A. and Calne, D. B. (1984). Essential tremor. *Clin. Neuropharmacol.* **6**, 185–206.

Larsen, T. A. and Teravainen, H. (1983). β_1 versus nonselective blockade in therapy of essential tremor. *Adv. Neurol.* **37**, 247–51.

Lee, T., Seeman, P., Rajput, A., Farley, I., and Hornykiewicz, O. (1978). Receptor basis for dopaminergic supersensitivity in Parkinson's disease. *Nature* **273**, 59–61.

Lees, A. J. (1985). *Tics and related disorders.* Churchill, Livingstone, Edinburgh.

Lees, A. J., Shaw, K. M., and Stern, G. M. (1976). Bromocriptine and spasmodic torticollis. *Br. med. J.* **1**, 1343.

Lorden, J. F., McKeon, T. W., Baker, H. J., Cox, N., and Walkley, S. U. (1984). Characterization of the rat mutant dystonic (dt): a new animal model of dystonia musculorum deformans. *J. Neurosci.* **4**, 1925–32.

Lundh, H. and Tunving, K. (1981). An extrapyramidal choreiform syndrome caused by amphetamine addiction. *J. Neurol. Neurosurg. Psychiat.* **44**, 728–30.

MacKay, A. V. P. (1982). Clinical controversies in tardive dyskinesia. In *Movement disorders* (ed. C. D. Marsden and S. Fahn), pp. 249–62. Butterworths, London.

Marsden, C. D. (1982). The mysterious motor function of the basal ganglia: the Robert Wartenberg lecture. *Neurology* **32**, 514–39.

Marsden, C. D. and Parkes, J. D. (1976). "On–off" effects in patients with Parkinson's disease on chronic levodopa therapy. *Lancet* **i**, 292–6.

Marsden, C. D., Hallett, M., and Fahn. S. (1982*a*). The nosology and pathophysiology of myoclonus. In *Movement disorders* (ed. C. D. Marsden and S. Fahn), pp. 196–248. Butterworths, London.

Marsden, C. D., Parkes, J. D., and Quinn, N. (1982*b*). Fluctuations of disability in

Parkinson's disease: clinical aspects. In *Movement disorders* (ed. C. D. Marsden and S. Fahn), pp. 96–122. Butterworths, London.

Marsden, C. D., Obeso, J. A., and Rothwell, J. C. (1983). Benign essential tumor is not a single entity. In *Current concepts of Parkinson's disease and related disorders* (ed. M. D. Yahr), pp. 31–42.

Marsden, C. D., Marion, M. H., and Quinn, N. (1984). The treatment of severe dystonia in children and adults. *J. Neurol. Neurosurg. Psychiat.* **47**, 1166–73.

Marsden, C. D., Obeso, J. A., Zarranz, J. J., and Lang, A. E. (1985). The anatomical basis of symptomatic hemidystonia. *Brain* **108**, 463–83.

Martin, W. R. W., Stoessl, A. J., Palmer, M. R., Adam, M. J., Ruth, T. J., Grierson, J., Pate, B. D., and Calne, D. B.(1987). PET scanning in dystonia. *Adv. Neurol.* **50**, 223–9.

Mauborgne, A., Javoy-Agid, F., Legrand, J. G., Agid, Y., and Cesselin, F. (1983). Decrease of substance P-like immunoreactivity in the substantia nigra and pallidum of parkinsonian brains. *Brain Res.* **268**, 167–70.

McGeer, P. L. and McGeer, E. G. (1976). Enzymes associated with the metabolism of catecholamines, acetylcholine and GABA in human controls and patients with Parkinson's disease and Huntington's chorea. *J. Neurochem.* **26**, 65–76.

McGeer, P. L., Boulding, J. E., Gibson, W. C., and Foulks, R. G. (1961). Drug-induced extrapyramidal reactions. Treatment with diphenhydramine hydrochloride and dihydroxyphenylalanine. *J. Am. med. Ass.* **177**, 665–70.

McGeer, P. L., McGeer, E. G., and Suzuki, J. S. (1977). Aging and extrapyramidal function. *Arch. Neurol.* **34**, 33–5.

Melamed, E. (1979). Early morning dystonia: a late side effect of long term levodopa therapy in Parkinson's disease. *Arch. Neurol.* **36**, 308–10.

Meldrum, B. S., Anlezark, G. M., and Marsden, C. D. (1977). Acute dystonia as an idiosyncratic response to neuroleptics in baboons. *Brain* **100**, 313–26.

Mesulam, M. M. (1986). Cocaine and Tourette's syndrome. *N. Engl. J. Med.* **315**, 398.

Micheli, F., Pardal, N. M. F., and Leiguarda, R. C. (1982). Beneficial effects of lisuride in Meige disease. *Neurology* **32**, 432–4.

Muenter, M. D., Sharpless, N. S., Tyce, G. M., and Darley, F. L. (1977). Patterns of dystonia ('I-D-I' and 'D-I-D') in response to L-dopa therapy for parkinson's disease. *Mayo Clin. Proc.* **52**, 163–74.

Nielsen, E. B. and Lyon, M. (1978). Evidence for cell loss in corpus striatum after long term treatment with a neuroleptic drug (flupenthixol) in rats. *Psychopharmacology* **59**, 85–89.

Nishikawa, T., Tanaka, M., Tsuda, A., Kuwahara, H., Koga, I., and Uchida, Y. (1986). Effect of ceruletide on tardive dyskinesia: a pilot study of quantitative computer analyses on electromyogram and microvibration. *Psychopharmacology* **90**, 5–8.

Nutt, J. G., Woodward, W. R., Hammerstad, J., Carter, J. H., and Anderson, J. L. (1984). The "on–off" phenomenon in Parkinson's disease. Relation to levodopa absorption and transport. *N. Engl. J. Med.* **310**, 483–8.

Obeso, J. A., Rothwell, J. C., and Marsden, C. D. (1981). Simple tics in Gilles de la

Tourette's syndrome are not prefaced by a normal premovement EEG potential. *J. Neurol. Neurosurg. Psychiat.* **44**, 735-8.

Obeso, J.A., Rothwell, J.C., Lang, A.E., and Marsden, C.D. (1983a). Myoclonic dystonia. *Neurology* **33**, 825-30.

Obeso, J.A., Rothwell, J.C., Quinn, N.P., Lang, A.E., Thompson, C., and Marsden, C.D. (1983a). Cortical reflex myoclonus respond to intravenous lisuride. *Clin. Neuropharmacol.* **6**, 231-40.

Obeso, J.A., Luquin, M.R., and Martinez-Lage, J.M. (1986). Lisuride infusion pump: a device for the treatment of motor fluctuations in Parkinson's disease. *Lancet* i, 467-70.

O'Brien, M.D., Upton, A.R., and Toseland, P.A. (1981). Benign familial tremor treated with primidone. *Br. med. J.* **282**, 178-80.

Orme, M.L.E. and Tallis, R.C. (1984). Metoclopramide and tardive dyskinesia in the elderly. *Br. med. J.* **289**, 397-8.

Pakkenberg, H.F.R., Fog, R., and Nilakantan, B. (1973). The long term effect of perphenazine enanthate on the rat brain. Some metabolic and anatomical observations. *Psychopharmacologia* **29**, 85-9.

Parkes, J.D. (1979). Bromocriptine in the treatment of Parkinsonism. *Drugs* **17**, 365-82.

Parkes, J.D., Bedard, P., and Marsden, C.D. (1976). Chorea and torsion in parkinsonism. *Lancet* ii, 155.

Parkinson, J. (1817). *An essay on the shaking palsy.* Sherwood, Neely, and Jones, London.

Pauls, D.L. and Leckman, J.F. (1986). The inheritance of Gilles de la Tourette's syndrome and associated behaviours. Evidence for autosomal dominant transmission. *N. Engl. J. Med.* **315**, 993-7.

Pauls, D.L., Hurst, C.R., Kruger, S.D., Leckman, J.F., Kidd, K.K., and Cohen, D.J. (1986a). Gilles de la Tourette's syndrome and attention deficit disorder with hyperactivity. Evidence against a genetic relationship. *Arch. Gen. Psychiat.* **43**, 1177-9.

Pauls, D.L., Towbin, K.E., Leckman, J.F., Zahner, G.E.P., and Cohen, D.J. (1986b). Gilles de la Tourette's syndrome and obsessive–compulsive disorder. Evidence supporting a genetic relationship. *Arch. Gen. Psychiat.* **43**, 1180-2.

Perry, E.K., Curtis, M., Dick, D.J., Candy, J.M., Atack, J.R., Bloxham, C.A., Blessed, G., Fairbairn, A., Tomlinson, B.E., and Perry, R.H. (1985). Cholinergic correlates of cognitive impairment in Parkinson's disease: comparisons with Alzheimer's disease. *J. Neurol. Neurosurg. Psychiat.* **48**, 413-21.

Perry, T.L., Hansen, S., and Kloster, M. (1973). Huntington's chorea. Deficiency of γ-aminobutyric acid in brain. *N. Engl. J. Med.* **288**, 337-42.

Perry, T.L., Wright, J.M., Hansen, S., Baker Thomas, S.M., Allan, B.M., Baird, P.A., and Diewold, P.A. (1982). A double-blind clinical trial of isoniazid in Huntington's disease. *Neurology* **32**, 354-8.

Phillips, A.G., Lane, R.F., and Blaha, C.D. (1986). Inhibition of dopamine release by cholecystokinin: relevance to schizophrenia. *Trends pharmacol. Sci.* **7**, 126-7.

Quinn, N., Parkes, J.D., and Marsden, C.D. (1984). Control of on/off phenomenon by continuous intravenous infusion of levodopa. *Neurology* **34**, 1131-6.

Quinn, N.P., Lang, A.E., Sheehy, M.P., and Marsden, C.D. (1985). Lisuride in dystonia. *Neurology* **35**, 766-9.

Randrup, A. and Munkvad, I. (1967). Stereotyped activities produced by amphetamine in several animal species and man. *Psychopharmacologia* **11**, 300-10.

Rao, S.K. and Calne, D.B. (1973). Studies with carbidopa (MK 486). *Adv. Neurol.* **3**, 73-7.

Rascol, A., Guiraud, B., Montastruc, J.L., David, J., and Clanet, M. (1979). Long term treatment of Parkinson's disease with bromocriptine. *J. Neurol. Neurosurg. Psychiat.* **42**, 143-50.

Richardson, E.P. (1982). Neuropathological studies of Tourette syndrome. *Adv. Neurol.* **35**, 83-8.

Rivera-Calimlim, L., Tandon, D., Anderson, F., and Joynt, R. (1977). The clinical picture and plasma levodopa metabolite profile of parkinsonism non-responders. Treatment with levodopa and decarboxylase inhibitor. *Arch. Neurol.* **34**, 228-32.

Rothwell, J.C., Obeso, J.A., Day, B.L., and Marsden, C.D. (1983). Pathophysiology of dystonias. *Adv. Neurol.* **39**, 851-64.

Rupniak, N.M.J., Jenner, P., and Marsden, C.D. (1986). Acute dystonia induced by neuroleptic drugs. *Psychopharmacology* **88**, 403-19.

Sacks, O. (1982). Acquired Tourettism in adult life. *Adv. Neurol* **35**, 89-92.

Schenk, G. and Leijnse-Ybema, H.J. (1974). Huntington's chorea and levodopa. *Lancet* **i**, 364.

Schott, G.D. (1986). Induction of involuntary movements by peripheral trauma: an analogy with causalgia. *Lancet* **ii**, 712-16.

Schwab, R.S., Chafetz, M.E., and Walker, S. (1954). Control of two simultaneous voluntary motor acts in normals and in parkinsonism. *Arch. Neurol. Psychiat.* **72**, 591-8.

Sedman, G. (1976). Clonazepam in treatment of tardive oral dyskinesia. *Br. med. J.* **2**, 583.

Segawa, M., Hosaka, A., Miyagawa, F., Nomura, Y., and Imai, H. (1976). Hereditary progressive dystonia with marked diurnal fluctuation. *Adv. Neurol.* **14**, 215-33.

Seizinger, B.R., Liebisch, D.C., Kish, S.J., Arendt, R.M., Hornykiewicz, O., and Herz, A. (1986). Opioid peptides in Huntington's disease: alterations in prodynorphin and proenkephalin system. *Brain Res.* **378**, 405-8.

Shapiro, A.K., Shapiro, E., and Wayne, H. (1973). Treatment of Tourette's syndrome with haloperidol, review of 34 cases. *Arch. gen. Psychiat.* **28**, 92-7.

Sheehy, M.P. and Marsden, C.D. (1982). Writer's cramp: a focal dystonia. *Brain* **105**, 461-80.

Shoulson, I., Chase, T.N., Roberts, E., and Van Balgooy, J.N.A. (1975). Huntington's disease: treatment with imidazole-4-acetic acid. *N. Engl. J. Med.* **293**, 504-5.

Shoulson, I., Kartzinel, R., and Chase, T. N. (1976). Huntington's disease: treatment with dipropylacetic acid and gamma-aminobutyric acid, Neurology 26, 61-3.

Singer, H. S., Wong, D. F., Tiemeyer, M., Whitehouse, P., and Wagner, H. N. (1984). Pathophysiology of Tourette syndrome: a PET and postmortem analysis. Ann. Neurol. 18, 416.

Spitz, M. C., Jankovic, J., and Killian, J. M. (1985). Familial tic disorder, parkinsonism, motor neuron disease and acanthocytosis—a new syndrome. Neurology 35, 366-77.

Spokes, E. G. S. (1980). Neurochemical alterations in Huntington's chorea. A study of post mortem brain tissue. Brain 103, 179-210.

Stahl, S. M. (1980). Tardive Tourette syndrome in an autistic patient after long-term neuroleptic administration. Am. J. Psychiat. 137, 1267-9.

Stahl, S. M. (1985). Akathisia and tardive dyskinesia. Changing concepts. Arch. gen. Psychiat. 42, 915-17.

Stahl, S. M. and Berger, P. A. (1980). Physostigmine in Gilles de la Tourette's syndrome. N. Engl. J. Med. 302, 298.

Stahl, S. M. and Berger, P. A. (1981). Physostigmine in Tourette syndrome: evidence for cholinergic underactivity. Am. J. Psychiat. 138, 240-2.

Stahl, S. M. and Berger, P. A. (1982). Bromocriptine, physostigmine, and neurotransmitter mechanisms in the dystonia. Neurology 32, 889-92.

Stahl, S. M., Davis, K. L., and Berger, P. A. (1982). The neuropharmacology of tardive dyskinesia, spontaneous dyskinesia, and other dystonia. J. clin. Psychopharmacol. 2, 321-8.

Stahl, S. M., Thornton, J. E., Simpson, M. L., Berger, P. A., and Napoliello, M. J. (1985). Gamma-vinyl-GABA treatment of tardive dyskinesia and other movement disorders. Biol. Psychiat. 20, 888-93.

Stibe, C. M. H., Lees, A. J., Kempster, P. A., and Stern, G. M. (1988). Subcutaneous apomorphine in parkinsonian on-off oscillations. Lancet i, 403-6.

Stoessl, A. J., Dourish, C. T., and Iversen, S. D. (1989). Chronic neuroleptic-induced mouth movements in the rat: suppression by CCK and selective dopamine D_1 and D_2 receptor antagonists. Psychopharmacology 98, 372-9.

Stoessl, A. J., Martin, W. R. W., Clark, C., Adam, M. J., Ammann, W., Beckman, J. H., Bergstrom, M., Harrop, R., Rogers, J. G., Ruth, T. J., Sayre, C. I., Pate, B. D., and Calne, D. B. (1986a). PET studies of cerebral glucose metabolism in idiopathic torticollis. Neurology 36, 653-7.

Stoessl, A. J., Martin, W. R. W., Hayden, M. R., Adam, M. J., Ruth, T. J., Rajput, A., Pate, D. D., and Calne, D. B. (1986b). Dopamine in Huntington's disease: studies using positron emission tomography. Neurology 36, (Suppl. 1), 310.

Studler, J. M., Javoy-Agid, F., Legrand, J. C., Agid, Y., and Cesselin, F. (1982). CCK-8-immunoreactivity in human brain: selective decrease in the substantia nigra from parkinsonian patients. Brain Res 243, 176-9.

Svensson, T. H., Bunney, B. S., and Aghajanian, G. K. (1975). Inhibition of both noradrenergic and serotonergic neurons in brains by the α-adrenergic agonist clonidine. Brain Res. 92, 291-306.

Swash, M., Roberts, A. H., Zakko, H., and Heathfield, K. W. G. (1972). Treatment of involuntary movement disorders with tetrabenazine. J. Neurol. Neurosurg. Psychiat. 35, 186-91.

Sweet, R.D., Solomon, G.E., Wayne, H., Shapiro, E., and Shapiro, A.K. (1973). Neurological features of Gilles de la Tourette's syndrome. *J. Neurol. Neurosurg. Psychiat.* **36**, 1–9.

Tamminga, C.A., Crayton, J.W., and Chase, T.N. (1979). Improvement in tardive dyskinesia after muscimol therapy. *Arch. gen. Psychiat.* **36**, 595–8.

Tanner, C.M., Goetz, C.G., and Klawans, H.L. (1980). Cholinergic and anticholinergic effects in Tourette syndrome. *Neurology* **30**, 384.

Taquet, H., Javoy-Agid, F., Hanon, M., Legrand, J.C., Agid, Y., and Cesselin, F. (1983). Parkinson's disease affects differently Met^5 and Leu^5-enkephalin in the human brain. *Brain Res.* **280**, 379–82.

Tell, G.P., Schechter, P.J., Koch-Weser, J., Cantimaux, P., Chabannes, J-P., and Lambert, P.A. (1981). Effects of γ-vinyl GABA. *N. Engl. J. Med.* **305**, 581–2.

Tolosa, E.S. and Montserrat, L. (1985). Decreased blink reflex habituation in dystonic blepharospasm. *Neurology* **35**, (Suppl. 1), 271.

Truong, D.D., Pranzatelli, M.R., Jackson-Lewis, V., and Fahn, S. (1986). Intracerebroventricular glycine blocks myoclonus induced by p,p'-DDT in the rat. *Ann. Neurol.* **20**, 149.

Uhr, S.B., Pruitt, B., Berger, P.A., and Stahl, S.M. (1986). Improvement of symptoms in Tourette syndrome by piquindone, a novel dopamine-2 receptor antagonist. *Int. Clin. Psychopharmacol.* **1**, 216–20.

Van Woert, M.H. and Chung, E. (1986). Possible mechanisms of action of valproic acid in myoclonus. *Adv. Neurol.* **43**, 653–60.

Van Woert, M.H., Rosenbaum, D., Howieson, J., and Bowers, M.B. (1977). Long-term therapy of myoclonus and other neurologic disorders with L-5-hydroxytryptophan and carbidopa. *N. Engl. J. Med.* **296**, 70–5.

Waddington, J.L., Youssef, H.A., Molloy, A.G., O'Boyle, K.M., and Pugh M.T. (1985). Association of intellectual impairment, negative symptoms, and aging with tardive dyskinesia: clinical and animal studies. *J. clin. Psychiat.* **46**(4), 29–33.

Ward, CD., Duvoisin, R.C., Ince, S.E., Nutt, J.D., Eldridge, R., and Calne, D.B. (1983). Parkinson's disease in 65 pairs of twins and in a set of quadruplets. *Neurology* **33**, 815–24.

Weilburg, J.B., Mesulam, M.-M., Weintraub, S., Buonanno, Jenike, M., and Stakes, J.W. (1989). Focal striatal abnormalities in a patient with obsessive–compulsive disorder. *Arch. Neurol.* **46**, 233–5.

Weiner, W.J. and Luby, E.D. (1983). Tardive akathisia. *J. clin. Psychiat.* **44**, 417–19.

Weiner, W.J., Carvey, P.M., Nausieda, P.A., and Klawans, H.L. (1979). Dopaminergic antagonism of L-5-hydroxytryptophan-induced myoclonic jumping behaviour. *Neurology* **29**, 1622–5.

Whitehouse, P.H., Hedreen, J.C., White, C.L., and Price, D.L. (1983). Basal forebrain neurones in the dementia of Parkinson's disease. *Ann. Neurol.* **13**, 243–8.

Wolfson, L.I., Sharpless, N.S., Thal, L.J., Waltz, J.M., and Shapiro, K. (1983). Decreased ventricular fluid norepinephrine metabolite in childhood-onset dystonia. *Neurology* **33**, 369–72.

Young, R.R., Growdon, J.H., and Shahani, B.T. (1975). Beta-adrenergic mechanisms in action tremor. *N. Engl. J. Med.* **293**, 950–3.

Zeman, W. and Dyken, P. (1968). Dystonia musculorum deformans. In *Handbook of clinical neurology.* Vol. 6. *Diseases of the basal ganglia* (ed. P.J. Vinken and G.W. Bruyn), pp. 517–43. North-Holland, Amsterdam.

Subject Index

Page numbers in *italic* type refer to figures and tables; those in **bold** type refer to whole chapters.

acetylcholine
  yawning and 93–5
ACTH
  -induced grooming
    environmental influences on 123
    periaqueductal grey and 126
    structure of 119, *120*, 121
    temporal characteristics of 121
  -induced yawning 90–3, *92*
action tremor 264
akinesia
  selective disinhibition of components of forward locomotion 187–9
amphetamine
  conditioned reinforcement enhanced by 32
  -induced psychosis 1–2
  -induced stereotyped behaviour 2, 174, *175–6*
    co-ordinated functioning of caudate putamen and n. accumbens 45–9
    differences from apomorphine-induced stereotypy 40, *41–2*, 43, *44*, 45
    dopamine and 38–40
    limbic and cortical influences on 50–1, *52*, 53–4
    Lyon and Robbins hypothesis of 27–8, *29*, 30–2
    mediation at neuronal level 40
    neural substrates of 5–7
    perseverative switching and 31
    striatal efferents mediating 49–50
  microinjection into n. accumbens and caudate putamen *42*, *46*, *48*
  as a stressor 35–6
anticonvulsant drug action
  5-HT syndrome and 158
antipsychotic drugs, *see* dopamine antagonists, neuroleptics
apomorphine
  -induced gnawing 2–3
  -induced stereotyped behaviour 171, *172–4*
    differences from amphetamine-induced stereotypy 40, *41–2*, 43, *44*, 45

dopamine D–2 antagonists block 71, *72*, 73
  Eshkol-Wachman movement notation applied to 171, *172–3*
  neural substrates of 5–8
  -induced yawning 102, *103*, 104
  microinjection into caudate-putamen *42*
atropine
  disinhibits 'head-led' locomotion 188
  -induced stereotyped locomotion 185, *186*

backward walking
  dopamine's involvement in 154
  striatal 5-HT and 148–9
baseline-dependent effects
  in amphetamine-induced stereotypy 28
behavioural competition
  in amphetamine-induced stereotypy 28
behavioural processes
  in drug-induced stereotyped behaviour 11–6
'behavioural trap' method
  for revealing disintegration of exploratory locomotion 184–5, *186*
'behavioural trapping'
  induced by drugs is reversed by prior experience 189, *190*, 191
'body-initiated' locomotion
  released by methysergide 187–9

caudate nucleus
  apomorphine-induced yawning in 100–1
caudate-putamen
  amphetamine microinjected into *42*
  apomorphine microinjected into *44*
  co-ordinated functioning with the n. accumbens 45–9
cephalocaudal recruitment
  for scanning without locomotion 178, *179–80*
chewing mouth movements
  yawning and 94–5

cholinergic
   involvement in Tourette's syndrome 268
chorea
   of Huntington's disease 264–5
classification of dopamine receptors 65–8
components of movements
   in stereotyped behaviour 14–5
conditioned reinforcement
   enhancement by amphetamines 32
coping with stress
   stereotyped behaviour in terms of 33–8
corpus striatum
   dopamine and stereotyped behaviour 5–8

definitions of stereotyped behaviour in
      psychiatry and neurology 232–5
dementia
   stereotyped behaviour associated with 245
discovery of dopamine-containing
      pathways 3–4
disinhibition
   of components of forward locomotion in
      akinetic animals 187–9
disintegration into stereotypy
   induced by drugs or brain
      damage 169–199
dopamine
   amphetamine-induced stereotypy and
      38–40
   excessive grooming and 127, 128, 129
   involvement in 5-HT syndrome 151–2,
      153, 154–5, 156
   stereotyped behaviour and brain 1–24
   yawning and 95–104
dopamine agonists
   movement disorders induced by 274
   yawning induced by 95, 96, 100–2
dopamine antagonists
   blockade of stimulant-induced stereotypy
      identifies 9
dopamine autoreceptors
   yawning mediated by 96–8
dopamine D-1 and D-2 receptors
   D-1 agonists
      non-induction of stereotyped behaviour
         by 75–6
   D-1 antagonists
      stereotyped behaviour and 76, 77, 78
   D-2 agonists
      stereotyped behaviour induced by 73,
         74, 75
      yawning induced by 98–9
   D-2 antagonists
      apomorphine-induced stereotypy
         blocked by 71, 72, 73

   in the treatment of Tourette's
      syndrome 268
dopamine deficiency
   in Parkinson's disease 4, 261
dopamine movement subsystems
   gradient of integration in 177–82
   hierarchy of activation thresholds for
      182–4
dopamine neuroanatany
   stereotyped behaviour and 3–8
dopamine receptors
   classification of 9–10, 65–8
   stereotyped and non-stereotyped
      behaviour in relation to 64–90
   supersensitivity as model for tardive
      dyskinesia 277
dopamine-induced stereotyped behaviour
   neural substrates of 5–8
dorsal striatum
   neural connections of 39
drug-induced movement disorders 272–8
dysregulation of neural systems 133–4
dystonia 270–2

elicited stereotyped behaviour
   in normal adults 236–8
   in retarded and autistic individuals 240–1
   in schizophrenia 249–51
entrainment of running
   by periodic reward schedules 201, 203
environmental influence
   on ACTH-induced grooming 123
   on amphetamine-induced stereotypy
      28–32
   on apomorphine-induced yawning 102,
      103, 104
Eshkol-Wachman Movement Notation
   applied to stereotyped behaviour 14, 171
essential tremor 263
exploratory locomotion
   disintegrated forms of 184–9

frontal lobe lesions
   perseveration following 243–5
frontal cortex
   involvement in novel and spontaneous
      actions 255
full catalepsy
   body stability isolated from exploration
      177–8
function or purpose
   in stereotyped behaviour 26–8

Gilles de la Tourette syndrome 241, 266–8
gnawing
   induced by apomorphine 2–3

gradient of integration
    in dopaminergic movement subsystems
        177–82
grooming
    dopaminergic components of 127, *128*,
        129
    homeostatic mechanisms and 135–6
    induced by
        ACTH 119–29
        neuropeptides 121, *122*, 123
        SK&F 38393 80, *81*, 82
    neural substrates for 124–7
    reduction in activation correlated
        with 123–4

hallucinogenic drugs
    5-HT-dependent behaviour and 158
haloperidol
    catalepsy induced by 177
'head-led' locomotion
    anticholinergic disinhibtion of 187–8
Herrnstein's matching relation 206–7
hierarchy of activation thresholds
    in dopamine movement subsystems 182–4
hippocampal lesions
    stereotyped behaviour and *52*, 53
homeostatic mechanisms
    grooming and 135–6
Huntington's disease
    chorea in 264–5
8-hydroxy-2-(di-*n*-propylamino) tetralin
    (8-OH-DPAT)
    5-HT syndrome induced by 150–1
5-hydroxytryptamine (5-HT)
    receptors
        anticonvulsant drugs and 158
        hallucinogenic drugs and 158
        immobilization stress and 157
        stimulation, effects as experimental
            tools 157–9
        syndrome produced by stimulation
            of 149–51
    requirement in 5-HT syndrome 146–9
    stereotyped responses and **142–68**
    syndrome
        description of the 142
        dopamine's involvement in the 151–2,
            153, 154–5, *156*
        drugs which induce the 142–3
        5-HT receptors in 149–51
        5-HT requirement for 146–3
        mechanisms mediating the 146–57
        methods to evaluate the 144–146, *147*
        noradrenalin's involvement in 155–7
        yawning and 104

immobilization stress
    5-HT syndrome and 157

lateral hypothalamic damage
    spontaneous recovery from 182–3
L-dopa
    movement disorders induced by 272–4
    treatment of Parkinson's disease with 4,
        262–3
limbic and cortical influences
    on amphetamine-induced stereotypy
        50–1, *52*, 53–4
locomotor stimulation
    nucleus accumbens dopamine and 6–8
    olfactory tubercle dopamine and 8
Lyon-Robbins hypothesis 27–8, 29, 30–2,
        193

madness and health
    stereotyped behaviour in **232–59**
mechanisms of schedule entrainment **200–31**
5-methoxy-N, N-dimethyltryptamine
    (5-MeODMT)
    5-HT syndrome induced by *147*, 148,
        150–1
methysergide
    'body-initiated' locomotion disinhibited
        by 188–9
microdescriptive behavioural analysis
    of stereotyped behaviour **169–99**
motor perseverations
    after frontal lobe lesions 243
movement disorders
    induced by
        L-dopa 272–4
        dopamine agonists 274
MPTP model
    of Parkinson's disease 262
myoclonus 269–70

narrowing of response repertoire
    in stereotyped behaviour 27
neural bases of
    dopamine agonist-induced yawning
        100–1, 102
    excessive grooming 124–7
    stimulant-induced stereotypy 5–8, 38–54
    yawning **91–116**
neuroleptics
    akathesia induced by 275
    dystonia induced by 274
    parkinsonism induced by 274
    tardive dyskinesia and chronic treatment
        with 275–8
    (*see also* dopamine antagonists, dopamine
        D-1 and D-2 receptors)

neurological disease
  stereotyped motor phenomena in **260-92**
neuropeptides
  grooming induced by**117-141**
neuropsychological significance
  of stimulant-induced stereotypy **25-63**
neurotransmitter interactions
  yawning mediated by 105, *106-7*, 108
non-schedule-induced activities
  effects of absolute food frequency on
    204-5
noradrenalin
  involvement in the 5-HT syndrome 155-7
  yawning and 104-5
nucleus accumbens
  co-ordinated functioning with caudate-
    putamen 45-9
  dopamine and locomotor stimulation 6-8

Obsessive-compulsive disorder
  relationship to Tourette's syndrome 267
olfactory tubercle dopamine
  locomotor hyperactivity 8
onset of stereotypy
  behavioural characteristics 15-6

paraventricular nucleus of hypothalamus
  apomorphine-induced yawning in 102
Parkinson's disease
  dopamine loss in 4, 261
  L-dopa treatment for 262-3
  MPTP model for 262
  stereotyped behaviour and 242-3
  tremor in 261
partial catalepsy
  with head-orienting *181*, 182
  with head-scanning 178, *179-80*
  with pivoting 179-81
peptide hormones
  grooming and 118-27
  yawning and 91, *92*, 93
periacqueductal grey
  ACTH-induced grooming and 126
perseverative responses
  after frontal lobe lesions 243-5
perseverative switching
  after amphetamine 31
pharmacological analysis
  of stereotyped behaviour 9-11
pharmacological tools
  to investigate D-1 and D-2 receptor-
    mediated effects 68, *69*, 70
prefrontal cortex
  dopamine systems and 130-1
  stereotyped behaviour and 53-4

prior experience
  drug-induced 'behavioural trapping'
    reversed by 189, *190*, 191
psychomotor stimulant
  -induced stereotyped behaviour 170-1,
    172-6, 177
  neural bases of 5-8, 38-54
  neuropsychological significance of
    25-63
psychosis
  amphetamine-induced 1-2

random sequence generation 236-7
reduction in activation
  grooming as a correlate of 123-4
relativity matching
  applied to schedule-induced behaviour
    209, *210-1*, 212-3, *214*, 215-6
relative food frequency
  in relation to schedule-induced
    activities 208-16
repetitive behaviour
  cultural significance of 254-5
  in schizophrenia 246-51
repetitive movements
  in normal adults 235-8
  in retarded and autistic individuals
    238-41
repetitive speech and writing
  in schizophrenia 248-9
reward
  stereotyped behaviour as 32-3
reward frequency
  differential effects on induced and non-
    induced activities 203-18

SCH 23390
  antagonism of drug-induced stereotypy
    by 76, *77*, 78-80, 83-4
schedule entrainment
  of activities 218-25
  Staddon's model 224
schedule-induced activites
  absolute food frequency and 205-8
  relativity matching applied to 209-16
  schedule entrainment of 218-25
  temporal distributions of 220-1
schedule-induced drinking 202-3, 207
schedule non-induced activities
  schedule entrainment of *218*, 219-25
  temporal distributions of 219-20
schizophrenia
  elicited stereotyped behaviour in 249-51
  repetitive behaviour in 246-51
  repetitive speech and writing in 248-9

spontaneous involuntary movement
    disorders in 246
serotonin (see 5-hydroxytryptamine)
sexual arousal
    yawning accompanied by 99-100
SK&F 38393
    grooming induced by 80, 81, 82
    non-induction of stereotyped behaviour
        75
spinal 5-HT
    Straub tail mediated by 148
spontaneous involuntary movement
        disorders
    in schizophrenia 246-7
spontaneous stereotypies
    in normal adults 235
    in retarded and autistic individuals 238
stereotyped behaviour
    amphetamine-induced 2, 5-7, 27-38, 174,
        175-6
    apomorphine-induced 5-8, 171, 172-4
    baseline-dependent effects in 28
    behavioural competition in 28
    behavioural process involved in 11-6
    concept of 1-24
    coping response to stress 33-8
    definitions in psychiatry and neurology
        232-5
    dementia and 245
    as disintegration induced by drugs or
        brain damage 169-99
    dopamine-induced 5-8
    dopamine
        neuroanatomy and 3-8
        receptor subtypes and 64-90
    environmental control of 28-32
    Eshkol-Wachman Movement Notation
        applied to 14, 171
    function or purpose in 26-38
    hippocampal lesions and 52, 53
    5-HT receptor activation and 142-68
    madness and health 232-259
    narrowing of response repertoire 27
    neuropsychological significance of
        stimulant-induced 25-63
    organic aetiologies and 241-5
    origins in the retarded 238-40
    pharmacological analysis of 9-11
    prefrontal cortex and 53-4
    reward associated with 32-3
stereotyped locomotion
    induced by atropine 185, 186
stereotyped motor phenomena
    in neurological disease 260-92
Straub tail
    spinal 5-HT mediation of 148

stress
    forebrain dopamine and 129
    termination associated with yawning 10
striatal efferents
    mediating amphetamine-induced
        stereotypy 49-50
striatal 5-HT
    'wet dog' shakes, backward walking
        and 148-9
structure of ACTH-induced grooming 119,
    120, 121
substitutability
    between schedule-entrained activities
        221-3

tardive dyskinesia
    adverse effect of neuroleptic treatment
        275-8
    ameliorated by ceruletide 227
    dopamine receptor supersensitivity model
        of 227
temporal characteristics
    of ACTH-induced grooming 119, 120,
        121
temporal distributions
    of non-schedule induced activities 219-20
    of schedule-induced activities 220-1
tic 266-9
tremor 260-4

ventral striatum
    neural corrections of the 39

'wet dog' shakes
    striatal 5-HT and 148-9

yawning
    acetylcholine and 93-5
    chewing mouth movements and 94-5
    dopamine agonists induce 95, 96
    dopamine receptor mediation of
        autoreceptors 96-8
        D-2 receptors 98-9
    5-HT and 104
    neural basis of drug-induced 91-116
    neurotransmitter interactions
        mediate 105, 106-7, 108
    noradrenalin and 104-5
    peptide hormones and 91, 92, 93
    recovery from stress and 110
    sexual arousal accompanies 99-100

Zenith radio experiment 249